# Portal Hypertension in the 21st Century

# Portal Hypertension
# in the
# 21st Century

Edited by

**R. J. Groszmann**
Yale University School of Medicine
New Haven, CT, USA

**J. Bosch**
Hepatic Hemodynamic Laboratory
Liver Unit, Hospital Clínic
University of Barcelona, Spain

*The proceedings of a symposium sponsored by Axcan Pharma Inc. and*
*NicOx S.A., held in Montréal, Canada, April 2–4, 2004*

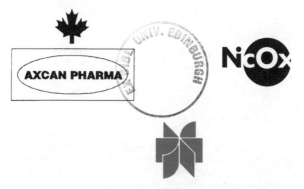

**KLUWER ACADEMIC PUBLISHERS**
DORDRECHT / BOSTON / LONDON

Library of Congress Cataloging-in-Publication Data is available.

ISBN 0-7923-8797-X

Published by Kluwer Academic Publishers BV,
PO Box 17, 3300 AA Dordrecht, The Netherlands

Sold and distributed in North, Central and South America
by Kluwer Academic Publishers, PO Box 358,
Accord Station, Hingham, MA 02018-0358, USA

In all other countries, sold and distributed
by Kluwer Academic Publishers, Distribution Center
PO Box 322, 3300 AH Dordrecht, The Netherlands

*Printed on acid-free paper*

Printed in Great Britain by MPG Books Limited, Bodmin, Cornwall.

# Contents

CONTENTS

CONTENTS

# List of principal contributors

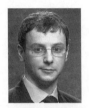

**J.G. ABRALDES**
VA Healthcare System
Hepatic Hemodynamic Laboratory/111J
950 Campbell Avenue
West Haven, CT 06516
USA

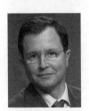

**A. ALBILLOS**
Department of Gastroenterology
Hospital Universitario Ramón y Cajal
University of Alcalá
Ctra. de Colmenar, km. 9,100
28034 Madrid
Spain

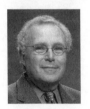

**A.T. BLEI**
Northwestern University Feinberg School of Medicine
303 E Chicago
Seale 10–573
Chicago, IL 60611
USA

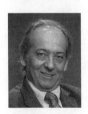

**J. BOSCH**
Hepatic Hemodynamic Laboratory, Liver Unit
Hospital Clinic
Villaroel 170
08036 Barcelona
Spain

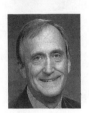

**T.D. BOYER**
Liver Research Institute
University of Arizona
AHSC 245136, Rm 6309
1501 N Campbell Avenue
Tucson, AZ 85724
USA

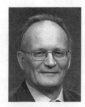

**A. BURROUGHS**
Liver Transplantation
Hepato-Biliary Medicine
Royal Free Hospital
Pond Street
Hampstead, London
NW3 2QG
UK

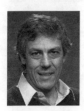

**G. D'AMICO**
Department of Gastroenterology
Ospedale V Cervello
Via Trabucco 180
90146 Palmero
Italy

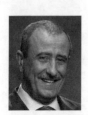

**R. DE FRANCHIS**
University of Milan
IRCCS Ospedale Maggiore
Department of Internal Medicine
Gastroenterology and Gastrointestinal Endoscopy Service
Via Pace 9
20122 Milan
Italy

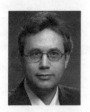

**S. FIORUCCI**
Department of Gastroenterology
University of Perugia
Via E dal Pozzo
06122 Perugia
Italy

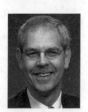

**S.L. FRIEDMAN**
Mount Sinai School of Medicine
Box 1123, Room 1170 F
1425 Madison Avenue
New York, NY 10029
USA

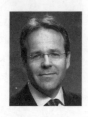

**J.C. GARCÍA-PAGÁN**
Hepatic Hemodynamic Laboratory
Liver Unit
Hospital Clinic
Villaroel 170
08036 Barcelona
Spain

# LIST OF PRINCIPAL CONTRIBUTORS

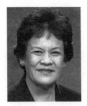

**G. GARCIA-TSAO**
Yale University School of Medicine
VA Connecticut Healthcare System
333 Cedar Street, 1080 LMP
New Haven, CT 06516
USA

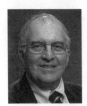

**N.D. GRACE**
Tufts University Medical School
Division of Gastroenterology
Brigham and Womens Hospital
Harvard University
75 Francis Street
Boston, MA 02115
USA

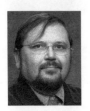

**R.J. GROSZMANN**
VA Connecticut Healthcare System
Hepatic Hemodynamic Laboratory/111J
950 Campbell Avenue
West Haven, CT 06516
USA

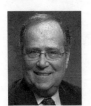

**W. JIMENEZ**
Laboratorio Hormonal
Hospital Clinic Universitari
Villaroel 170
08036 Barcelona
Spain

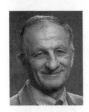

**D. LEBREC**
INSERM U-481 and Service d'Hepatologie
Hopital Beaujon
100 Bd du General Leclerc
92110 Clichy
France

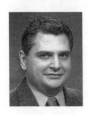

**M.R. LOUREIRO-SILVA**
Yale University School of Medicine
Hemodynamic Hepatic Laboratory
VA Connecticut Healthcare System
111H – 950 Campbell Avenue
West Haven, CT 06516
USA

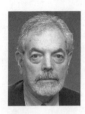

**N.E. MARCON**
The Center for Therapeutic Endoscopy and Endoscopic Oncology
St Michaels Hospital
30 Bond Street
Toronto, Ontario
M5B 1W8 CANADA

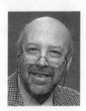

**C. MERKEL**
Department of Clinical and Experimental Medicine
University of Padua
Via Giustiniani, 2
35128 Padova
Italy

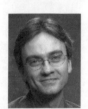

**M. MORALES-RUIZ**
Hormonal Laboratory
Hospital Clinic, IDIBAPS
University of Barcelona
Villaroel 170
08036 Barcelona
Spain

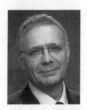

**R. MOREAU**
Service hepato-gastroenterologie
INSERM U-481
Hopital Beaujon
92118 Clichy
France

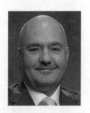

**M. PINZANI**
Dipartimento di Medicina Interna
Universita degli Studi di Firenze
Viale G.B. Morgagni, 85
I-50134 Firenze
Italy

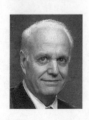

**G. POMIER-LAYRARGUES**
Liver Unit, Hôpital Saint-Luc
Centre Hospitalier de l'Université de Montréal
264 East Rene-Levesque Blvd
Montreal, Quebec H2X 1P1
Canada

# LIST OF PRINCIPAL CONTRIBUTORS

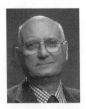

**J. RODÉS**
Catedrático de Patología Digestiva
Servicio de Gastroenterología y Hepatología
Hospital Clínico y Provincial
Casanova 143
08036 Barcelona
Spain


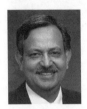

**S.K. SARIN**
Department of Gastroenterology
G.B. Pant Hospital
201–Academic Block
New Delhi 110 002
India


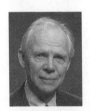

**T. SAUERBRUCH**
Department of Internal Medicine I
University of Bonn
Sigmund-Freud-Str. 25
D-53127 Bonn
Germany


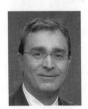

**W.C. SESSA**
Yale University School of Medicine
Boyer Center for Molecular Medicine
295 Congress Avenue
New Haven, CT 06536–0812
USA


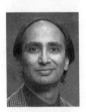

**V. SHAH**
Department of Medicine, Physiology and Tumor Biology
Mayo Clinic Foundation and School of Medicine
AL 2–435, GI Research Unit
200 First St SW
Rochester, MN 55903
USA


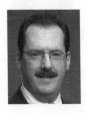

**B. SHNEIDER**
Division of Pediatric Hepatology
Mount Sinai Medical Center, Box 1656
One Gustave L. Levy Place
New York, NY 10029–8060
USA

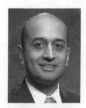

**J.A. TALWALKAR**
Division of Gastroenterology and Hepatology
Mayo Clinic and Foundation
200 First Street SW
Rochester, MN 55905
USA

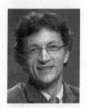

**C. VILLANUEVA**
Servei de Patologia Digestiva
Hospital de la Santa Creu I Sant Pau
Avgda. Sant Antoni Ma. Claret, 167
08025 Barcelona
Spain

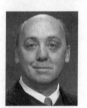

**J.L. WALLACE**
Departments of Pharmacology and Therapeutics
University of Calgary
3330 Hospital Drive NW
Calgary, Alberta T2N 4N1
Canada

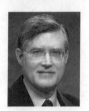

**I. WANLESS**
Department of Pathology
University of Toronto
Toronto General Hospital
E4–305–200 Elizabeth Street
Toronto, Ontario M5G 2C4
Canada

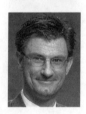

**R. WIEST**
Department of Internal Medicine I
University Hospital Regensburg
Franz-Josef-Strauss Allee 11
93042 Regensburg
Germany

# Preface

**J. RODÉS**

---

Portal hypertension is the most important complication of a great variety of both acute and chronic liver diseases. Nevertheless, hepatic cirrhosis is the most frequent cause of portal hypertension. Gastrointestinal bleeding due to rupture of oesophageal varices is, without doubt, the most severe complication of portal hypertension. At present, great advances are being made in the pathophysiology and in the development of new therapeutic tools for controlling and preventing this severe clinical event.

This book includes the papers presented and discussed during the Symposium held in Montréal, Canada, in April 2004. There are eight Sections covering basic mechanisms, new drugs, prevention and current treatment of variceal bleeding, prevention of recurrent bleeding and hepatic hemodynamic monitoring.

Portal hypertension is initially caused by distortion of the hepatic circulation. This obstruction is a consequence of the obliteration of small hepatic and portal venules. Furthermore, there is an increase in arterial flow that contributes to enhance portal pressure. At present, it has been well established that, in addition to this mechanical mechanism, there are other functional factors that may be implicated in the development of portal hypertension. All these mechanisms are discussed in depth in Sections 1 to 3. Knowledge of the biology of the endothelium and the endothelial dysfunction in the sinusoids has been essential to define the humoral factors such as the impaired activity of vasodilators (nitric oxide (NO), prostaglandins, anandamide) and the increased production of vasoconstrictors (endothelin, norepinephrine, angiotensin, vasopressin, leukotrienes and thromboxane A2) which play a key role in favoring the increased intrahepatic vascular resistance in cirrhosis. In addition to these vascular factors, hepatic fibrosis is also one of the most important phenomena in producing an increase in portal pressure. Therefore, control of hepatic fibrogenesis may, in the future, be a very useful therapeutic tool in the treatment and prevention of portal hypertension. Up to now, several drugs have proven to be useful in controlling fibrogenesis in experimental animals with hepatic cirrhosis. However, these results have not yet been reproduced in human beings.

In Section 4 there is a very interesting discussion regarding the therapeutic effect of new drugs in the treatment of patients with portal hypertension. Clinical studies have shown that the use of nitrates produces a reduction in portal pressure; unfortunately this therapy causes vasodilation in both the systemic arterial and venous vascular beds which, in turn, aggravates the vasodilatory syndrome in cirrhotic patients. Consequently, the ideal drug should act by decreasing intrahepatic vascular resistance without worsening the splanchnic and systemic vasodilation. The development of liver-selective NO-donors using bile acids (ursodeoxycholic acid) as a carrier is based on this idea. Preclinical studies have shown that the administration of this drug to rats with chronic liver injury impairs the development of portal hypertension, suggesting that it may provide a new therapy for this syndrome.

As indicated previously, in cirrhosis there is a decreased endothelial NO production at the sinusoids, which contributes to the increase in hepatic resistance and portal hypertension. Statins may correct endothelial dysfunction in cirrhosis because it has been demonstrated that they are able to increase NO production in endothelial cells. In a recent study, performed in cirrhotic patients, the administration of a single dose of simvastatin was followed by an acute reduction in hepatic sinusoidal resistance and an increase in hepatic blood flow with no changes in portal pressure. These findings may have a potential role in the treatment of these patients. However, new studies are required to confirm these results and to determine whether the chronic administration of simvastatin may be useful in patients with portal hypertension.

Other potential therapeutic agents are also discussed. Akt is the major activator of the endothelial NO-synthase enzyme and it has been shown to be reduced in cirrhotics rats. In an experimental study it was found that myr-Akt gene therapy restored Akt activation and NO production in the cirrhotic liver. On the other hand, the NO synthase gene transfer and inhibition of NO-mediated vasodilation with the use of several drugs (apamin, woutmannin, L-arginine analogs and terlipressin) were able to produce an increased production of NO and, consequently, all these agents could be considered in the future as a new therapeutic tool in the treatment of portal hypertension.

Section 5 is devoted to natural history of esophageal varices, portal hypertension in childhood and the pathophysiology of variceal bleeding. It is well established that, once formed, varices tend to increase in size progressively and they rupture when the variceal wall tension increases above the elastic limit of the vessels. This is directly related to the intravariceal pressure and the radius of the varix and inversely to the thickness of the variceal wall. The role of increased intravascular pressure is underscored by the finding that the hepatic venous pressure gradient (HVPG) increases above 12 mmHg for varices to bleed. Increased radius explains why large varices are at higher risk than small ones, and decreased variceal wall thickness explains the prognostic value of endoscopic red color signs.

In Sections 6 to 8, the current therapy and prevention of esophageal bleeding, and hepatic hemodynamic monitoring are discussed. It is fully accepted that the use of beta-blockers is an excellent treatment for preventing the first episode of variceal bleeding and recurrent bleeding in cirrhotic patients. More recently vasodilators (nitrates, prazosin, losartan, irbesastan and endothelin receptor blockers) have been proven in both experimental animals and in patients with cirrhosis. To date, only organic nitrates have shown any clinical use when applied in combination with beta-blockers to increase their effectiveness at lowering portal pressure. In addition to drugs, endoscopic treatment with band ligation or intravariceal injection of glue has been widely used in these patients. At present, there is great discussion among hepatologists and endoscopists about which of these treatments should be applied in cirrhotics with portal hypertension. As a hepatologist I prefer to use drugs! In my opinion, endoscopic procedures should be used when drug therapy fails. The transjugular intrahepatic portosystemic shunt (TIPS) is one of the most recent therapeutic tools to have been introduced in the management of these patients. At present, TIPS is used as a second-line therapy for variceal bleeding when pharmacologic and endoscopic treatment fails. The usefulness of TIPS is limited by two major problems: shunt dysfunction and hepatic encephalopathy. The use of polytetrafluoroethylene-covered stents may be useful to prevent the former complication.

The general management of patients with acute variceal bleeding consists in the correction of hypovolemia and the prevention of infections with antibiotic prophylaxis. Hemostatic treatment should aim at controlling bleeding and preventing early rebleeding. Pharmacologic therapy with vaso-active drugs (terlipressin, vasopressin associated with nitrates, somatostatin and octreotide) and endoscopic treatment (sclerotherapy and band ligation) are effective in controlling acute bleeding. The combination of drugs and endoscopic treatment is probably the best approach for the management of these patients. It seems that the adjuvant administration of recombinant activated factor VII may be useful in Child B and C variceal bleeding patients. However, although this information is very encouraging, it is evident that further confirmation is required.

The prevention of recurrent bleeding in cirrhotics is mandatory, since 65–70% of patients rebleed within 6 months of the index bleed. First-line treatment consists in the administration of beta-blockers. When this pharmacologic treatment fails, band ligation is the next therapy to be used. Band ligation seems more effective when associated with beta-blockers. It is important to point out that a reduction in HVPG greater than 20% or a reduction below 12 mmHg are the best predictors of clinical efficacy for the prevention of rebleeding. When this combination therapy fails there are other therapeutic options such as surgical shunts, TIPS or liver transplantation.

In these Sections there are several important clinical chapters – cirrhotic patients with no varices and with small varices, the management of gastric variceal bleeding and patients who cannot receive beta-blockers – which are, without doubt, very useful for hepatologists treating patients.

At the end of the Section there is a very interesting discussion regarding the need for hepatic hemodynamic monitoring in cirrhotic patients. In this sense the most important question is: should measurement of WHVP be incorporated in clinical practice? My answer is yes, because this measurement will allow us to predict the risk for bleeding in cirrhotic patients and to know whether a vasoactive drug may be useful to prevent the first episode and the recurrence of variceal bleeding in these patients.

In finishing, I would like to congratulate all the speakers – now authors – for their outstanding scientific level in the presentation and discussion of their papers in the meeting. And last but not the least, I would like to express my sincere admiration to Profs. Roberto Groszmann, Jaime Bosch and Guido Tytgat for organizing this excellent meeting on portal hypertension in Montréal.

# Section I
# Introductory lectures

# 1
# Portal hypertensive syndrome: its importance and complications

**ANDRES T. BLEI**

## INTRODUCTION

The management of portal hypertension continues to be a critical clinical problem for hepatologists and gastroenterologists. At one end of the spectrum of this clinical activity there is increasing interest in approaches to prevent the development of portal hypertension in chronic liver disease[1]. At the other end patients who are candidates for liver transplantation may develop all the complications of portal hypertension while waiting for an organ, as the current MELD (Model for End-stage Liver Disease) system has resulted in a higher priority for sicker patients. A rational approach, centered on evidence-based medicine, is needed to guide the practitioner through complex decisions.

Underlying this clinical complexity is an increase in our understanding of the pathophysiology of the syndrome[2]. Studies in experimental animals and humans have provided deeper insight into the mechanisms that result in the rise in portal pressure, the opening of portal–systemic collaterals and the repercussions of a systemic hemodynamic abnormality on the structure and function of numerous organs that are affected in the portal hypertensive syndrome. All chronic liver diseases go through two stages: the first reflects the alterations caused by the original injury; the second is a new disease, which we can term the portal hypertensive syndrome.

## PATHOPHYSIOLOGY

The development of the portal hypertensive syndrome in cirrhosis can be sequentially described in three steps. (Other etiologies of portal hypertension are not discussed in these introductory remarks, including the most common cause of portal hypertension worldwide, hepatosplenic schistosomiasis.)

### An increase in intrahepatic resistance

The increase in intrahepatic resistance is related to the development of hepatic fibrosis. Original descriptions focused on distortions of the intrahepa-

3

tic vasculature as a result of scar tissue. Popper et al. noted specific changes in the anatomy of the sinusoids[3], where their "capillarization" was the result of the loss of fenestrae and the development of a basement membrane. The demonstration that the increased intrahepatic resistance can be altered by pharmacological means, as shown in studies in the isolated perfused rat liver[4], indicated the presence of a contractile element in this increased resistance. Interest grew in the role of hepatic stellate cells after liver injury. These cells, residing in the Disse space, become activated after liver injury and acquire the phenotype of smooth muscle cells. Isoforms of actin and myosin can be identified, with the resulting acquisition of contractile properties[5].

As a result of these anatomical changes the balance between pro- and anticontractile elements is altered. Hepatic sinusoids can respond to physiological stimuli by constriction[6]. In models of cirrhosis it has been shown that endothelin-1 production in stellate cells is increased; other procontractile forces exist in this condition, such as the increase in angiotensin and α-adrenergic stimulation. More specifically, alterations in the production of cysteinyl-leukotrienes[7] and thromboxane[8] (the latter by Kupffer cells) may contribute to sinusoidal constriction. On the other hand, the release of nitric oxide from sinusoidal endothelial cells is reduced[9]. The decreased hepatic production of nitric oxide has also been shown in human disease[10].

The net balance of this profound change is one that favors contraction, with its implications on hepatic sinusoidal diameter and its repercussions on intrahepatic resistance. Considerable interest has arisen regarding the mechanisms for the decreased production of nitric oxide by sinusoidal endothelial cells. Endothelial nitric oxide synthase (eNOS) activity is decreased and may reflect post-translational alterations in the intracellular regulation of eNOS[11–13]. In addition to its inability to counteract vasoconstrictive stimuli, the decreased production of nitric oxide by sinusoidal endothelial cells may favor the development of thrombosis in the portal and hepatic veins, an event that has been proposed to result in hepatic extinction[14].

This paradigm has led to novel views on potential pharmacological means to reduce intrahepatic vascular resistance. These include antagonism of the effects of vasoconstrictive stimuli as well as increasing the provision of nitric oxide to the sinusoidal endothelial cells. The latter has included the use of adenoviral vectors of eNOS[15] or of activated Akt, a key step in eNOS phosphorylation[16], in order to transduct whole livers; studies in experimental animals have been promising, though clinical applicability is still uncertain. Of greater immediacy is the demonstration that coupling of nitric oxide to molecules that can specifically target the liver can result in a clinically favorable effect[17]. A recent study in humans indicated the ability of simvastatin, a compound that enhances Akt-dependent eNOS phosphorylation, to increase hepatic blood flow and decrease intrahepatic resistance[18]. Manipulation of the abnormal intrahepatic resistance in chronic liver disease should be an area of fertile development over the coming years.

## The opening of portal–systemic collaterals

Once a critical portal pressure is reached, portal–systemic collaterals open. The existence of a threshold value of portal pressure has been extensively

4

studied in humans. A portal pressure gradient between 10 and 12 mmHg is seen in patients who develop esophageal varices[19] as well as those who develop bleeding from gastroesophageal varices[20]. Further proof of the importance of this threshold value comes from clinical studies in which a reduction of pressure to values below 12 mmHg is associated with the disappearance of the risk of bleeding (reviewed in ref. 21).

Measurements of portal pressure in humans are obtained in static conditions, in a supine position and in the fasting state. Ambulation, and most importantly feeding, will result in transient changes in splanchnic hemodynamics. Several times a day, postprandial hyperemia will increase splanchnic inflow and result in a transient rise in portal pressure in patients with well-established portal hypertension[22]. The role of such events at the early stage of the progression of the syndrome has not been examined, but may be one additional factor contributing to the opening of portal–systemic collaterals.

The prevailing view on the nature of such collaterals includes the passive opening of closed vessels or a redirection of flow in the splanchnic area. More recently this view has been challenged with the hypothesis that active angiogenesis may be involved in this process. Mediators of this active vessel neo-formation may be similar to factors involved in the systemic hemodynamic alteration of the portal hypertensive syndrome, including the production of nitric oxide via an increased activity of eNOS[23]. An anti-vascular endothelial growth factor receptor-2 monoclonal antibody decreased the formation of collaterals in mice and rats with partial portal vein ligation[24]. The role of such angiogenesis in human disease is less clear, as the nature of collateralization in rodent models is different from that seen in humans.

## The portal hypertensive syndrome

In its full expression the syndrome includes alterations of several organs.

### The gastrointestinal tract

Anatomical alterations predominate, with esophagogastric varices, portal hypertensive gastropathy and colopathy keeping busy clinicians even busier. Pathophysiological studies have been performed on the mechanisms that underlie variceal rupture[25], of the alterations that exist in the gastric mucosa[26] and of changes in intestinal function[27]. An area of particular interest is the phenomenon of bacterial translocation, shown to occur in rats with cirrhosis and ascites[28] and in patients with advanced liver disease[29]. Release of cytokines, such as TNF, may be an important factor in the progression of the portal hypertensive syndrome. The pathways by which bacterial translocation occurs, as well as the timing of this event within the evolution of the portal hypertensive syndrome, remain to be determined.

### Systemic and splanchnic circulation

The characteristic feature of the portal hypertensive syndrome is the development of a hyperdynamic circulation, with a decrease in systemic vascular resistance and a rise in cardiac output with a lower mean arterial pressure. In the splanchnic territory the increase of portal vein inflow maintains the portal hypertensive state. The combination of an increased resistance and increased flow generates the unique hemodynamic feature of the portal hypertensive state, in which both variables affect the development of portal hypertension.

The search for the mediator of this vasodilated state occupies several decades of research. From the original interest in bile acids and glucagon[30], to the current interest in cannabinoids[31], and carbon monoxide[32] a putative mediator of arteriolar vasodilation is still actively sought. An increased splanchnic production of nitric oxide, the result of an increased activity of eNOS, is well supported by experiments in which specific inhibitors of this enzyme are administered[33]. The complexity of the pathogenesis of vasodilation is illustrated by experiments in portal hypertensive mice. In eNOS knockout animals with partial portal vein ligation the hyperdynamic circulation also develops[34]. It is clear that multiple variables, including humoral, endothelial and neural factors, contribute to this profound hemodynamic alteration. Liver dysfunction underlies this phenomenon, as the hyperdynamic state is more prominent in patients with Child class C cirrhosis.

What remains to be elucidated is the initial event that leads to the vasodilatory state. Because the hyperdynamic circulation can be improved in humans with the administration of antibiotics[35], it is tempting to speculate that bacterial translocation, with the subsequent release of cytokines, plays an important role in the development of vasodilation. Antagonism of TNF with thalidomide[36] or anti-TNF antibody[37] ameliorates the hyperdynamic circulation in animal models. However, the development of the hyperdynamic state in animal models without bacterial translocation suggests the presence of other explanations. Recently, Groszmann proposed that the initial response to a rise in portal pressure, mesenteric arterial vasoconstriction, is the trigger that up-regulates eNOS activity in the superior mesenteric artery of rats with prehepatic portal hypertension[38]. This attractive hypothesis awaits confirmation in other experimental models.

*The kidney*

Systemic vasodilation will result in relative arterial underfilling, stimulating baroreceptors and volume receptors as well as compensatory neural and humoral responses, including activation of the sympathetic nervous system, renin–angiotensin system and vasopressin release (reviewed in ref. 39). Sodium and water is retained by the kidney and plasma volume expands. Such expansion of plasma volume is required for the full expression of the hyperdynamic circulatory state, which cannot be simply equated with vasodilation.

The clinical expression of the effects on the kidney will vary according to the ability of intrarenal mechanisms to compensate for the changes imposed by systemic vasodilation. Progressive arterial vasodilation results in renal arterial vasoconstriction, which in its most severe manifestation results in renal failure, the hepatorenal syndrome. The favorable clinical response of patients with the hepatorenal syndrome to vasoconstrictor therapy[40] supports the role of systemic arterial vasodilation as a key pathophysiological event in the renal abnormality of cirrhosis, as postulated 15 years ago[41].

6

*The lung*

Unique clinical syndromes develop in the lungs of patients with cirrhosis. The hepatopulmonary syndrome, reflecting the effects of pulmonary arterial vasodilation and subsequent hypoxemia, can develop in other etiologies (prehepatic, posthepatic) of portal hypertension. The search for the mechanisms responsible for this pulmonary vasodilation parallels those discussed in the systemic circulation, although the isoform of nitric oxide synthase involved in the generation of NO is still controversial. Recent studies also involve the heme-oxygenase-1/carbon monoxide system in the genesis of pulmonary vasodilation[42]. Endothelin-1 production by the liver, with subsequent activation of endothelin receptors mediating vasodilation, may also exert synergistic effects with TNF in causing pulmonary arterial vasodilation[43]. From a clinical perspective it is striking that the manifestations of pulmonary and systemic vasodilation do not progress in parallel. The reasons for this discrepancy are unclear.

Of even greater interest is the development of pulmonary arterial hypertension, a feared complication of the portal hypertensive state. The mechanisms responsible for this change are less well understood, in part as a result of the lack of an experimental model that combines features of portal and pulmonary arterial hypertension. Extrapolating from the experience of patients with primary pulmonary hypertension, clinical improvement with bosentan, an endothelin antagonist[44], suggests a pathogenic role for this vasoconstrictor system. The favorable effects of sildenafil, an oral phosphodiesterase type-5 inhibitor, whose effects are mediated by an increase in the local availability of nitric oxide[45], also points to a deficiency of the generation of this vasodilator in the pulmonary vasculature. Intravenous prostacyclin has been used in patients, though its use is cumbersome and costly.

*The brain*

The importance of portal–systemic shunting in the pathogenesis of hepatic encephalopathy is well established. Toxins that escape liver uptake reach the systemic circulation and, once in the brain, result in a cascade of neurochemical alterations whose scope is beyond the limits of this review. The reader is referred to other sources[46,47]. What is less clear is the role of circulatory abnormalities in the pathogenesis of an abnormal mental state. Most studies have shown a decrease of cerebral blood flow in patients with cirrhosis[48]. The close relation between the increase of cerebrovascular and cerebral resistance in human disease[49] suggests the brain also responds to the systemic vasodilatory state by vasoconstriction. It is tempting to speculate on a potential role for this change in flow on the manifestations of encephalopathy. However, a reduction in brain metabolic activity as a result of specific toxins, such as ammonia, can also lead to a reduction in blood flow.

*Other organs*

The existence of a cirrhotic cardiomyopathy is still subject of controversy. A state of high-output cardiac failure can be seen in other chronically

7

vasodilated conditions, such as Paget's disease or thiamine deficiency. An intrinsic abnormality of the myocardium, as postulated[50], has been recently questioned with the results obtained in experimental models[51]. A role for an intrinsic cardiac defect has been recently postulated to explain in part the renal failure associated with spontaneous bacterial peritonitis[52].

Platelet dysfunction in liver disease can aggravate an already complex picture. A prolonged bleeding time in experimental cirrhosis can be corrected with inhibitors of nitric oxide synthesis[53], suggesting that nitric oxide generated in the arterial circulation will affect platelet adhesion and aggregation. More recently the development of hepatic osteodystrophy has been linked to the development of portal–systemic shunting[54].

## CLINICAL IMPORTANCE

The review of the pathophysiological changes in the portal hypertensive syndrome indicates the wide range of alterations, the disparity in the responses between different organs as well as the complexity of their interplay. However, it is in the sheer volume of clinical work, use of resources, morbidity and mortality that portal hypertension leaves its mark.

It has been estimated that approximately 5.5 million Americans have cirrhosis[55]. It is difficult to obtain data on prevalence of portal hypertension, but some approximations can be made on the overall prevalence of varices, as well as the yearly development of varices and encephalopathy (reviewed in ref. 56). A special report from the American Gastroenterological Association estimates the yearly cost of treatment of cirrhosis at $1.4 billion, 90% of which is related to inpatient care[57].

Multiple well-designed, randomized controlled studies have examined the optimal treatment of portal hypertension. Of all areas of hepatology, portal hypertension is the one in which decisions can be best made following the principles of evidence-based medicine. It is not the goal of these introductory remarks to review this experience. Much of it will be covered in other chapters. Rather, I would like to highlight two important developments in recent years.

1. TIPS (transjugular intrahepatic portal–systemic shunt) can correct portal hypertension by bypassing all portal blood through the radiologically placed metal stent[58]. It does not solve, and in some occasions worsens, the degree of liver failure. While it can improve the management of gastrointestinal hemorrhage and ascites, it can worsen hepatic encephalopathy. Portal hypertension and portal–systemic shunting are very different sides of the same coin.

2. Liver transplantation is the ultimate therapy for patients with cirrhosis and portal hypertension. In 1999 more than 14000 patients were listed by UNOS, slightly over 4000 transplants were performed and more than 1000 patients died in the waiting list (reviewed in ref. 56). The current adjudication system for transplantation, the MELD score, prioritizes patients with poor hepatic and renal function. Treating the portal hypertensive syndrome in the age of MELD carries a greater complexity as

liver failure dominates the clinical picture.

Prevention of infections, TIPS for intractable ascites and measures to deal with recurrent encephalopathy are among the major problems faced by the hepatologist when dealing with patients on the waiting list. Interest in hyponatremia, recognized for many years as a poor prognostic manifestation in cirrhosis with ascites[59], has been rekindled with the observation that it may also affect brain function in these patients[60]. The type of encephalopathy seen in patients with acute-on-chronic liver failure, deep and resistant to therapy, is very different from that seen in patients with acute, precipitant-induced encephalopathy.

## CONCLUSION

Much insight has been provided into the mechanisms responsible for the development and progression of portal hypertension. For a clinical problem that is so prevalent, the clinical armamentarium is not so abundant. It is anticipated that more studies will focus on the ability of pharmacological agents to reduce intrahepatic resistance. Antagonism of peripheral vasodilation with oral vasoconstrictors is another logical extension of this line of investigation. Newer drugs based on newer concepts are in stages of development. While prevention of the development of portal hypertension could not be demonstrated with timolol[61], the large NIH-sponsored trial showed that this goal should be sought by clinical researchers. In the future one can envision therapy of chronic liver disease based on such prophylactic measures.

## References

1. Boyer TD. Pharmacological treatment of portal hypertension: past, present, and future. Hepatology. 2001;34:834–9.
2. Bosch J, Garcia-Pagan JC. Complications of cirrhosis. I. Portal hypertension. J Hepatol. 2000;32:141–56.
3. Popper H, Paronetto F, Schaffner F, Perez V. Studies on hepatic fibrosis. Lab Invest. 1961;10:265–90.
4. Bhatal PS, Grossman HJ. Reduction of the increased portal vascular resistance of the isolated cirrhotic perfused rat liver by vasodilators. J Hepatol. 1985;1:325–9.
5. Iredale JP. Cirrhosis: new research provides a basis for rational and targeted treatments. Br Med J. 2003;327:143–7.
6. Bauer M, Zhang JX, Bauer I et al. ET-1 induced alterations of hepatic microcirculation: sinusoidal and extrasinusoidal sites of action. Am J Physiol. 1994;267:G143–9.
7. Graupera M, Garcia-Pagan JC et al. 5-Lipoxygenase inhibition reduces intrahepatic vascular resistance of cirrhotic rat livers: a possible role of cysteinyl-leukotrienes. Gastroenterology. 2002;122:387–93.
8. Yokoyama Y, Xu H, Kresge N et al. Role of thromboxane A2 in early BDL-induced portal hypertension. Am J Physiol Gastrointest Liver Physiol. 2003;284:G453–60.
9. Rockey DC. Vascular mediators in the injured liver. Hepatology. 2003;37:4–12.
10. Sarela AI, Mihaimeed FM, Batten JJ et al. Hepatic and splanchnic nitric oxide activity in patients with cirrhosis. Gut. 1999;44:749–53.
11. Shah V, Haddad FG, Garcia-Cardena G et al. Liver sinusoidal endothelial cells are responsible for nitric oxide modulation of resistance in the hepatic sinusoids. J Clin Invest. 1997;100:2923–30.

12. Gupta TK, Toruner M, Chang MK et al. Endothelial dysfunction and decreased production of nitric oxide in the intrahepatic microcirculation of cirrhotic rats. Hepatology. 1998;28:926–31.
13. Hendrickson H, Chatterjee S, Cao S et al. Influence of caveolin on constitutively activated recombinant eNOS: insight into eNOS dysfunction in BDL rat liver. Am J Physiol Gastrointest Liver Physiol. 2003;285:G652–60.
14. Wanless IR, Wong F, Blendis LM et al. Hepatic and portal vein thrombosis in cirrhosis: possible role in development of parenchymal extinction and portal hypertension. Hepatology. 1995;21:1238–47.
15. Van de Casteele M, Omasta A, Janssens S et al. In vivo gene transfer of endothelial nitric oxide synthase decreases portal pressure in anaesthetized carbon tetrachloride cirrhotic rats. Gut. 2002;51:440–5.
16. Morales-Ruiz M, Cejudo-Martin P, Fernandez-Varo G et al. Transduction of the liver with activated Akt normalizes portal pressure in cirrhotic rats. Gastroenterology. 2003;125:522–31.
17. Fiorucci S, Antonelli E, Morelli O et al. NCX-1000, a NO-releasing derivative of ursodeoxycholic acid, selectively delivers NO to the liver and protects against development of portal hypertension. Proc Natl Acad Sci USA. 2001;98:8897–902.
18. Zafra C, Abraldes JG, Turnes J et al. Simvastin enhances hepatic nitric oxide production and decreases the hepatic vascular tone in patients with cirrhosis. Gastroenterology. 2004;126:749–55.
19. Garcia-Tsao G, Grozsmann RJ, Fisher RL et al. Portal pressure, presence of gastroesophageal varices and variceal bleeding. Hepatology. 1985;5:419–24.
20. Viallet A, Marleau D, Huet M et al. Hemodynamic evaluation of patients with intrahepatic portal hypertension. Relationship between bleeding varices and the portohepatic gradient. Gastroenterology. 1975;69:1297–300.
21. Boyer TD. Changing clinical practice with measurements of portal pressure. Hepatology. 2004;39:283–5.
22. Sabba C, Ferraioli G, Buonamico P et al. A randomized study of propranolol on postprandial portal hypertension in cirrhotic patients. Gastroenterology. 1992;102:1009–16.
23. Lee FY, Colombato LA, Albillos A et al. Administration of N omega-nitro-L-arginine ameliorates portal–systemic shunting in portal-hypertensive rats. Gastroenterology. 1993;105:1464–70.
24. Fernandez M, Vizzutti F, Garcia-Pagan JC et al. Anti-VEGF receptor-2 monoclonal antibody prevents portal–systemic collateral vessel formation in portal hypertensive mice. Gastroenterology. 2004;126:886–94.
25. Polio J, Groszmann RJ. Hemodynamic factors involved in the development and rupture of esophageal varices: a pathophysiologic approach to treatment. Semin Liver Dis. 1986;6:318–31.
26. Kawanaka H, Jones MK, Szabo IL et al. Activation of eNOS in rat portal hypertensive gastric mucosa is mediated by TNF-alpha via the PI 3-kinase-AKT signaling pathway. Hepatology. 2002;35:393–402.
27. Chesta J, Defilippi C, Defilippi C. Abnormalities in proximal small bowel motility in patients with cirrhosis. Hepatology. 1993;17:828–32.
28. Wiest R, Das S, Cadelina G et al. Bacterial translocation in cirrhotic rats stimulates eNOS-derived NO production and impairs mesenteric vascular contractibility. J Clin Invest. 1999;104:1223–33.
29. Cirera I, Bauer TM, Navasa M et al. Bacterial translocation of enteric organisms in patients with cirrhosis. J Hepatol. 2001;34:32–7.
30. Benoit JN, Barrowman JA, Harper SL et al. Role of humoral factors in the intestinal hyperemia associated with chronic portal hypertension. Am J Physiol. 1984;247:G486–93.
31. Batkai S, Jarai Z, Wagner JA et al. Endocannabonoids acting as vascular CB1 receptors mediate the vasodilated state in advanced liver cirrhosis. Nat Med. 2001;7:827–32.
32. Chen YC, Gines P, Yang J et al. Increased vascular heme oxygenase-1 expression contributes to arterial vasodilation in experimental cirrhosis in rats. Hepatology. 2004;39:1075–87.
33. Wiest R, Groszmann RJ. The paradox of nitric oxide in cirrhosis and portal hypertension: too much, not enough. Hepatology. 2002;35:478–91.
34. Iwakiri Y, Cadelina G, Sessa WC et al. Mice with targeted deletion of eNOS develop hyperdynamic circulation associated with portal hypertension. Am J Physiol Gastrointest Liver Physiol. 2002;283:G1074–81.

35. Rasaratnam B, Kaye D, Jennings G et al. The effect of selective intestinal decontamination on the hyperdynamic circulatory state in cirrhosis. A randomized trial. Ann Intern Med. 2003;139:186–93.
36. Lopez-Talavera JC, Cadelina G, Olchowski J et al. Thalidomide inhibits tumor necrosis factor alpha, decreases nitric oxide synthesis, and ameliorates the hyperdynamic circulatory syndrome in portal hypertensive rats. Hepatology. 1996;23:1616–21.
37. Lopez-Talavera JC, Merrill WW, Groszmann RJ. Tumor necrosis factor alpha: a major contributor to the hyperdynamic circulation in prehepatic portal-hypertensive rats. Gastroenterology. 1995;108:761–7.
38. Tsai MH, Iwakiri Y, Cadelina G et al. Mesenteric vasoconstriction triggers nitric oxide overproduction in the superior mesenteric artery of portal hypertensive rats. Gastroenterology. 2003;125:1452–61.
39. Arroyo V, Colmenero J. Ascites and hepatorenal syndrome in cirrhosis: pathophysiological basis therapy and current management. J Hepatol. 2003;38:S69–89.
40. Ortega R, Gines P, Uriz J et al. Terlipressin therapy with and without albumin for patients with hepatorenal syndrome: results of a prospective, nonrandomized study. Hepatology. 2002;36:941–8.
41. Schrier RW, Arroyo V, Bernardi M et al. Peripheral arterial vasodilation hypothesis: a proposal for the initiation of renal sodium and water retention in cirrhosis. Hepatology. 1988;8:1151–7.
42. Zhang J, Ling Y, Luo B et al. Analysis of pulmonary heme oxygenase-1 and nitric oxide synthase alterations in experimental hepatopulmonary syndrome. Gastroenterology. 2003;125:1441–51.
43. Luo B, Liu L, Tang L et al. ET-1 and TNF-alpha in HPS: analysis in prehepatic portal hypertension and biliary and nonbiliary cirrhosis in rats. Am J Physiol Gastrointest Liver Physiol. 2004;286:G294–303.
44. Kim NH, Rubin LJ. Endothelin in health and disease: enothelin receptor antagonists in the management of pulmonary artery hypertension. J Cardiovasc Pharmacol Ther. 2002;7:9–19.
45. Michelakis ED, Tymchak W, Noga M et al. Long-term treatments with oral sildenafil is safe and improves functional capacity and hemodynamics in patients with pulmonary arterial hypertension. Circulation. 2003;108:2066–9.
46. Butterworth RF. Hepatic encephalopathy: a neuropsychiatric disorder involving multiple neurotransmitter systems. Curr Opin Neurol. 2000;13:721–7.
47. Blei AT. Diagnosis and treatment of hepatic encephalopathy. Baillieres Best Pract Res Clin Gastroenterol. 2000;14:959–74.
48. Larsen FS. Cerebral circulation in liver failure: Ohm's law in force. Semin Liver Dis. 1996;16:282–92.
49. Guevara M, Bru C, Gines P et al. Increased cerebrovascular resistance in cirrhotic patients with ascites. Hepatology. 1998;28:39–44.
50. Myers PP, Cerini R, Sayegh R et al. Cardiac hepatopathy: clinical, hemodynamic, and histologic characteristic correlations. Hepatology. 2003;37:393–400.
51. Inserte J, Perello A, Agullo L et al. Left ventricular hypertrophy in rats with biliary cirrhosis. Hepatology. 2003;38:589–98.
52. Ruiz-del-Arbol L, Urman J, Fernandez J et al. Systemic, renal, and hepatic hemodynamic derangement in cirrhotic patients with spontaneous bacterial peritonitis. Hepatology. 2003;38:1210–18.
53. Kim WR, Brown RS, Terrault NA, El-Serag H. Burden of liver disease in the United States: Summary of a workshop. Hepatology. 2002;36:227–42.
54. Adams PC, Arthur MJ, Boyer TD et al. Screening in liver disease: report of an AASLD clinical workshop. Hepatology. 2004;39:1203–12.
55. Sandler RS, Everhart JE, Donowitz M et al. The burden of the selected digestive diseases in the United States. Gastroenterology. 2002;122:1500–11.
56. Boyer TD. Transjugular intrahepatic portosystemic shunt: current status. Gastroenterology. 2003;124:1700–10.
57. Arroyo V, Rodes J, Gutierrez-Lizarraga MA, Revert L. Prognostic value of spontaneous hyponatremia in cirrhosis with ascites. Am J Dig Dis. 1976;21:249–56.
58. Restuccia T, Gomez-Anson B, Guevara M et al. Effects of dilutional hyponatremia on brain organic osmolytes and water content in patients with cirrhosis. Hepatology. 2004 (in press).

59. Groszmann RJ, Garcia-Tsao G, Makuch R et al. Multicenter randomized placebo-controlled trial of non-selective beta blockers in the prevention of the complications of portal hypertension: final results and identification of a predictive factor. Hepatology. 2003;38:206A.
60. Albornoz L, Bandi JC, Otaso JC et al. Prolonged bleeding time in experimental cirrhosis: role of nitric oxide. J Hepatol. 1999;30:456–60.
61. Van der Merwe SW, van den Bogaerde, Goosen C et al. Hepatic osteodystrophy in rats results mainly from portosystemic shunting. Gut. 2003;52:580–5.

# 2
# The vascular endothelium and nitric oxide

JOHN L. WALLACE

## INTRODUCTION

The endothelium is a single layer of cells lining blood and lymphatic vessels. The endothelium separates the contents of the lumen of blood vessels from the underlying connective tissue and vascular smooth muscle. It therefore serves as a semi-permeable barrier, regulating the movement of substances from the lumen of the blood vessel to the interstitium, and vice-versa. The endothelium also acts as a transducer of signals from the lumen to the vascular smooth muscle, and plays a crucial role in regulating inflammatory responses and regulating the growth of new blood vessels. Nitric oxide (NO) is produced via the metabolism of L-arginine by a family of enzymes known as nitric oxide synthases (NOS). Endothelial NO production occurs primarily via the appropriately named endothelial NOS (eNOS). In recent years a great deal has been learned about the molecular regulation of eNOS activity. Moreover, the availability of selective NOS inhibitors and of genetically modified mice that lack eNOS has aided in gaining a better understanding of the physiological and pathophysiological roles of eNOS. NO is an important regulator of blood pressure and of local tissue blood flow. Along with prostacyclin, endothelial NO production is crucial to the regulation of platelet aggregation, as well as in regulating leukocyte adherence to endothelium (thus modulating inflammatory responses). In situations of endothelial dysfunction the impairment of NO synthesis contributes to elevated blood pressure, enhanced inflammatory reactions, impaired tissue blood flow and thrombogenesis. Controlled delivery of NO from exogenous sources may represent an attractive approach to the treatment of disorders characterized by endothelial dysfunction.

As in many tissues, the actions of NO on endothelial function can appear to be inconsistent, causing stimulation of a function in some instances and inhibition of the same function in other instances. Usually these differences are related to the concentration of NO produced. This chapter is focused on the physiological effects of NO (generated by eNOS), rather than the pathophysiological effects associated with high concentrations of NO.

## THE ENDOTHELIUM AS A BARRIER

Throughout the body the endothelium acts as a barrier to restrict movement of materials between the interstitium and the lumen of blood vessels. The regulation of the permeability of this barrier can be crucial for survival of an organism. For example, the "blood–brain barrier" consists of the endothelial cells in the brain that restrict movement of potentially noxious blood-borne substances from gaining entry to the central nervous system. The permeability of the blood–brain barrier is, at least in part, regulated by NO[1].

Endothelial permeability is regulated by contractile elements within these cells. Contraction of these elements opens the gaps between neighboring cells, facilitating the movement of fluid or cells between the lumen and the interstitium. Thus, endothelial contraction contributes to edema formation in the context of inflammation. Various chemical mediators can increase endothelial permeability and promote edema formation, including histamine, leukotriene $C_4$ and platelet-activating factor. NO, in physiological concentrations, acts to diminish endothelial permeability (i.e. an anti-inflammatory action). Moreover, NO donors have been found to reduce edema formation in various experimental models, while inhibitors of NO synthesis can exacerbate edema formation[2–4].

## THE ENDOTHELIUM AS A TRANSDUCER

In 1980 Furchgott and Zawadzki[5] reported the existence of what they termed an "endothelium-derived relaxing factor" or "EDRF". It had been known for many years that acetylcholine caused relaxation of vascular smooth muscle. What Furchgott and Zawadzki demonstrated was that, if they removed the endothelium from their blood vessel preparations, acetylcholine could no longer produce a relaxation of the vascular smooth muscle. They proposed that acetylcholine stimulated the production by the endothelium of a substance (EDRF) that diffused to the adjacent vascular smooth muscle where it induced relaxation. This stimulated a vigorous race among cardiovascular physiologists and pharmacologists for the identification of EDRF. At a conference on EDRF in 1986, Louis Ignarro and Robert Furchgott independently proposed that EDRF was NO, and in the following year, Ignarro et al.[6] and Palmer et al.[7] independently demonstrated that this was indeed the case. Furchgott and Ignarro received the Nobel Prize for Medicine/Physiology in 1998 for their pioneering work on the biology of EDRF and NO.

It is now recognized that many vasodilators produce their effects via stimulation of NO synthesis by the endothelium, including histamine, calcitonin gene-related peptide and bradykinin. These mediators bind to specific receptors on the luminal surface of endothelial cells and trigger the activation of eNOS (discussed in more detail below). This enzyme converts L-arginine plus oxygen to L-citrulline plus NO. The NO is able to freely diffuse from the endothelial cells. From the basolateral side of the endothelial cell NO can diffuse to the neighboring smooth muscle cells, where it can bind to and activate soluble guanylate cyclase. The subsequent generation of cyclic guanosine monophosphate (GMP) leads to relaxation of the smooth muscle cell.

## THE ENDOTHELIUM AS A REGULATOR OF LEUKOCYTE INFILTRATION

To get to a site of injury or infection a leukocyte must first leave the vasculature, and to do this it must cross the endothelium. The process of "diapedesis" is therefore crucial to inflammatory reactions, and is tightly regulated. Leukocytes are normally travelling within the blood stream at the same rate as the erythrocytes. The first step in their recruitment to a site of injury or infection involves "trapping" the leukocyte so that it begins to make contact with the endothelium. This is accomplished through up-regulation of selectins, a family of "Velcro"-like adhesion molecules. Endothelial cells contain P-selectin within Weibel–Palade bodies in the cytoplasm. When appropriately stimulated, such as by histamine, the P-selectin is expressed on the luminal surface of the endothelium where it can bind to complementary leukocyte selectins (e.g. L-selectin). This binding is of fairly low affinity, so the leukocyte continues to move through the blood vessel, but it does so in such a way that it is described as "rolling" along the endothelium. The velocity of the leukocyte is reduced sufficiently such that it can bind, via the CD11/CD18 family of adhesion molecules, to endothelial integrins, such as ICAM-1. The process of migration of the leukocyte through gaps between adjacent endothelial cells is coordinated, in part, by another endothelial adhesion molecule, PECAM-1[8].

NO plays role in regulation of P-selectin expression. NO reduces P-selectin expression, and inhibitors of NO synthase elicit an increase in P-selectin expression, and a corresponding increase in leukocyte adherence to the endothelium.[9,10] Like the relaxant effects of NO on vascular smooth muscle, the down-regulation of P-selectin expression by NO is mediated via soluble guanylate cyclase/cGMP[11]. Endothelial adhesion molecules other than P-selectin do not appear to be regulated, in terms of their expression, by NO.

## THE ENDOTHELIUM AS A MODULATOR OF PLATELET FUNCTION AND HEALING

Platelets play a crucial role not only in blood clotting, but also in inflammatory processes and in thrombosis. Platelets contain or can generate numerous proinflammatory mediators, including serotonin, thromboxane and lipoxins, which can be released at sites of injury. Platelets also contain a number of factors capable of regulating the process of new blood vessel growth (angiogenesis), including vascular endothelial growth factor (VEGF) and endostatin. VEGF is one of the most potent pro-angiogenic factors, while endostatin is a powerful anti-angiogenic factor. The ability of platelets to adhere to the vascular endothelium and to aggregate is under the control of many soluble mediators, including NO. Thus, endothelial NO acts to down-regulate platelet aggregation and adherence, and therefore plays an important role in down-regulating inflammatory processes and thrombus formation. NO is a potent inhibitor of platelet aggregation[12] and of platelet adherence[13]. The role of NO in the regulation of platelet function has been reviewed by Moncada et al.[14].

NO also mediates at least some of the pro-angiogenic effects of VEGF[15]. A recent series of studies from my laboratory illustrated some of the interactions among the endothelium, platelets, NO and angiogenic factors in the context of gastric ulcer healing. We first demonstrated an important role of endothelial NO synthesis in the healing of experimental gastric ulcers[16]. Inhibition of eNOS, but not of iNOS, delayed gastric ulcer healing. Platelets played a critical role in the ulcer healing process, apparently through their ability to deliver pro-angiogenic factors, such as VEGF, to the site of damage[17]. Interestingly, experimentally altering the levels of VEGF versus endostatin in the platelet could alter the rate of ulcer healing. When endostatin levels were increased relative to VEGF levels, ulcer healing was retarded. Treatment with an experimental anti-inflammatory drug that releases NO was found to produce the opposite effect; that is, VEGF levels were increased relative to endostatin levels, and gastric ulcer healing was accelerated[18].

## HOW IS ENDOTHELIAL NO PRODUCTION REGULATED?

Expression of eNOS can be altered in several pathophysiological circumstances. Physiological regulation of eNOS activity occurs through many different mechanisms, and has been the subject of several excellent reviews[19-22]. Immunohistochemical staining for eNOS reveals that it is expressed in close association with caveolin-1, adjacent to the plasma membrane of endothelial cells. Upon appropriate stimulation, such as by the binding of bradykinin, acetylcholine or histamine to their receptors on the luminal surface of the endothelial cell, an influx of calcium and its binding to calmodulin leads to activation of eNOS. One of the events that permits eNOS to catalyze the conversion of L-arginine to L-citrulline and NO is the dissociation of the enzyme from caveolin-1. The activity of eNOS can be further enhanced by the association of the enzyme to heat-shock protein 90. This can be stimulated by a number of factors, including shear stress and bradykinin. The dissociation of the bradykinin receptor from eNOS also facilitates the catalytic activity of the enzyme, as does phosphorylation of certain serine residues on eNOS and association of the enzyme with dynamin-2.

As stated at the outset, the focus of this chapter is the physiological functions of the endothelium, and the role of NO in those functions. It is worth noting, however, that impaired endothelial synthesis of NO has been associated with a number of common diseases, including heart failure, hypertension, atherosclerosis, diabetes and hypercholesterolemia[22-24]. Delivery of NO in appropriate amounts, and at an appropriate rate, may offer a therapeutic approach to the treatment of these disorders. Indeed, this has been proposed for a number of NO-releasing derivatives of common anti-inflammatory drugs, including aspirin[25].

## Acknowledgements

Dr Wallace's research is supported by grants from the Canadian Institutes of Health Research. Dr Wallace holds a Canada Research Chair in Inflammation and is an Alberta Heritage Foundation for Medical Research Senior Scientist.

## References

1. Krizanac-Bengez L, Kapural M, Parkinson F et al. Effects of transient loss of shear stress on blood–brain barrier endothelium: role of NO and IL-6. Brain Res. 2003;977:239–46.
2. Persson J, Ekelund U, Grande PO. Endogenous nitric oxide reduces microvascular permeability and tissue oedema during exercise in cat skeletal muscle. J Vasc Res. 2003;40:538–46.
3. Mundy AL, Dorrington KL. Inhibition of nitric oxide synthesis augments pulmonary oedema in isolated perfused rabbit lung. Br J Anaesth. 2000;85:570–6.
4. Hinder F, Stubbe HD, Van Aken H, Waurick R, Booke M, Meyer J. Role of nitric oxide in sepsis-associated pulmonary edema. Am J Respir Crit Care Med. 1999;159:252–7.
5. Furchgott RF, Zawadzki JV. The obligatory role of endothelial cells in the relaxation of arterial smooth muscle by acetylcholine. Nature. 1980;288:373–6.
6. Ignarro LJ, Buga GM, Wood KS, Byrns RE, Chaudhuri G. Endothelium-derived relaxing factor produced and released from artery and vein is nitric oxide. Proc Natl Acad Sci USA. 1987;84:9265–9.
7. Palmer RM, Ferrige AG, Moncada S. Nitric oxide release accounts for the biological activity of endothelium-derived relaxing factor. Nature. 1987;327:524–6.
8. Liao F, Huynh HK, Eiroa A, Greene T, Polizzi E, Muller WA. Migration of monocytes across endothelium and passage through extracellular matrix involve separate molecular domains of PECAM-1. J Exp Med. 1995;182:1337–43.
9. Armstead VE, Minchenko AG, Schuhl RA, Hayward R, Nossuli TO, Lefer AM. Regulation of P-selectin expression in human endothelial cells by nitric oxide. Am J Physiol. 1997;273:H740–6.
10. Kubes P, Suzuki M, Granger DN. Nitric oxide: an endogenous modulator of leukocyte adhesion. Proc Natl Acad Sci USA. 1991;88:4651–5.
11. Ahluwalia A, Foster P, Scotland RS et al. Antiinflammatory activity of soluble guanylate cyclase: cGMP-dependent down-regulation of P-selectin expression and leukocyte recruitment. Proc Natl Acad Sci USA. 2004;101:1386–91.
12. Radomski MW, Palmer RM, Moncada S. Endogenous nitric oxide inhibits human platelet adhesion to vascular endothelium. Lancet. 1987;2:1057–8.
13. Sneddon JM, Vane JR. Endothelium-derived relaxing factor reduces platelet adhesion to bovine endothelial cells. Proc Natl Acad Sci USA. 1988;85:2800–4.
14. Moncada S, Radomski MW, Palmer RM. Endothelium-derived relaxing factor. Identification as nitric oxide and role in the control of vascular tone and platelet function. Biochem Pharmacol. 1988;37:2495–501.
15. Ziche M, Morbidelli L, Choudhuri R et al. Nitric oxide synthase lies downstream from vascular endothelial growth factor-induced but not basic fibroblast growth factor-induced angiogenesis. J Clin Invest. 1997;99:2625–34.
16. Ma L, Wallace JL. Endothelial nitric oxide synthase modulates gastric ulcer healing in rats. Am J Physiol. 2000;279:G341–6.
17. Ma L, Elliott SN, Cirino G, Buret A, Ignarro LJ, Wallace JL. Platelets modulate gastric ulcer healing: role of endostatin and vascular endothelial growth factor release. Proc Natl Acad Sci USA. 2001;98:6470–5.
18. Ma L, del Soldato P, Wallace JL. Divergent effects of new cyclooxygenase inhibitors on gastric ulcer healing: shifting the angiogenic balance. Proc Natl Acad Sci USA. 2002;99:13243–7.
19. Cirino G, Fiorucci S, Sessa WC. Endothelial nitric oxide synthase: the Cinderella of inflammation? Trends Pharmacol Sci. 2003;24:91–105.
20. Fulton D, Gratton J-P, Sessa WC. Post-translational control of endothelial nitric oxide synthase: why isn't calcium/calmodulin enough? J Pharm Exp Ther. 2001;299:818–24.

21. Solomonson LP, Flan BR, Pendleton LC, Goodwin BL, Eichler DC. The caveolar nitric oxide synthase/arginine regeneration system for NO production in endothelial cells. J Exp Biol. 2003;206:2083–7.
22. Govers R, Rabelink T. Cellular regulation of endothelial nitric oxide synthase. Am J Physiol. 2001;280:F193–206.
23. Maxwell AJ. Mechanisms of dysfunction of the nitric oxide pathway in vascular diseases. Nitric Oxide. 2002;6:101–24.
24. Vallance P, Chan N. Endothelial function and nitric oxide: clinical relevance. Heart. 2001;85:342–50.
25. Wallace JL, Ignarro LJ, Fiorucci S. Potential cardioprotective actions of nitric oxide-releasing aspirin. Nature Rev Drug Discov. 2002;1:375–82.

# 3
# Endothelial-derived nitric oxide as a marker for healthy endothelium

WILLIAM C. SESSA

## INTRODUCTION

In the past decade the importance of the vascular endothelium as a multi-functional regulator of vascular smooth muscle physiology and pathophysio-logy has been appreciated. Indeed, the endothelium responds to hemodynamic stimuli (pressure, shear stress and wall strain) and locally manufactured mediators (such as bradykinin, prostaglandins and angio-tensin) and in turn can release factors that can influence the adhesion and aggregation of circulating cells to the endothelium and the tone of vascular smooth muscle. In many diseases, including cirrhosis, atherosclerosis or diabetes, endothelial dysfunction manifested as an impairment of nitric oxide (NO) production may be an early hallmark of disease and a treatable entity. In this chapter the importance of NO as a mediator of vascular function and potential mechanisms leading to endothelial dysfunction will be discussed.

## REGULATION OF VASCULAR TONE BY ENDOGENOUS NO

Endothelial nitric oxide synthase (eNOS) is the NOS isoform responsible for producing the classical endothelium-derived relaxing factor as originally described by Furchgott and Zawadski[1]. Evidence for the importance of eNOS-derived NO in the regulation of vascular tone is based on experiments in animals and in humans demonstrating that L-arginine-based inhibitors of NOS increase blood or perfusion pressure and vascular resistance and reduce blood flow *in vivo* and *in vitro*. More recently this has been unequivocally confirmed using mice with targeted disruption of the eNOS gene locus. eNOS knockout mice (−/−) are mildly hypertensive relative to wild-type littermate control mice (+/+) of the same generation. Importantly, the pressor effect of nitro-L-arginine, a NOS inhibitor, is attenuated in the −/− mice and endothelium-dependent relaxation in response to acetylcholine is abrogated in isolated vessels[2,3]. This fundamental finding is direct "proof-of-principle" for the major contribution of NO in vasomotor control in large blood vessels.

## PHYSIOLOGICAL ACTIVATION OF eNOS AND NO RELEASE

Typically, endothelial cells release NO in response to autacoids that mobilize intracellular calcium such as thrombin, vascular endothelial growth factor (VEGF) or adenosine diphosphate (ADP). The proposed mechanism for eNOS activation is that the released calcium will bind to calmodulin (CaM) and the calcium/CaM complex will bind to the CaM site in the enzyme to promote NO synthesis. However, the most physiological agonist for NO release is fluid shear stress. Shear stress *in vitro*, or shear rate *in vivo*, is the tangential vector of force elicited by the flow of blood over the endothelial cell surface. Exposure of endothelial cells to shear stress results in a burst of NO release, followed by a sustained phase. *In vivo*, increasing shear rate due to high blood flow or vasoconstriction will cause flow-dependent dilations of certain vascular beds including the splanchnic circulation. Shear-induced NO release *in vitro* and flow-dependent vasodilation *in vivo* can be blocked with NOS inhibitors. Interestingly, shear-induced NO release appears to be "independent" of fluctuations of calcium since shear causes a rapid burst of calcium release that does not parallel the sustained release of NO; chelation of intracellular calcium does not influence the rate of NO production elicited by shear and CaM antagonists can block bradykinin-induced NO release but not shear-induced release[4,5]. These data collectively suggest a fundamental difference in the signal transduction mechanisms for agonist versus shear- or growth factor-induced activation of eNOS.

## REGULATION OF NO PRODUCTION BY PROTEIN INTERACTIONS AND DISEASE

eNOS is a membrane-associated NOS isoform that is modified by co-translational *N*-myristoylation at glycine 2 and post-translational cysteine palmitoylation at positions 15 and 26[6], and these fatty acids are important for its tarageting in the Golgi region and plasmalemmal caveolae. The proper localization of eNOS is necessary for its interactions with other regulatory proteins (scaffolds, chaperones, kinases) that fine-tune the cycles of eNOS activation and inactivation.

The major negative regulatory protein for eNOS is caveolin-1. Caveolin-1 is the major coat protein of caveolae, and has several faces that may influence the biology of proteins that localize to cholesterol-rich plasmalemma caveolae. Indeed caveolin-1 is necessary for the biogenesis of caveolae through an unknown mechanism[7]. In addition, caveolin-1 can serve as a cholesterol-binding protein and traffic cholesterol from the endoplasmic reticulum through the Golgi to the plasma membrane. Finally, caveolin has the capacity to directly interact with other intracellular proteins such as c-Src and H-Ras through amino acids 82–101, the putative scaffolding domain. Indeed, three groups independently demonstrated that eNOS could directly interact with caveolin-1 or caveolin-3[8–10]. The primary binding region of caveolin-1 for eNOS is within amino acids 60–101 and to lesser extent amino acids 135–178. Furthermore, the caveolin–eNOS immunocomplex is disrupted in the presence of caveolin scaffolding peptides (amino acids 82–101).

*In-vivo* evidence supporting the role of caveolin-1 as a negative regulator of eNOS is emerging. Recent work using the caveolin scaffolding domain as a surrogate for caveolin has demonstrated that eNOS can be regulated *in situ*. Exposure of permeabilized cardiac myocytes to the caveolin-3 scaffolding domain peptide (amino acids 55–74), but not a scrambled version, antagonized the negative chronotropic actions of carbachol[11]. Our group recently used a membrane-permeable form of the caveolin-1 scaffolding domain (amino acids 82–101) by fusing it to a cell-permeable leader sequence[12]. Exposure of the peptide to blood vessels blocked acetylcholine-induced relaxations, with no effect on relaxant responses to sodium nitro-prusside or the release of prostacyclin showing that, in an intact blood vessel, the caveolin peptide is a potent inhibitor of eNOS. In addition, the peptide also blocked inflammation in two different models by influencing vascular permeability, suggesting that peptidomimetics may be useful thera-peutically. Most recently this peptide has been shown to block microvascular permeability in tumors and hyperpermeability of postcapillary venules[13]. Finally, genetic evidence from caveolin-1 knockout mice strongly supports the concept that eNOS is negatively regulated by caveolin-1 *in vivo*. Both basal and stimulated eNOS activation and relaxations are enhanced in vessels from caveolin-1 $(-/-)$ mice[14,15]. In addition, the vessels in the microcirculation are hyperpermeable from NO-dependent vascular leakage[16].

With respect to disease mechanisms that may influence the caveolin/eNOS interaction, there is evidence that, in a rat model of cirrhosis, caveolin-1 is overexpressed, more caveolin-1 interacts with eNOS and the basal and stimulated production of NO is depressed[17], suggesting that this interaction may increase portal pressures and contribute to the disease state. More recently, in cholestatic models of disease, the up-regulation of sinusoidal caveolin-1 and a decrease in eNOS activity is seen[18]. Most importantly, elevated expression of caveolin-1 has been found in patients with hepatocellu-lar carcinoma and hepatitis C-related cirrhosis, suggesting that the up-regulation of caveolin-1 may contribute to endothelial dysfunction in the liver[19,20].

Another protein interaction that regulates eNOS is via heat-shock protein 90 (hsp90). Blockade of hsp90-mediated signaling with geldanamycin (GA), or more recently radidicol (RAD), attenuates histamine and VEGF-stim-ulated cGMP production in cultured endothelial cells and blocked acetylcho-line-induced vasorelaxation of rat aortic rings, middle cerebral artery and flow-induced dilation, indicating that hsp90 signaling was crucial for NO release and endothelial function[21,22]. Further support for the relevance of hsp90/eNOS interactions *in vivo* was demonstrated in a model of portal vein ligation (PVL) in rats[23], and in a model of inflammation[24]. In the former study the physical interaction of hsp90 with eNOS isolated from the mesen-teric microcirculation was documented and GA attenuated acetylcholine-dependent vasodilation to the same extent as conventional NOS inhibitors.

In portal hypertensive rats eNOS protein levels are not changed compared to control rats, but NOS activity is markedly enhanced in the mesenteric tissue of hypertensive rats. The enhanced activity correlated with hypo-responsiveness to the vasoconstrictor methoxamine (MTX) and GA potentiated the MTX-induced vasoconstriction after PVL, partially reversing the hyporeactivity to this agent, indicating that hsp90 can act as a signaling component leading to NO-dependent responses in the mesenteric microcirculation. In the latter study GA dose-dependently inhibited inflammation, an effect as potent as a steroid. Since GA blocks NO release, and NOS inhibitors reduce edema formation, it is possible that drugs that specifically inhibit hsp90 will be good anti-inflammatory drugs.

## FUTURE DIRECTIONS TO CORRECT ENDOTHELIAL DYSFUNCTION

In many vascular-based diseases endothelial dysfunction, characterized by an impairment of eNOS funtion or inactivation of NO by oxidative stress, will result in a deficit in bioavailable NO. Insights into how eNOS is regulated, and the development of novel NO donors to supplant the "NO-deficient state", will hopefully lead to improvements in blood flow in the intrahepatic circulation during cirrhosis.

## Acknowledgements

I apologize to colleagues whose references were omitted for the sake of brevity, or whose contributions were cited in reviews. This work is supported by grants from the National Institutes of Health and the American Heart Association.

## References

1. Furchgott RF, Zawadski JV. The obligatory role of the endothelial cells in the relaxation of arterial smooth muscle by acetylcholine. Nature 1981;288:373–6.
2. Huang PL, Huang Z, Mashimo H et al. Hypertension in mice lacking the gene for endothelial nitric oxide synthase [See comments]. Nature 1995;377:239–42.
3. Shesely EG, Maeda N, Kim HS et al. Elevated blood pressures in mice lacking endothelial nitric oxide synthase. Proc Natl Acad Sci USA. 1996;93:13176–81.
4. Kuchan MJ, Frangos JA. Role of calcium and calmodulin in flow-induced nitric oxide production in endothelial cells. Am J Physiol. 1994;266:C628–36.
5. Fleming I, Bauersachs J, Fisslthaler B, Busse R. $Ca^{2+}$-independent activation of the endothelial nitric oxide synthase in response to tyrosine phosphatase inhibitors and fluid shear stress. Circ Res. 1998;82:686–95.
6. Fulton D, Gratton JP, Sessa WC. Post-translational control of endothelial nitric oxide synthase: why isn't calcium/calmodulin enough? J Pharmacol Exp Ther. 2001;299:818–24.
7. Smart EJ, Graf GA, McNiven MA et al. Caveolins, liquid-ordered domains, and signal transduction. Mol Cell Biol. 1999;19:7289–304.
8. Feron O, Belhassen L, Kobzik L, Smith TW, Kelly RA, Michel T. Endothelial nitric oxide synthase targeting to caveolae. Specific interactions with caveolin isoforms in cardiac myocytes and endothelial cells. J Biol Chem. 1996;271:22810–14.
9. Garcìa-Cardeña G, Fan R, Stern DF, Liu J, Sessa WC. Endothelial nitric oxide is regulated by tyrosine phosphorylation and interacts with caveolin-1. J Biol Chem. 1996;271:27237–40.
10. Ju H, Zou R, Venema VJ, Venema RC. Direct interaction of endothelial nitric-oxide synthase and caveolin-1 inhibits synthase activity. J Biol Chem. 1997;272:18522–5.

11. Feron O, Dessy C, Opel DJ, Arstall MA, Kelly RA, Michel T. Modulation of the endothelial nitric-oxide synthase–caveolin interaction in cardiac myocytes. Implications for the autonomic regulation of heart rate. J Biol Chem. 1998;273:30249–54.
12. Bucci M, Gratton JP, Rudic RD et al. *In vivo* delivery of the caveolin-1 scaffolding domain inhibits nitric oxide synthesis and reduces inflammation. Nat Med. 2000;6:1362–7.
13. Gratton JP, Lin MI, Yu J et al. Selective inhibition of tumor microvascular permeability by cavtratin blocks tumor progression in mice. Cancer Cell. 2003;4:31–9.
14. Razani B, Engelman JA, Wang XB et al. 2001. Caveolin-1 null mice are viable but show evidence of hyperproliferative and vascular abnormalities. J Biol Chem. 2001; 276:38121–38.
15. Drab M, Verkade P, Elger M et al. 2001. Loss of caveolae, vascular dysfunction, and pulmonary defects in caveolin-1 gene-disrupted mice. Science. 2001;293:2449–52.
16. Razani B, Woodman SE, Lisanti MP et al. Caveolae: from cell biology to animal physiology. Pharmacol Rev. 2002;54:431–67.
17. Shah V, Toruner M, Haddad F et al. Impaired endothelial nitric oxide synthase activity associated with enhanced caveolin binding in experimental cirrhosis in the rat. Gastroenterology. 1999;117:1222–8.
18. Shah V, Cao S, Hendrickson H, Yao J, Katusic ZS et al. Regulation of hepatic eNOS by caveolin and calmodulin after bile duct ligation in rats. Am J Physiol Gastrointest Liver Physiol. 2001;280:G1209–16.
19. Yokomori H, Oda M, Ogi M, Sakai K, Ishii H. Enhanced expression of endothelial nitric oxide synthase and caveolin-1 in human cirrhosis. Liver. 2002;22:150–8.
20. Yokomori H, Oda M, Yoshimura K et al. Elevated expression of caveolin-1 at protein and mRNA level in human cirrhotic liver: relation with nitric oxide. J Gastroenterol. 2003;38:854–60.
21. Garcia-Cardena G, Fan R, Shah V et al. Dynamic activation of endothelial nitric oxide synthase by Hsp90. Nature. 1998;392:821–4.
22. Ou J, Fontana JT, Ou Z et al. Heat shock protein 90 and tyrosine kinase regulate eNOS NO* generation but not NO* bioactivity. Am J Physiol Heart Circ Physiol. 2004; 286:H561–9.
23. Shah V, Wiest R, Garcia-Cardena G, Cadelina G, Groszmann RJ, Sessa WC. Hsp90 regulation of endothelial nitric oxide synthase contributes to vascular control in portal hypertension. Am J Physiol. 1999;277:G463–8.
24. Bucci M, Roviezzo F, Cicala C, Sessa WC, Cirino G. Geldanamycin, an inhibitor of heat shock protein 90 (Hsp90) mediated signal transduction has anti-inflammatory effects and interacts with glucocorticoid receptor *in vivo*. Br J Pharmacol. 2000; 131:13–16.

# Section II
# Mechanism of disease progression

# 4
# Mechanisms of hepatic fibrogenesis

SCOTT L. FRIEDMAN

## GENERAL ASPECTS OF FIBROSIS AND CIRRHOSIS

Cirrhosis represents the end-stage consequence of fibrosis of the hepatic parenchyma resulting in nodule formation and altered hepatic function. Mounting evidence has now established that even advanced fibrosis and cirrhosis are reversible. Examples include alcohol abstinence, lamivudine treatment for chronic hepatitis B[1], treatment of hepatitis C with interferon/ribavirin[2], surgical decompression of biliary obstruction[3,4], immunosuppressive therapy for autoimmune hepatitis, and phlebotomy for hemochromatosis. Fibrosis and cirrhosis represent the consequences of a sustained wound-healing response to chronic liver injury from a variety of causes. Cirrhosis affects hundreds of millions of patients worldwide. In the USA, it is the most common non-neoplastic cause of death among hepatobiliary and digestive diseases, accounting for approximately 30 000 deaths per year. In addition 10 000 deaths occur due to liver cancer, the majority of which arise in cirrhotic livers, with mortality rate steadily rising[5,6].

The molecular composition of the scar tissue in cirrhosis is similar regardless of etiology, and consists of the extracellular matrix constituents, collagen types I and III (i.e. "fibrillar" collagens), sulfated proteoglycans, and glycoprotein. These scar constituents accumulate from a net increase in their deposition in liver, and not simply collapse of existing stroma.

## HEPATIC FIBROSIS IS THE LIVER'S WOUND-HEALING RESPONSE TO INJURY

There has been steady progress in defining the cells responsible for accumulation of scar, or extracellular matrix (ECM), the signals that drive ECM production, and the enzymes that can degrade scar. Even after acute injury the fibrogenic pathways are already being harnessed, but in order for these to eventuate in scar, the injury must be sustained.

Stellate cells also make a major contribution to the regulation of intrahepatic blood flow. The microvascular unit of the liver, the sinusoid, is remarkably similar to peripheral capillary beds. Sinusoids are lined by endothelial cells, and on their basal surface are stellate cells within the space of Disse. Hepatic stellate cells resemble tissue pericytes, a cell population that has smooth muscle features and is thought to regulate blood flow by modulating pericapillary resistance[8]. During stellate cell activation they increase their expression of the contractile protein alpha smooth muscle actin. Incubation of isolated human stellate cells with vasoconstrictors such as angiotensin-II and thrombin, leads to phenotypic changes including cellular rounding, which are associated with increased intracellular calcium[9]. Furthermore, studies using *in-vivo* microscopy to co-localize sinusoidal constriction with associated autofluorescence[10–13], provide more direct evidence that stellate cells are contractile and can regulate intrahepatic blood flow. The increased intrahepatic vascular resistance characteristic of cirrhosis is thought to arise from an imbalance between vasodilator/vasoconstrictor forces that regulate hepatic vascular tone, as reviewed in related chapters in this book. In summary, the contractile phenotype and perisinusoidal orientation of stellate cells make them ideally positioned to regulate sinusoidal blood flow.

## REGULATION OF HEPATIC FIBROSIS – THE ROLE OF THE HEPATIC STELLATE CELL

Hepatic stellate cells represent one-third of the non-parenchymal (i.e. non-hepatocyte) population, or about 15% of the total number of resident cells in liver. In normal liver they are the principal cell for storing vitamin A, primarily as retinyl esters within perinuclear cytoplasmic droplets. "Stellate cells" actually represent a heterogeneous group of cells which are functionally and anatomically similar, but may differ in the types of cellular filaments they express and their potential for activation into more fibrogenic "myofibroblasts"[14].

Because stellate cells are wrapped around the sinusoid they are able to interact readily through long cytoplasmic processes with all neighboring cell types, including Kupffer cells, hepatocytes, sinusoidal endothelial cells, and immune cells. This orientation facilitates paracrine (i.e. cell-to-cell) interactions that are essential for both normal liver function and the fibrotic response to injury.

The hepatic stellate cell (previously called lipocyte, Ito, fat-storing, or perisinusoidal cell) is the primary source of the extracellular matrix in normal and fibrotic liver. Hepatic stellate cells are resident perisinusoidal cells in the subendothelial space between hepatocytes and sinusoidal endothelial cells. They are the primary site for storing retinoids and therefore can be recognized by their vitamin A autofluorescence in normal unfixed liver and following their isolation. In addition, their perisinusoidal orientation and expression of the cytoskeletal proteins desmin, glial acidic fibrillary protein and smooth muscle actin (in injured liver) facilitate their identification *in situ*[14].

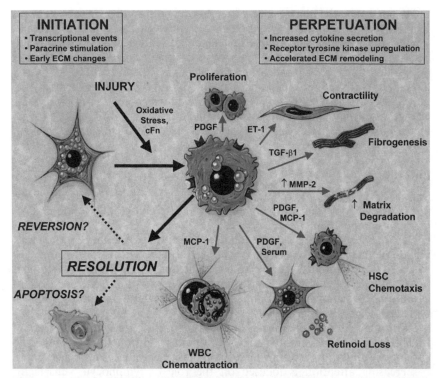

**INITIATION**
* Transcriptional events
* Paracrine stimulation
* Early ECM changes

**PERPETUATION**
* Increased cytokine secretion
* Receptor tyrosine kinase upregulation
* Accelerated ECM remodeling

**Figure 1.** Pathways of stellate cell activation and its resolution. Hepatic stellate cells (HSC) undergo activation in which they acquire many features that contribute to their fibrogenic and proliferative phenotype. Early activation ("Initiation") is followed by major phenotype changes ("Perpetuation") that includes proliferation, contractility, fibrogenesis, matrix degradation, chemotaxis, retinoid loss, and WBC chemotaxis. Finally, when liver injury ceases ("Resolution"), stellate cells may either reverse or undergo apoptosis, thereby reducing the fibrogenic population in liver (reprinted from ref. 14, with permission)

Studies in both animals and humans with progressive injury have defined a gradient of changes within stellate cells that collectively are termed "*activation*"[15] (Figure 1). Stellate cell activation refers to the transition from a quiescent vitamin A-rich cell to a highly fibrogenic cell type characterized morphologically by enlargement of rough endoplasmic reticulum, diminution of vitamin A droplets, ruffled nuclear membrane, appearance of contractile filaments, and proliferation. Proliferation of stellate cells generally occurs in regions of greatest injury, which is typically preceded by an influx of inflammatory cells and is associated with subsequent extracellular matrix (ECM) accumulation.

Stellate cell activation, the central event in hepatic fibrosis, can be conceptualized as occurring in at least two stages: initiation and perpetuation. Initiation refers to early events encompassing rapid changes in gene expression and phenotype that render the cells responsive to cytokines and other stimuli. It results from paracrine stimulation due to rapid, disruptive effects of liver injury on the homeostasis of neighboring cells and from early changes in ECM composition. Perpetuation incorporates those cellular events that amplify the activated phenotype through enhanced cytokine expression and responsiveness and involves at least seven discrete changes in cell behavior: (a) proliferation, (b) chemotaxis, (c) fibrogenesis, (d) contractility, (e) matrix degradation, (f) retinoid loss, and (g) white blood cell (WBC) chemoattractant and cytokine release. Either directly or indirectly the net effect of these changes is accumulation of ECM, architectural distortion, and gradual increase in intrahepatic resistance ultimately leading to clinically significant portal hypertension.

## Initiation

Stimuli initiating stellate cell activation derive from injured hepatocytes and neighboring endothelial and Kupffer cells in addition to rapid, subtle changes in ECM composition.

Hepatocytes, as the most abundant cell in liver by number and volume, are a potent source of reactive oxygen intermediates (ROI), or free radicals, when they are injured[16]. Kupffer cells also generate ROI in response to liver injury. These compounds exert paracrine stimulation of stellate cells. Moreover, their activity is amplified *in vivo* by depletion of antioxidants as typically occurs in diseased liver.

Sinusoidal endothelial cells play a dual role in early stellate cell activation. Injury to sinusoidal endothelial cells stimulates production of a specific variant of cellular fibronectin which has an activating effect on stellate cells[17].

Increasing attention is focused on the role of lymphocyte subsets on hepatic fibrosis, and specifically on hepatic stellate cell activation. Genetic determinants of fibrosis are being uncovered in mice[18], many of which regulate the type and vigor of the inflammatory response. These animal studies are complemented by human data that emphasize the impact of immune suppression on accelerating fibrosis progression, for example in HIV infection[19] or following liver transplantation[20]. Stellate cells express key molecules that participate in the inflammatory response, including CD40, which enables direct interaction with lymphocytes expressing CD40 ligand[21]. Our own studies have begun to explore the impact of specific T cell subsets in animal models of fibrosis using adoptive transfer methods. These efforts may help define new points of attack in modulating fibrosis therapeutically.

## Perpetuation

Perpetuation of stellate cell activation involves key phenotypic responses mediated by effects of cytokines (i.e. soluble growth factors) and degradation of ECM. Enhanced cytokine responses occur at many levels, including increased expression of cell membrane receptors and enhanced signaling. In particular, a family of receptors known as receptor tyrosine kinases (RTK) mediate many of the stellate cell's responses to cytokines, and are broadly up-regulated during liver injury.

Fibrillar or scar ECM also accelerates stellate cell activation. These effects are mediated not only through interactions with integrins, the classic ECM receptors, but also through binding to at least one RTK. We have recently found that a subfamily of receptor tyrosine kinases, discoidin domain receptors (DDR), are up-regulated during stellate cell activation[22-24]. What makes DDR unique is that, unlike other RTK, DDR signal in response to fibrillar collagens rather than soluble growth factors. The identification of discoidin domain receptor-2 (DDR-2) in stellate cells explains why fibril-forming matrix (especially collagen type I) provokes activation of stellate cells during sinusoidal fibrosis. The receptors contribute to a positive feedback loop in which activated stellate cells generate increased fibrillar collagen at a time when the cells are beginning to express a receptor that signals in response to this collagen. As a result of DDR-2 activation by collagen ligand, the cells generate more MMP-2 (matrix metalloproteinase-2), which in turn hastens pathologic matrix degradation by MMP-2. Thus, as the subendothelial basement membrane is replaced by fibrillar collagen, stellate cell activation may be perpetuated via binding of collagen to the DDR-2 receptor.

Successful efforts to reverse fibrosis and cirrhosis must include the degradation of excess ECM in order for normal liver architecture to be restored. Fortunately, there has been significant progress in understanding how scar is degraded in liver by specific enzymes whose activities and specificities are tightly regulated. There are broadly two kinds of matrix degradation in liver: one that disrupts the low-density matrix of normal liver ("pathologic matrix degradation") and may therefore worsen liver disease; the other the degradation of excess scar that may help restore the architecture of the injured liver to normal.

In liver "pathologic" matrix degradation refers to the early disruption of the normal subendothelial matrix which occurs through the actions of at least four enzymes: MMP-2 (also called "gelatinase A" or "72 kDa type IV collagenase") and MMP-9 ("gelatinase B" or "92 kDa type IV collagenase"), which degrade type IV collagen, membrane-type MMP-1 or MMP-2, which activates latent MMP-2, and stromelysin-1, which degrades proteoglycans and glycoproteins, and also activates latent collagenases (see ref. 25 for review).

Failure to degrade the accumulated scar matrix is a major reason why fibrosis will progress to cirrhosis. MMP-1 is the main protease which can degrade type I collagen, the principal collagen in fibrotic liver, although it is not clear which cell(s) in liver produce this important enzyme. More importantly, progressive fibrosis is associated with marked increases in TIMP-1 and TIMP-2 (tissue inhibitor of metalloproteinases 1 and 2), leading to a net decrease in protease activity, and therefore more unopposed matrix accumulation[26]. Stellate cells are the major source of these inhibitors. Sustained TIMP-1 expression is emerging as a key reason why fibrosis progresses.

## PHENOTYPIC RESPONSES OF ACTIVATED STELLATE CELLS

Discrete phenotype responses of stellate cells can be identified as their activation in response to liver injury is perpetuated. These include: (a) proliferation, (b) contractility, (c) fibrogenesis, (d) matrix degradation, (e) chemotaxis, (f) retinoid loss, (g) cytokine release and WBC chemoattraction. A review of these features is instructive to illustrate how their integration leads to sustained ECM production and liver disease.

## Proliferation

Increased numbers of stellate cells in injured liver arise in part from local proliferation in response to polypeptide growth factors, most of which signal through receptor tyrosine kinases[27]. Platelet-derived growth factor (PDGF) is the best-characterized and most potent among these proliferative factors in hepatic fibrosis. Injury is associated with both increased autocrine PDGF and up-regulation of PDGF receptor. PDGF signaling in activated stellate cells includes activation of the ERK/MAP kinase pathway as well as calcium, changes in intracellular pH and phosphoinositol 3 kinase (PI3-kinase).

A large number of other mitogens can provoke stellate cell proliferation, but none is as potent as PDGF. These include thrombin, fibroblast growth factor, and vascular endothelial growth factor. For most of these cytokines, induction of their specific cell membrane receptors parallels their increased growth stimulation.

## Contractility

Contractility by activated stellate cells represents an important mechanism underlying increased portal resistance during liver injury[28]. The key contractile stimulus towards stellate cells is endothelin 1 (ET-1). Up-regulation of ET-1 production is accompanied by increased endothelin-converting enzyme-1, which activates the latent ET-1. ET-1, in addition to its potent contractile effect, also regulates stellate cell proliferation.

At least two G-protein-coupled receptors mediate the effects of ET-1. Unlike receptor tyrosine kinases, which are generally induced during activation, ET receptor types A and B are expressed on both quiescent and activated stellate cells. However, the relative prevalence of ETA and ETB receptors changes with the cellular activation, and each mediates divergent responses.

## Fibrogenesis

Transforming growth factor beta 1 (TGF-$\beta_1$) is the dominant stimulus to ECM production by stellate cells[29]. TGF-$\beta_1$ is increased in experimental and human hepatic fibrosis. There are many sources of this cytokine; however, autocrine expression is most important. Regulation of TGF-$\beta$ activity is highly complex, with multiple levels including activation of the latent cytokine, binding to circulating proteins, as well as a complex signaling cascade within cells following binding to their receptors. Up-regulation of collagen synthesis during activation is among the most striking molecular responses of stellate cells to injury, and is mediated by both transcriptional and post-transcriptional mechanisms, not all of which can be ascribed to TGF-$\beta_1$. Recently, fibrogenic stimulation of stellate cells has also been ascribed to connective tissue growth factor (CTGF), a widely expressed growth factor[30].

## Matrix degradation

As noted above, changes in matrix protease activity lead to remodeling of the hepatic ECM during liver injury, which both directly and indirectly accelerates stellate cell activation.

Through the up-regulation of TIMP-1 and TIMP-2, activated stellate cells can also inhibit the activity of interstitial collagenases, which additionally favors the accumulation of scar. Up-regulation of TIMP-1 gene expression requires a high-mobility activator protein-1 (AP-1) binding activity which is absent from quiescent stellate cells; this mode of regulating TIMP-1 gene expression has not previously been described.

## Stellate cell chemotaxis

The directed migration of activated stellate cells enhances their accumulation in areas of injury[31]. PDGF and monocyte chemotactic protein-1 (MCP-1) can stimulate directed migration of activated but not quiescent stellate cells. Chemotaxis of activated stellate cells towards areas of injury explains why scar begins to develop in linear septae, since this is the region where activated stellate cells are aligned.

## Retinoid loss

Loss of intracellular vitamin A is a notable feature of stellate cell activation, yet it remains unknown whether retinoid loss is required for stellate cells to activate, and which retinoids might accelerate or prevent activation *in vivo*.

## Cytokine release and leukocyte chemoattraction

Increased production and/or activity of cytokines are critical for perpetuation of stellate cell activation[27]. Almost all features of stellate cell activation can be attributed to autocrine cytokines. ECM in liver is an important reservoir of bound growth factors, many of which are likely to be derived from stellate cells.

Stellate cells can also amplify inflammation through the release of neutrophil and monocyte chemoattractants. Key inflammatory chemokines are colony-stimulating factor and MCP-1. Up-regulation of adhesion molecules accompanying stellate cell activation further amplifies inflammation during liver injury.

## SUMMARY

Progress in understanding intracellular signaling, transcriptional gene regulation and genetic determinants of fibrosis offers optimism for continued advances in understanding hepatic stellate cell activation and fibrosis. The field has advanced to a critical stage in which there are now realistic expectations for treatment of hepatic fibrosis in patients with chronic liver disease built upon this increased understanding.

## References

1. Dienstag JL, Goldin RD, Heathcote EJ et al. Histological outcome during long-term lamivudine therapy. Gastroenterology. 2003;124:105–17.

2. Poynard T, McHutchison J, Manns M et al. Impact of pegylated interferon alfa-2b and ribavirin on liver fibrosis in patients with chronic hepatitis C. Gastroenterology. 2002;122:1303–13.
3. Bonis PA, Friedman SL, Kaplan MM. Is liver fibrosis reversible? N Engl J Med. 2001;344:452–4.
4. Hammel P, Couvelard A, O'Toole D et al. Regression of liver fibrosis after biliary drainage in patients with chronic pancreatitis and stenosis of the common bile duct. N Engl J Med. 2001;344:418–23.
5. El-Serag HB, Mason AC. Risk factors for the rising rates of primary liver cancer in the United States. Arch Intern Med. 2000;160:3227–30.
6. Befeler AS, Di Bisceglie AM. Hepatocellular carcinoma: diagnosis and treatment. Gastroenterology. 2002;122:1609–19.
7. Rojkind M, Giambrone MA, Biempica L. Collagen types in normal and cirrhotic liver. Gastroenterology. 1979;76:710–19.
8. Sims D. Recent advances in pericyte biology and implications for health and disease. Can J Cardiol. 1991;7:431–43.
9. Pinzani M, Failli P, Ruocco C et al. Fat-storing cells as liver-specific pericytes. Spatial dynamics of agonist-stimulated intracellular calcium transients. J Clin Invest. 1992;90:642–6.
10. Bauer M, Paquette N, Zhang J et al. Chronic ethanol consumption increases hepatic sinusoidal contractile response to endothelin-1 in rat. Hepatology. 1994;22:1565.
11. Bauer M, Zhang J, Bauer I et al. ET-1 induced alterations of hepatic microcirculation: sinusoidal and extrasinusoidal sites of actions. Am J Physiol. 1994;267:143–9.
12. Bhathal P, Grossman H. Reduction of the increased portal vascular resistance of the isolated perfused cirrhotic rat liver by vasodilators. J Hepatol. 1985;1:325–37.
13. Okumura S, Takei Y, Kawano S. Vasoactive effect of endothelin-1 on rat liver in vivo. Hepatology. 1994;19:155–61.
14. Geerts A. History and heterogeneity of stellate cells, and role in normal liver function. Semin Liver Dis. 2001;21:311–36.
15. Friedman SL. Molecular regulation of hepatic fibrosis, an integrated cellular response to tissue injury. J Biol Chem. 2000;275:2247–50.
16. Tsukamoto H, Horne W, Kamimura S et al. Experimental liver cirrhosis induced by alcohol and iron. J Clin Invest. 1995;96:620–30.
17. Jarnagin WR, Rockey DC, Koteliansky VE, Wang SS, Bissell DM. Expression of variant fibronectins in wound healing: cellular source and biological activity of the EIIIA segment in rat hepatic fibrogenesis. J Cell Biol. 1994;127:2037–48.
18. Shi Z, Wakil AE, Rockey DC. Strain-specific differences in mouse hepatic wound healing are mediated by divergent T helper cytokine responses. Proc Natl Acad Sci USA. 1997;94:10663–8.
19. Benhamou Y, Di Martino V, Bochet M et al. Factors affecting liver fibrosis in human immunodeficiency virus- and hepatitis C virus-coinfected patients: impact of protease inhibitor therapy. Hepatology. 2001;34:283–7.
20. Schluger LK, Sheiner PA, Thung SN et al. Severe recurrent cholestatic hepatitis C following orthotopic liver transplantation. Hepatology. 1996;23:971–6.
21. Schwabe RF, Schnabl B, Kweon YO, Brenner DA. CD40 activates NF-kappa B and c-Jun N-terminal kinase and enhances chemokine secretion on activated human hepatic stellate cells. J Immunol. 2001;166:6812–19.
22. Ikeda K, Wang LH, Torres R et al. Discoidin domain receptor 2 interacts with Src and Shc following its activation by type I collagen. J Biol Chem. 2002;277:19206–12.
23. Olaso E, Ikeda K, Eng FJ et al. DDR2 receptor promotes MMP-2-mediated proliferation and invasion by hepatic stellate cells. J Clin Invest. 2001;108:1369–78.
24. Olaso E, Labrador JP, Wang L et al. Discoidin domain receptor 2 regulates fibroblast proliferation and migration through the extracellular matrix in association with transcriptional activation of matrix metalloproteinase-2. J Biol Chem. 2002;277:3606–13.
25. Benyon D, Arthur MJP. Extracellular matrix degradation and the role of stellate cells. Semin Liver Dis. 2001;21:373–84.
26. Iredale JP. Stellate cell behavior during resolution of liver injury. Semin Liver Dis. 2001;21:427–36.
27. Pinzani M, Marra F. Cytokine receptors and signaling during stellate cell activation. Semin Liver Dis. 2001;21:397–416.

28. Rockey DC. Vascular mediators in the injured liver. Hepatology. 2003;37:4–12.
29. Gressner AM, Weiskirchen R, Breitkopf K, Dooley S. Roles of tgf-beta in hepatic fibrosis. Front Biosci. 2002;7:D793–807.
30. Paradis V, Dargere D, Bonvoust F, Vidaud M, Segarini P, Bedossa P. Effects and regulation of connective tissue growth factor on hepatic stellate cells. Lab Invest. 2002;82:767–74.
31. Marra F. Chemokines in liver inflammation and fibrosis. Front Biosci. 2002;7:d1899–914.

# 5
# The role of hepatic stellate cells/myofibroblasts

MASSIMO PINZANI

## HEPATIC STELLATE CELLS (HSC) AND OTHER CONTRACTILE CELLS

The recognition that HSC are provided with contractile properties represents a key acquisition in the knowledge of the biology of this cell type[1]. Contraction of activated HSC occurs *in vitro* in response to different vaso-constrictors. This experimental evidence is representative of HSC contractile status in fibrotic liver, where contraction of activated HSC in response to various stimuli may have important implications in the pathogenesis of portal hypertension and in the contraction of mature scar tissue. Following the demonstration that culture-activated human and rat HSC are able to contract in response to different vasoconstrictors[2,3], the potential involvement of this cell type in the genesis and progression of portal hypertension has been postulated. The presence of a contractile cell type operating in liver sinusoids and in developing scar tissue reinforced the concept of a dynamic component for the increased intrahepatic resistance in cirrhotic liver modifiable by vasodilators[4].

The potential consequences of the contractile attitude of HSC are still a matter of controversy and some key questions should be addressed for an objective assessment of this theme. These include: (1) Do HSC play a role in the regulation of sinusoidal tone in normal liver? (2) Do HSC influence portal pressure in conditions of developing fibrosis and "capillarization" of sinusoids? (3) Do HSC influence portal pressure in cirrhotic liver?

Although several lines of evidence suggest a role of HSC in the regulation of sinusoidal blood flow in normal liver, this issue is still matter of substantial controversy. From the morphological standpoint some observations argue against the role of HSC in the regulation of sinusoidal blood flow[5]. First, in their *in-vivo* tridimensional disposition HSC do not have a stellate form (typical of their aspect in bidimensional culture on plastic) but rather a "spider-like" appearance ("arachnocytes") in respect of their small cell body with a series of radiating and parallel slender processes. According to the authors of these observations, cells with this tridimensional disposition are not likely to be "contraction-ready". Additional limitations to effective cell contraction are offered by the spatial limitation of the space of Disse, by the intracytoplasmic presence of lipid droplets that prevent microfilaments from assembly in a long span, and by the ultrastructural evidence of a limited development of contractile filaments in quiescent HSC. However, recent work from the same group of investigators has highlighted how HSC disposed along sinusoidal structures are highly pleomorphic, with morphological aspects resembling true myofibroblasts at the periphery of portal tracts[6]. It is therefore possible that only a subpopulation of HSC, with contraction-ready features, contribute to the regulation of sinusoidal blood flow in normal liver.

Regardless, studies evaluating the hepatic microcirculation by intravital microscopy techniques have suggested that HSC could be involved in the regulation of sinusoidal tone in normal liver[7,8]. An additional matter of debate is provided by studies aimed at estimating HSC contraction with techniques able to detect the development of contractile forces in response to vasoconstrictors[9]. The results of these studies indicate that the magnitude and kinetics of contraction and relaxation are consistent with the hypothesis that HSC may affect sinusoidal resistance. However, for understandable technical reasons, these data were obtained in rat HSC in primary culture 7 days after isolation, when a certain degree of activation in culture has occurred. In conclusion, although HSC could be proposed as liver-specific pericytes by reason of their location, spatial distribution, relationship with the peripheral nervous system, and ultrastructural features, no conclusive evidence is presently available concerning their role in the regulation of sinusoidal blood flow in physiological conditions.

As stated previously, a remarkable increase in HSC contractile properties is likely a key feature of their activated state[2,3,10,11]. At this stage HSC have been shown to express a large number of voltage-operated calcium channels, the activation of which is associated with an increased intracellular calcium concentration followed by marked cell contraction[12]. These changes are possibly dependent on intracellular and extracellular factors. First, the transition to the "myofibroblast-like" phenotype is ultrastructurally characterized by the appearance of massive contractile structures including dense bodies and patches of myofilaments throughout the cytoplasm. Second, HSC activation is accompanied by increased expression of α-SMA (alpha-smooth muscle actin), and it is likely that this cytoskeletal protein is, at least in part, responsible for increased cell contractility. Interestingly, both pro-fibrogenic agents and vasoconstrictors represent potential regulators of the α-SMA gene, and, in this context, the transcription factor c-myb has been shown to form complexes with a regulatory element of the α-SMA gene, suggesting that induction of this gene may be transcriptionally regulated[13]. Among "external" factors that could affect HSC contractility, the modified extracellular matrix (ECM) pattern typical of fibrotic liver is also likely to play an important role. The presence of a microenvironment rich in fibrillar ECM, and the expression of integrin receptors specific for the constitutive components of this ECM (particularly collagen type I and III)[14,15], lead to a structural configuration of activated HSC characterized by cytoskeletal tension or stress. This feature of activated HSC is likely to be relevant for the modulation of different cell functions including proliferation and migration in response to growth factors and contraction in response to vasoconstrictors. It is indeed logical to hypothesize that HSC contractile status could be conditioned by the presence of vasoactive substances present in the microenvironment of hepatic tissue undergoing active fibrogenesis.

As a consequence of their activated state, HSC contribute to profound alteration of the sinusoidal structure during the early stages of hepatic fibrogenesis. Capillarized sinusoids are characterized by accumulation of fibrillar ECM in the space of Disse. In this context endothelial cells are characterized by a loss of their fenestrations, thus acquiring a "generic" endothelial cell phenotype (denoted by the positivity for factor VIII). These changes are associated with: (a) impairment in the metabolic exchange between blood and hepatocytes, (b) impairment in the natural dispersion of hydrostatic forces that occurs in the normal sinusoidal sieve. For these reasons capillarization of sinusoids is likely to represent an initial cause of portal hypertension during the early development of hepatic fibrosis. In conditions characterized by portal tract expansion and periportal fibrosis, such as chronic viral hepatitis and primary biliary cirrhosis, HSC activation occurs in periportal sinusoids, thus contributing to the so-called "early presinusoidal resistance locus". In other conditions, such as chronic alcoholic hepatitis and non-alcoholic steatohepatitis, capillarization of sinusoids is initially limited to the center of the liver lobule, around the centrilobular vein, resulting in obstruction to sinusoidal blood flow.

It is likely that activated HSC, together with other contractile cells present in the liver tissue, play an important role in the development of portal hypertension only during initial fibrotic transformation. However, at these early stages in the fibrogenic evolution of chronic liver diseases portal hypertension is not yet clinically relevant. This is likely due to the substantial integrity of hepatic angioarchitecture and to the compensatory adjustments occurring at the presinusoidal level in the intrahepatic portal circulation.

The hallmark of any form of cirrhosis is a profound alteration of the liver angioarchitecture with two prominent features: (a) development of septal fibrosis establishing portal–central anastomoses, and (b) arterialization and capillarization of sinusoids due to both reduction of portal flow and formation of "feeding vessels" derived from the hepatic artery. These changes *per se* could be sufficient to explain the increase in portal pressure typical of liver cirrhosis[16]. Indeed, portal–central anastomoses, although representing direct connections between the portal and the systemic circulation, follow irregular patterns and are embedded in a developing scar tissue undergoing, to a certain extent, spontaneous retraction. In addition, these neoformed vessels could be the site of thrombosis, thus aggravating the intrahepatic hemodynamic disturbances[17]. These general alterations are typical of postnecrotic cirrhosis. In other types of cirrhosis, additional factors may play a role. In alcoholic cirrhosis, compression of hepatic venules by scar tissue that develops around the central vein (pericentral fibrosis) and marked hepatocellular swelling may aggravate portal hypertension. In primary or secondary biliary cirrhosis, distortion of portal vein branches secondary to a progressive portal–portal fibrosis, may represent a "presinusoidal" cause of portal hypertension.

It is very clear that all these potential causes of portal hypertension are likely irreversible and not likely affected by pharmacologic intervention. Particularly in the case of septal fibrosis, the establishment of portal–central anastomoses likely represents a "point of no-return" for the fibrogenic process as the profound derangement of hepatic angioarchitecture causes additional liver tissue damage perpetuating and aggravating the fibroproliferative process. However, this view bears the same defect of the classic concept of fibrosis, considered as a simple deposition of fibrillar extracellular matrix in a tissue context. Indeed, the altered angioarchitecture of cirrhotic liver is characterized by neoformed venous vessels (i.e. portal–central anastomoses) embedded in an actively evolving scar tissue where a complex interplay occurs between several cell types and soluble mediators. This new biological microenvironment may support the experimental evidence indicating the existence of a "reversible" intrahepatic tissue component responsible for portal hypertension. Several classes of vasodilators administered in the portal vein of cirrhotic rats have been shown to decrease portal pressure and to favorably influence microvascular exchange and function[4,18,19]. In agreement with the role of activated HSC in the progression of liver fibrosis, their topographical distribution, and their biological features, there is no doubt that this cellular element may constitute a key element in this context. However, several other contractile cell types may contribute to the contraction of the evolving scar tissue typical of cirrhotic liver. In particular, while activated HSC may be important at the edge and within cirrhotic nodules where sinusoids are capillarized, activated portal myofibroblasts and smooth muscle cells, derived from portal arterial vessels, are likely to strongly affect the neoformed vascular structures located in the inner part of fibrous septa. It should be stressed that all these cell types contribute to the progression of liver fibrosis and that no major differences in their contractile potential are likely to occur.

## VASOACTIVE AGENTS AS PLEIOTROPIC CYTOKINES IN PORTAL HYPERTENSION

Because of the close relationship occurring between progressive fibrosis and portal hypertension, any cytokine shown to be involved in the progression of hepatic fibrogenesis (i.e. factors that are mitogenic, chemoattractant or able to induce a regulation of genes involved in ECM deposition) could be considered important also for the development of portal hypertension[1]. However, factors generally defined as "vasoactive" may be provided with effects which are not simply limited to cell contraction or relaxation. Indeed, many of these factors are characterized by effects on cell functions relevant for the progression of fibrosis, and therefore could be regarded as cytokines. Several vasoactive agents have been shown to be effective in modulating activated HSC contractility in culture. Among other vasoconstrictors, the role of endothelin 1 (ET-1) has been particularly highlighted. ET-1, a potent vasoactive 21-amino-acid peptide secreted by endothelial as well as other cell types, has been shown to exert a multifunctional role in a variety of tissues and cells[20], including the liver.

Endothelins (ET-1, ET-2, and ET-3) bind to G-protein-coupled receptors, termed $ET_A$, $ET_B$, and to a still not-well-characterized $ET_C$ receptor. The $ET_A$ receptor binds ET-1 with a higher affinity than ET-3, the $ET_B$ receptor displays similar affinity for both peptides, and the $ET_C$ receptor exhibits a higher affinity for ET-3 than ET-1. Activation of ET receptors originates intracellular signals leading to differentiation, proliferation, growth inhibition, cell contraction and a variety of metabolic effects. However, it is increasingly clear that activation of a given ET receptor does not necessarily lead to identical biologic effects in different cell types. This intriguing and peculiar feature is currently explained in terms of receptor structure, since the ET receptor is a typical heptahelical G-protein-coupled receptor. In ligand binding to the heptahelical receptor the receptor has two functions, i.e. "address" (address domain: regulates the affinity for the ligand) and "message" (message domain: regulates the activation of different G proteins and their downstream effectors). A different part of the ligand structure also corresponds to each domain of the receptor. Although ET receptors are currently classified according to their affinity for the three known forms of ET, it has been proposed that they should be classified according to their message domain. Indeed, each $G\alpha$ protein acts on different target molecules, resulting in different responses. In addition, the activation of each $G\alpha$ protein presumably depends on its intracellular level. Therefore, although the same ET receptor is activated by the same ligand, the resulting final response may be different from cell to cell[21]. This complex organization of ET-related intracellular signaling may explain at least some of the discrepancies in the biologic effects of this class of peptides reported in the literature.

Infusion of ET-1 in the isolated perfused rat liver causes a sustained and dose-dependent increase in portal pressure associated with increased glycogenolysis and oxygen consumption[22–24]. ET-1 stimulates glycogenolysis, phosphoinositide turnover and repetitive, sustained intracellular calcium transients in isolated rat hepatocytes[25,26]. Other studies indicate that ET-1 may also have important interactions with liver non-parenchymal cells. Cultured sinusoidal endothelial cells isolated from rat liver have been shown to release ET-1[27], and preferential binding sites for ET-1 have been identified, both in vivo and in vitro[28,29], on HSC. Importantly activated rat and human HSC have been shown to express pre-proET-1 mRNA[30,31] and to release ET-1 in cell supernatants in response to agonists such as angiotensin II, PDGF, TGF-β and ET-1 itself[31], thus raising the possibility of a paracrine and autocrine action of ET-1[32,33]. Consolidated experimental evidence indicates that ET-induced ET-1 synthesis in HSC is regulated through modulation of endothelin-converting enzyme-1 (ECE-1), rather than by modulation of the precursor pre-proET-1[34]. Overall, it is increasingly evident that the process of HSC activation and phenotypical modulation is characterized by a close and complex relationship with the ET system. The ability to synthesize and release ET-1 is associated with a progressive shift in the relative predominance of $ET_A$ and $ET_B$ receptors observed during serial subculture: $ET_A$ are predominant in the early phases of activation, whereas $ET_B$ become increasingly more abundant in "myofibroblast-like" cells[31,35]. This shift in the relative receptor densities may be directed at differentiating the possible paracrine and autocrine effects of ET-1 on HSC during the activation process. Indeed, when HSC are provided with a majority of $ET_A$ receptors (early phases of activation), stimulation with ET-1 causes a dose-dependent increase in cell growth, ERK activity and expression of c-*fos*. These effects, likely related to the activation of the Ras-ERK pathway, are completely blocked by pre-treatment with BQ-123, a specific $ET_A$ receptor antagonist[31], and are in agreement with studies performed in other vascular pericytes such as glomerular mesangial cells[36]. Conversely, in later stages of activation, when the number of $ET_B$ receptors increases, ET-1 appears to induce a prevalent antiproliferative effect linked to the activation of this receptor subtype[37]. In this setting the activation of the $ET_B$ receptor stimulates the production of prostaglandins, leading to an increase in intracellular cAMP, which in turn reduces the activation of both ERK and JNK[38]. In addition, both cAMP and prostaglandins up-regulate $ET_B$ binding sites, thus suggesting the possibility of a positive feedback regulatory loop. In this context it is important to note that, at least in human HSC, ET-1-induced cell contraction occurs at any stage of HSC activation[31]. Since HSC contraction is always blocked by $ET_A$ receptor antagonists, and never reproduced by selective $ET_B$ agonists, it is conceivable that the signaling pathways regulating HSC contraction require the activation of a small number of $ET_A$ receptors and are somehow divergent from those regulating cell growth.

In aggregate these observations suggest that ET-1 may act as a potent vasoconstrictor agonist regulating intrahepatic blood flow in cirrhotic liver with a potential role in the pathogenesis of portal hypertension. Along these lines, morphological studies have clearly indicated that ET-1 (both at mRNA and protein levels) is markedly overexpressed in different cellular elements present within cirrhotic liver tissue, and particularly in sinusoidal endothelial and HSC in their activated phenotype located in the sinusoids of the regenerating nodules, at the edges of fibrous septa, and in the ECM embedding neoformed vessels within fibrous bands[31]. In addition, clinical studies indicate that a direct relationship exists between ET receptor mRNA abundance and the degree of portal hypertension in cirrhotic patients[39]. The *in-vivo* relevance of the ET system during chronic fibrogenic disorders involving liver has been analyzed in animal models of hepatic fibrosis by employing pharmacological ET-receptor blockers. The use of mixed $ET_A/ET_B$ receptor blockers yielded conflicting results: Rockey and co-workers reported a significant reduction of ECM accumulation following the administration of Bosentan[40], whereas other investigators reported an increased ECM accumulation by employing RO 48-5695[41]. Based on the evidence obtained *in vitro*, it is conceivable that the simultaneous inhibition of two receptors mediating divergent effects on cell proliferation would likely lead to marginal effects on the progression of fibrosis. This interpretation is corroborated by a more recent study, performed in the bile duct ligation model, showing a remarkable inhibition of ECM accumulation following the administration of the non-peptide $ET_A$ receptor antagonist LU 135252[42]. Indeed, considering in aggregate all the potential effects (metabolic, proliferative, antiproliferative, contractile, etc.) of the ET system in fibrotic liver, it would be reasonable to reduce the negative effects of ET-1 (mediated through the $ET_A$ receptor), maximizing the potentially positive actions (mediated through the $ET_B$ receptor). The observation that ET-1 may exert direct pro-cholestatic effects on the biliary tree by inhibiting secretin-stimulated ductal secretion through interaction with $ET_A$ receptors[43], further reinforces this view.

Analogously to what is proposed for ET-1, angiotensin II, vasopressin, and thrombin, although generally referred to as "vasoconstrictors", promote pro-fibrogenic actions and are considered pleiotropic cytokines when viewed in the context of the chronic wound-healing process. Circulating levels of angiotensin II (A-II), a powerful vasoconstrictor, are frequently increased in cirrhotic patients, and have been implicated in the circulatory disturbances typical of this clinical condition. However, A-II, in addition to its action as vasoconstrictor, is provided with biologic properties potentially relevant for the progression of chronic fibrogenic disorders. These include increase in cell proliferation and cell hypertrophy, and accordingly A-II may be considered also as a pleiotropic cytokine. Bataller and co-workers reported that activated human HSC express A-II receptors of the AT1 subtype, and that an increased expression of this type of receptor may represent a feature of HSC activation[44]. Stimulation with A-II elicits a marked dose-dependent increase in $[Ca^{2+}]_i$ concentration associated with rapid cell contraction. Moreover, A-II stimulates DNA synthesis and cell growth. The involvement of AT1 receptors in these effects of A-II is confirmed by their complete abrogation following pre-incubation with the AT1 receptor antagonist losartan. Further work by this group of investigators has shown that, upon activation, HSC express the components of the renin–angiotensin system and synthesize A-II[45], and that NADPH oxidase mediates the biologic actions of A-II on HSC[46]. This *in-vitro* evidence is largely supported by the results of studies performed in animal models. By employing the bile duct ligated model, Paiziz and co-workers have demonstrated that the renin–angiotensin system, expressed also in normal rat liver, becomes markedly up-regulated during the fibrogenic process typical of this model[47]. In addition, these authors have shown that A-II type 1 receptor blockade in the same experimental model leads to a reduced expression of pro-fibrogenic genes[48].

Analogous effects on HSC biology have been described for arginine vasopressin (AVP). Human activated HSC express V1 receptors, and stimulation with AVP elicits a dose-dependent increase in intracellular $[Ca^{2+}]_i$ coupled with cell contraction. Moreover, AVP increases ERK activity, DNA synthesis, and cell growth[49].

The serine protease thrombin (THR) regulates platelet aggregation, endothelial cell activation and other important responses in vascular biology and in acute and chronic wound repair. Although THR is a protease, it acts as a traditional hormone or as a pleiotropic cytokine based on the nature of its receptors, the protease-activated receptors or PAR. PAR are G-protein-coupled receptors that use a fascinating mechanism to convert an extracellular proteolytic cleavage event into a transmembrane signal: these receptors carry their own ligands, which remain cryptic until unmasked by receptor cleavage[50]. Four PAR are known in mouse and human: human PAR1, PAR3, and PAR4 can be activated by THR, whereas PAR2 is activated by trypsin and tryptase as well as by coagulation factors VIIa and Xa, but not by THR. Studies by Marra and co-workers have shown that expression of PAR1 is markedly increased in chronic fibrogenic disorders involving liver. In addition human HSC express PAR1, and this expression increases during HSC activation[51,52]. Stimulation of human HSC with THR induces cell contraction[2], proliferation[51], synthesis and release of chemokines such as MCP-1[52], or platelet-activating factor[53]. The signaling mechanisms specifically regulating THR action in HSC have not been reported thus far.

In addition to ET-1, A-II and thrombin, the potential involvement of other vasoconstrictors synthesized and released within liver tissue has been suggested. Titos and co-workers[54] have recently reported that in cirrhotic rat liver there is an increased synthesis of cysteinyl leukotrienes (LT). In this context, hepatocytes exhibit the highest ability to generate cysteinyl-LT. Importantly, these compounds elicit a strong contractile response in activated HSC. Additional studies by the same investigators have demonstrated that 5-lipoxygenase inhibition reduces intrahepatic vascular resistance of cirrhotic rat livers, thus confirming a pathogenic role of cysteinyl-LT in this setting[55].

Taken together all these findings reinforce the concept of an imbalance between vasoconstrictor and vasodilator agents within the intrahepatic circulation of cirrhotic liver. Importantly, the concentration of vasoconstrictors acting on the intrahepatic microvasculature of cirrhotic liver may increase as a consequence of clinical or subclinical events such as infections in the peritoneal cavity, which are clearly associated with a worsening of portal hypertension and with an increased incidence of variceal bleeding[56]. Appropriate use of drugs currently indicated for the treatment of portal hypertension[57] should be carefully reconsidered in light of the current knowledge of the cellular and molecular mechanisms of portal hypertension.

## References

1. Pinzani M, Gentilini P. Biology of hepatic stellate cells and their possible relevance in the pathogenesis of portal hypertension in cirrhosis. Semin Liver Dis. 1999;19:397–410.
2. Pinzani M, Failli P, Ruocco C et al. Fat-storing cells as liver-specific pericytes: spatial dynamics of agonist-stimulated intracellular calcium transients. J Clin Invest. 1992;90:642–6.
3. Kawada N, Klein H, Decker K. Eicoesanoid-mediated contractility of hepatic stellate cells. Biochem J. 1992;285:367–71.
4. Bhathal PS, Grossman HJ. Reduction of the increased portal vascular resistance of the isolated perfused cirrhotic rat liver by vasodilators. J Hepatol. 1985;1:325–37.
5. Ekataksin W, Kaneda K. Liver microvascular architecture: an insight into the pathophysiology of portal hypertension. Semin Liver Dis. 1999;19:359–82.
6. Pattanapen G, Noriko K, McCuskey RS, Ekataksin W. The porcine arachnocyte spectrum: panzonal polymorphism of hepatic stellate cell population as revealed by extensive reconstruction of confocal optic imaging. Hepatology. 2003;38:784A (abstract).
7. Zhang JX, Pegoli W Jr, Clemens MG. Endothelin-1 induces direct constriction of hepatic sinusoids. Am J Physiol. 1994;266:G624–32.
8. Zhang JX, Bauer M, Clemens MG. Vessel- and target cell-specific actions of endothelin-1 and endothelin-3 in rat liver. Am J Physiol. 1995;269:G269–77.

9. Thimgan MS, Yee HF Jr. Quantitation of rat hepatic stellate cell contraction: stellate cells' contribution to sinusoidal tone. Am J Physiol. 1999;277:G137–43.
10. Rockey DC, Housset CN, Friedman SL. Activation-dependent contractility of rat hepatic lipocytes in culture and *in vivo*. J Clin Invest. 1993;92:1795–804.
11. Rockey DC, Weisiger RA. Endothelin induced contractility of stellate cells from normal and cirrhotic rat liver: implications for regulation of portal pressure and resistance. Hepatology. 1996;24:233–40.
12. Bataller R, Nicolas JM, Gines P et al. Contraction of human hepatic stellate cells activated in culture: a role for voltage-operated calcium channels. J Hepatol. 1998;29:398–408.
13. Buck M, Kim DJ, Houglum K, Hassanein T, Chojkier M. c-Myb modulates transcription of the α-smooth muscle actin gene in activated hepatic stellate cells. Am J Physiol. 2000;278:G321–8.
14. Carloni V, Romanelli RG, Pinzani M, Laffi G, Gentilini P. Expression and function of integrin receptors for collagen and laminin in cultured human hepatic stellate cells. Gastroenterology. 1996;110:1127–36.
15. Racine-Samson L, Rockey DC, Bissell DM. The role of alpha1beta1 integrin in wound contraction. A quantitative analysis of liver myofibroblasts *in vivo* and in primary culture. J Biol Chem. 1997;49:30911–17.
16. Shibayama Y, Nakata K. Significance of septal fibrosis for disturbance of hepatic circulation. Liver. 1992;12:22–5.
17. Wanless IR, Wong F, Blendis LM, Greig P, Heathcote EJ, Levy G. Hepatic and portal vein thrombosis in cirrhosis: possible role in the development of parenchymal extinction and portal hypertension. Hepatology. 1995;21:1238–47.
18. Reichen J, Le M. Verapamil favorably influences hepatic microvascular exchange and function in rats with cirrhosis of the liver. J Clin Invest. 1986;78:448–55.
19. Marteau P, Ballet F, Chazouilleres O et al. Effect of vasodilators on hepatic microcirculation in cirrhosis: a study in the isolated perfused rat liver. Hepatology. 1989;9:820–3.
20. Kedzierski RM, Yanagisawa M. Endothelin system: the double-edged sword in health and disease. Annu Rev Pharmacol Toxicol. 2001;41:851–76.
21. Masaki T, Ninomiya H, Sakamoto A, Okamoto Y. Structural basis of the function of endothelin receptor. Mol Cell Biochem. 1999;190:153–6.
22. Gandhi CR, Stephenson K, Olson MS. Endothelin, a potent peptide agonist in the liver. J Biol Chem. 1990;265:17432–5.
23. Roden M, Vierhapper H, Liener K, Waldhausl W. Endothelin-1-stimulated glucose production *in vitro* in the isolated perfused rat liver. Metabolism. 1992;41:290–5.
24. Thran-Thi T-A, Kawada N, Decker K. Regulation of endothelin-1 action on the perfused rat liver. FEBS Lett. 1993;318:353–7.
25. Gandhi CR, Behal RH, Harvey SA, Nouchi TA, Olson MS. Hepatic effects of endothelin. Receptor characterization and endothelin-induced signal transduction in hepatocytes. Biochem J. 1992;287:897–904.
26. Serradeil-Le Gal C, Jouneaux C, Sanchez-Bueno A et al. Endothelin action in rat liver. Receptors, free $Ca^{2+}$ oscillations, and activation of glycogenolysis. J Clin Invest. 1991;87:133–8.
27. Rieder H, Ramadori G, Meyer zum Buschenfelde KH. Sinusoidal endothelial liver cells *in vitro* release endothelin: augmentation by transforming growth factor β and Kupffer cell-conditioned media. Klin Wochenschr. 1991;69:387–91.
28. Furoya S, Naruse S, Nakayama T, Nokihara K. Binding of [125]I- endothelin-1 to fat-storing cells in rat liver revealed by electron microscopic radioautography. Anat Embryol. 1992;185:97–100.
29. Gondo K, Ueno T, Masaharu S, Sakisaka S, Sata M, Tanikawa K. The endothelin-1 binding site in rat liver tissue: light- and electron-microscopic autoradiographic studies. Gastroenterology. 1993;104:1745–9.
30. Housset CN, Rockey DC, Bissel DM. Endothelin receptors in rat liver: lipocytes as a contractile target for endothelin 1. Proc Natl Acad Sci USA. 1993;90:9266–70.
31. Pinzani M, Milani S, DeFranco R et al. Endothelin 1 is overexpressed in human cirrhotic liver and exerts multiple effects on activated hepatic stellate cells. Gastroenterology. 1996;110:534–48.
32. Rockey DC, Fouassier L, Chung JJ, Carayon A, Vallee P, Rey C, Housset C. Cellular localization of endothelin-1 and increased production in liver injury in the rat: potential for autocrine and paracrine effects on stellate cells. Hepatology. 1998;27:472–80.

33. Gabriel A, Kuddus RH, Rao AS, Watkins WD, Ghandi CR. Superoxide-induced changes in endothelin (ET) receptors in hepatic stellate cells. J Hepatol. 1998;29:614–27.
34. Shao R, Yan W, Rockey DC. Regulation of endothelin-1 synthesis by endothelin-converting enzyme-1 during wound healing. J Biol Chem. 1999;274:3228–34.
35. Reinehr RM, Kubitz R, Peters-Regehr T, Bode JG, Haussinger D. Activation of rat hepatic stellate cells in culture is associated with increased sensitivity to endothelin 1. Hepatology. 1998;28:1566–77.
36. Wang YZ, Pouyssegur J, Dunn MJ. Endothelin stimulates mitogen-activated protein kinase activity in mesangial cells through ET(A). J Am Soc Nephrol. 1994;5:1074–80.
37. Mallat A., Fouassier F, Preaux AM et al. Growth inhibitory properties of endothelin-1 in human hepatic myofibroblastic Ito cells: an endothelin B receptor-mediated pathway. J Clin Invest. 1995;96:42–9.
38. Mallat A, Preaux A-M, Serradeil-Le Gal C et al. Growth inhibitory properties of endothelin-1 in activated human hepatic stellate cells: a cyclic adenosine monophosphate-mediated pathway. J Clin Invest. 1996;98:2771–8.
39. Leivas A, Jimenez W, Bruix J et al. Gene expression of endothelin-1 and ET(A) and ET(B) receptors in human cirrhosis: relationship with hepatic hemodynamics. J Vasc Res. 1998;35:186–93.
40. Rockey DC, Chung JJ. Endothelin antagonism in experimental hepatic fibrosis. Implications for endothelin in the pathogenesis of wound healing. J Clin Invest. 1996;98:1381–8.
41. Poo JL, Jimenez W, Maria Munoz R et al. Chronic blockade of endothelin receptors in cirrhotic rats: hepatic and hemodynamic effects. Gastroenterology. 1999;116:161–7.
42. Cho JJ, Hocher B, Herbst H et al. An oral endothelin-A receptor antagonist blocks collagen synthesis and deposition in advanced rat liver fibrosis. Gastroenterology. 2000;118:1169–78.
43. Caligiuri A, Glaser S, Rodgers RE et al. Endothelin-1 inhibits secretin-stimulated ductal secretion by interacting with ET$_A$ receptors on large cholangiocytes. Am J Physiol. 1998;275:G835–46.
44. Bataller R, Gines P, Nicolas JM et al. Angiotensin II induces contraction and proliferation of human hepatic stellate cells. Gastroenterology. 2000;118:1149–56.
45. Bataller R, Sancho-Bru P, Gines P et al. Activated human hepatic stellate cells express the renin–angiotensin system and synthesize angiotensin II. Gastroenterology. 2003;125:117–25.
46. Bataller R, Schwabe RF, Choi YH et al. NADPH oxidase signal transduces angiotensin II in hepatic stellate cells and is critical in hepatic fibrosis. J Clin Invest. 2003;112:1383–94.
47. Paizis G, Cooper ME, Schembri JM, Tikellis C, Burrell LM, Angus PW. Up-regulation of components of the renin–angiotensin system in the bile duct-ligated rat liver. Gastroenterology. 2002;123:1667–76.
48. Paizis G, Gilbert RE, Cooper ME et al. Effect of angiotensin II type 1 receptor blockade on experimental hepatic fibrogenesis. J Hepatol. 2001;35:376–85.
49. Bataller R, Nicolas JM, Gines P et al. Arginine vasopressin induces contraction and stimulates growth of cultured human hepatic stellate cells. Gastroenterology. 1997;113:615–24.
50. Coughlin SR. Thrombin signalling and protease-activated receptors. Nature. 2000;407: 258–64.
51. Marra F, Grandaliano G, Valente AJ, Abboud HE. Thrombin stimulates proliferation of liver fat-storing cells and expression of monocyte chemotactic protein-1: potential role in liver injury. Hepatology. 1995;22:780–7.
52. Marra F, DeFranco R, Grappone C et al. Expression of the thrombin receptor in human liver: up-regulation during acute and chronic injury. Hepatology. 1998;27:462–71.
53. Pinzani M, Carloni V, Marra F, Riccardi D, Laffi G, Gentilini P. Biosynthesis of platelet-activating factor and its 10-acyl analogue by liver fat-storing cells. Gastroenterology. 1994;106:1301–11.
54. Titos E, Claria J, Bataller R et al. Hepatocyte-derived cysteinyl leukotrienes modulate vascular tone in experimental cirrhosis. Gastroenterology. 2000;119:794–805.
55. Graupera M, Garcia-Pagan JC, Titos E et al. 5-Lipoxygenase inhibition reduces intrahepatic vascular resistance of cirrhotic rat livers: a possible role of cysteinyl-leukotrienes. Gastroenterology. 2002;122:387–93.
56. Goulis J, Patch D, Burroughs AK. Bacterial infection in the pathogenesis of variceal bleeding. Lancet. 1999;353:139–42.
57. Wiest R, Tsai M-H, Groszmann R. Octreotide potentiates PKC-dependent vasoconstrictors in portal-hypertensive rats. Gastroenterology. 2001;120:975–83.

# 6
# Structural changes in the liver leading to cirrhosis and portal hypertension

IAN R. WANLESS

## INTRODUCTION

Portal hypertension is caused primarily by obstruction of the hepatic vasculature. In cirrhosis, the obstruction involves mostly obliteration of small hepatic venules and portal venules. There is a reflex increase in arterial flow that contributes to the portal hypertension. It is becoming known that cirrhosis is to some degree reversible. This chapter will review the pathogenesis of cirrhosis and its reversal from the perspective of hepatic vascular disease.

## DEFINITION OF CIRRHOSIS

Cirrhosis is a condition defined anatomically as the presence of fibrous septa throughout the liver that subdivide the hepatic parenchyma into hepatocellular nodules[1,2]. The nature of these fibrous septa is important for an understanding of what this definition really means. Fibrosis is often assumed, from this definition, to be the defining material for the progression to cirrhosis. Indeed, some staging systems, such as the METAVIR system, grade the progression to cirrhosis in terms of a fibrosis score. Attempts to objectify this progression in tissue samples have often quantified collagen histochemically or chemically. However, it is important to recognize that fibrous septa and fibrosis are not equivalent. Fibrosis is the accumulation of collagen and related macromolecules. Septa are the product of focal tissue loss, a process called parenchymal extinction.

Examination of the early phase of chronic liver disease reveals that tissue loss (parenchymal extinction) is concentrated in small units, generally 1–2 mm in diameter[1,3]. Areas of tissue loss are seen as collapsed stroma flattened into small sheets or discs of connective tissue that are seen in section as "septa". As many of these lesions accumulate they meet adjacent

47

lesions and thus become confluent by the time cirrhosis is easily recognizable. Cirrhosis is then said to be "established". Thus the diagnosis of cirrhosis depends on arbitrary quantitative limits. One feature that makes cirrhosis recognizable is the curved shape of the fibrous septa. The curved shape is a result of unequal tissue growth against the two sides of the collapsed tissue disc. This curved shape is not apparent until there are sufficient decrements of regenerative activity occasioned by abundant sublethal vascular lesions in the surviving tissue. Thus there is regeneration side-by-side with less vigorous regeneration or slight atrophy. Extinction lesions that are very small, involving only a few hepatocytes, heal rapidly and are not associated with apparent deformity of the tissue fabric. Slightly larger lesions, composed of a single acinus, are identified by the close approximation of a small hepatic vein and its adjacent portal tract. This short septum or "adhesion" may sometimes be recognized as fibrous portal tract expansion but with serial sections one may find the adjacent obliterated terminal hepatic venule, proving the lesion is a collapse lesion. Large extinction lesions may involve many acini or even a whole lobe. Large lesions may be recognized by regions of closely approximated portal tracts separated only by collapsed stroma and fibrosis.

The mechanism of parenchymal extinction can be deduced from a number of diseases in which the pathogenesis can be easily understood, for example in congestive heart failure[4], hepatic vein thrombosis (Budd-Chiari syndrome)[5], and sarcoidosis[6]. In these conditions, primary injury to the vessels is evident, especially the hepatic veins, through thrombosis or phlebitis. Obstruction of hepatic veins is particularly injurious because it leads to decompensation of the sinusoidal circulation through congestion, hemorrhage into the space of Disse, and eventual atrophy and apoptosis of the hepatocytes in the congested regions. Thus extinction occurs by a mechanism of ischemia secondary to obstruction of veins and sinusoids (Figure 1). Obstruction of portal veins may lead to atrophy but not to extinction, because the ischemic insult is compensated by arterial flow and injury to the sinusoidal walls is minimal or absent. In most of the frequent chronic liver diseases such as fatty liver disease and chronic viral hepatitis, vascular obstruction is a result of necroinflammation adjacent to small hepatic veins[7]. The veins are damaged as bystanders to the adjacent hepatocellular injury.

## REVERSIBILITY OF CIRRHOSIS

There is abundant evidence that cirrhosis is at least partially reversible. This was demonstrated in a large follow-up study where biopsies showing micronodular cirrhosis transformed into macronodular cirrhosis or absent cirrhosis when autopsy livers were examined[8]. Individual patients successfully treated for hemochromatosis[9], Wilson disease[10], autoimmune hepatitis[11], and biliary obstruction[12] were also shown to improve with follow-up biopsy examination. Recently, in large trials of antiviral or interferon treatment of chronic hepatitis, improved histology has repeatedly been reported[13,14].

Nine histologic features attributed to the process of regression were described that occurred together in the majority of low-activity cirrhotic

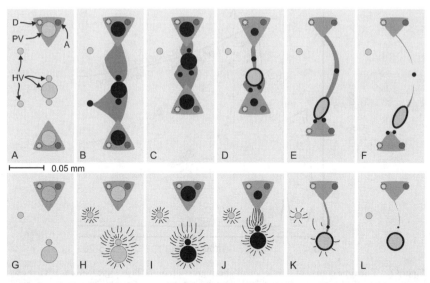

0.05 mm

**Figure 1.** Cirrhosis can be defined as the state of the liver after accumulation of many lesions of parenchymal extinction. The natural history of 3 small parenchymal extinctions is shown diagrammatically. Normal acini are shown in (A) and (G). Obstructed veins are shown as black circles. In chronic hepatitis (B–F) obliteration of small portal and hepatic veins occurs early in response to local inflammatory damage. The supplied parenchyma becomes ischemic, collapses, and is replaced by fibrosis (B–D). The collapse is accompanied by close approximation of adjacent vascular structures (D). Septa are deformed and stretched by unsymmetrical regeneration (E). Fibrous septa are resorbed (F), becoming progressively thinner and perforating. These septa may disappear or leave residual tags extending from portal tracts. Trapped portal structures and hepatic veins are released from the septa and are recognizable as remnants. Note the absence of portal veins. In alcoholic disease (G–L), the sequence of events may differ from other forms of chronic liver disease. (H) Sinusoidal fibrosis is often prominent prior to the development of parenchymal collapse, leading to a pericellular pattern of fibrosis. (I,J) Inflammation and fibrosis lead to hepatic and portal vein obliteration with secondary condensation of preformed sinusoidal collagen fibers into a septum. (K,L) After prolonged periods of inactivity, sinusoidal fibrosis and septa are resorbed. (Modified from Wanless IR, Nakashima E, Sherman M. Regression of human cirrhosis. Morphologic features and the genesis of incomplete septal cirrhosis. Arch Pathol Lab Med. 2000;124:1599–607, and Wanless IR. Physioanatomic considerations. In: Schiff ER, Sorrell MF, Maddrey WC, editors. Schiff's Diseases of the Liver. 9th ed. Philadelphia: Lippincott-Raven; 2003, page 43, with permission).

livers removed at transplantation[1] (see Figures 1 and 2). These features were labeled as the "hepatic repair complex". One of these features was the presence of delicate perforated septa. These septa extend from one portal tract to another or to an hepatic vein. Because these septa are very thin there is focal continuity between the microcirculation of adjacent cirrhotic nodules. These septa were formerly interpreted by many pathologists as newly formed septa. However, there is no physiologically likely mechanism for these septa to be newly formed because the chronic disease is often inactive without necroinflammation and migration of a linear array of fibers from one portal tract to another is unlikely to happen.

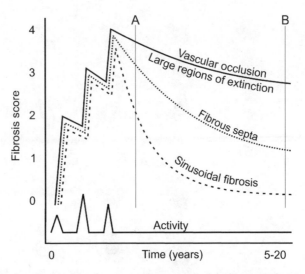

**Figure 2.** The time course of development and regression of the histologic features of cirrhosis. Small regions of fibrosis resorb quickly. Vascular obliteration is less able to return to normal. The diagnosis of cirrhosis is easy with biopsies taken close to the periods of activity (time A) but may be impossible after years of inactivity (time B). (From Wanless IR, Arch Pathol Lab Med. 2000;124:1592–3.)

Another important feature found in regressing liver disease is the presence of remnants of portal tracts and hepatic veins. These are damaged structures left behind after they have been released from fibrous septa. Portal tract remnants usually lack portal veins and may have an increase in arteries. The importance of remnants is that these structures appear to remain in tissue long after septa have resorbed and thus identify a liver that was once more severely altered. These remnants may also explain residual "non-cirrhotic" portal hypertension in patients with such livers[15].

## LIMITS TO REVERSIBILITY

The major impediments to the reversibility of cirrhosis are continuing primary activity, cholestatic decompensation, secondary thrombosis, and the arterialized state of the liver[3].

### Continuing activity

The morphology of cirrhosis is determined by the amount of time that has elapsed from the onset of parenchymal extinction. If active injury continues, new lesions of extinction will coexist with old lesions. If the primary disease is inactive and remote, the liver will contain only lesions in late stages of repair. Fresh extinction lesions can be recognized by bridging necrosis in highly active hepatitis or focal congestion and apoptosis in mild hepatitis. Cholestatic decompensation causes progression of the cirrhosis, likely through bile salt-induced vascular inflammation.

## Thrombosis

Once cirrhosis has developed, the hepatic blood flow is chaotic and sluggish. Portal vein flow may be reversed (hepatofugal). In addition, loss of anticoagulant function and prothrombotic effects of sepsis and cholestasis may contribute to the increased risk of thrombosis of the hepatic and portal vein. Portal vein thrombosis is found in up to 40% of cirrhotic livers examined at transplantation. Thrombosis of medium or large hepatic veins causes large regions of extinction to occur, explaining the markedly irregular capsular shapes found in a third of livers with late stage cirrhosis[16].

## Arterialization

When septa regress, the most visible evidence of cirrhosis disappears so that casual observation of a biopsy may suggest a normal liver. However, close approximation of portal tracts and hepatic veins can usually be identified if sufficient tissue is available for examination. Even in small biopsies, obliterated small portal and hepatic veins are found. Obliterated portal veins imply the tissue is arterialized.

The importance of arterialization has recently been indicated by a mouse model of angiogenesis[17]. In transgene mutated mice, angiopoietin-1 was conditionally expressed in hepatocytes. When the gene was active during development of the liver, there was marked arterial enlargement with terminal sprouting of arterioles and secondary dilation of the hepatic veins. Interestingly, the terminal portal vein radicles were undeveloped so that the distal portal tracts were incomplete, rather similar in form to the portal tract remnants seen in regressed human cirrhosis. These phenotypic changes were completely reversed within 14 days of turning off transgene expression. In particular, the terminal portal venules developed and complete portal tracts were present. This model implies that dominance of the arterial tree is incompatible with the presence of normal portal veins, possibly because of increased pressure in the sinusoids leading to retrograde portal flow and thrombosis of these delicate veins. A further implication of this study is that therapy to suppress arterial dominance in the human liver might allow terminal portal veins to develop after cirrhosis has otherwise regressed.

## STAGING SYSTEMS

Many staging systems are in wide use, including the METAVIR[18] and Ishak[19] systems, applicable for most forms of chronic liver disease, and the Scheuer[20] and Ludwig[21] systems for chronic biliary disease. These systems vary in the number of categories (0-to-4, 0-to-6, or 1-to-4) and the category definitions. These systems do not provide categories for the different severities of cirrhosis. The Laennec system attempts to standardize staging for all chronic liver disease on a scale of 0–4 with cirrhosis being grade 4 (Table 1)[3,22]. An extension divides cirrhosis into subgrades 4A, 4B, and 4C, in recognition of the variable severity among cirrhotic livers. The definitions of each grade are based on the number and width of fibrous septa. This simplification decreases the opportunity for interobserver variation. The

**Table 1.** Laennec scoring system for grading fibrosis in liver biopsies

| Grade | Name | Criteria: septa (thickness and number) | Descriptive examples |
|---|---|---|---|
| 0 | No definite fibrosis | | |
| 1 | Minimal fibrosis | +/− | No septa or rare thin septum, may have portal expansion or mild sinusoidal fibrosis |
| 2 | Mild fibrosis | + | Occasional thin septa. May have portal expansion or mild sinusoidal fibrosis |
| 3 | Moderate fibrosis | ++ | Moderate thin septa, up to incomplete cirrhosis |
| 4A | Cirrhosis, mild, definite or probable | +++ | Marked septation with rounded contours or visible nodules. Most septa are thin (one broad septum allowed) |
| 4B | Moderate cirrhosis | ++++ | At least two broad septa, but no very broad septa and less than half of biopsy length composed of minute nodules |
| 4C | Severe cirrhosis | +++++ | At least one very broad septum or more than half of biopsy length composed of minute nodules (micronodular cirrhosis) |

From reference 2, with permission.

expanded scale allows quantification of changes with time in patients with cirrhosis. As with other systems, the Laennec system also reports grade of activity on a scale of 0–4, as well as noting etiology-specific features.

Regressed cirrhosis may have no septa but detection of obliterated veins distinguishes the biopsy from normal (Figure 2). Immunostain for CD34 may detect arterialized sinusoids that would otherwise appear normal. However, another strategy is to quantitate the venous obliteration by counting the patent portal and hepatic veins and the arteries and expressing the data as total number of patent veins divided by the number of arteries (VA ratio)[23]. In cirrhosis the veins are reduced and the arteries are increased. This ratio does not return to normal during regression of cirrhosis. Thus the VA ratio is an expression of past chronic liver disease or cirrhosis even after fibrous septa have been resorbed and cirrhosis can no longer be diagnosed by classic histologic features. This ratio is a necessary supplement to other systems to allow proper assessment of highly regressed chronic liver disease.

## References

1. Wanless IR, Nakashima E, Sherman M. Regression of human cirrhosis: morphologic features and the genesis of incomplete septal cirrhosis. Arch Pathol Lab Med. 2000;124:1599–607.
2. Wanless IR. Cirrhosis. In: Johnson LR, ed. Encyclopedia of Gastroenterology. New York: Academic Press; 2003:356–62.
3. Wanless IR, Crawford JM. Cirrhosis. In: Odze RD, Goldblum JR, Crawford JM, eds. Surgical Pathology of the Alimentary Tract, Pancreas, Biliary Tree, and Liver. Philadelphia: Saunders; 2004:863–84.

4. Wanless IR, Liu JJ, Butany J. Role of thrombosis in the pathogenesis of congestive hepatic fibrosis (cardiac cirrhosis). Hepatology. 1995;21:1232–7.
5. Tanaka M, Wanless IR. Pathology of the liver in Budd-Chiari syndrome: portal vein thrombosis and the histogenesis of veno-centric cirrhosis, veno-portal cirrhosis, and large regenerative nodules. Hepatology. 1998;27:488–96.
6. Moreno-Merlo F, Wanless IR, Shimamatsu K, Sherman M, Greig P, Chiasson D. The role of granulomatous phlebitis and thrombosis in the pathogenesis of cirrhosis and portal hypertension in sarcoidosis. Hepatology. 1997;26:554–60.
7. Wanless IR, Shiota K. The pathogenesis of nonalcoholic steatohepatitis and other fatty liver diseases: a four-step model including the role of lipid release and hepatic venular obstruction in the progression to cirrhosis. Semin Liver Dis. 2004;24:99–106.
8. Fauerholdt L, Schlichting P, Christensen E, Poulsen H, Tygstrup N, Juhl E. Conversion of micronodular cirrhosis into macronodular cirrhosis. Hepatology. 1983;3:928–31.
9. Lewis DR, Burbige EJ, French SW. Reversal of cirrhosis in hemochromatosis following long-term phlebotomy. Gastroenterology. 1983;84:1382.
10. Grand RJ, Vawter GF. Juvenile Wilson disease: histologic and functional studies during penicillamine therapy. J Pediatr. 1975;87:1161–70.
11. Dufour JF, DeLellis R, Kaplan MM. Reversibility of hepatic fibrosis in autoimmune hepatitis. Ann Intern Med. 1997;127:981–5.
12. Bunton GL, Cameron R. Regeneration of liver after biliary cirrhosis. Ann NY Acad Sci. 1963;111:412–21.
13. Villeneuve JP, Condreay LD, Willems B et al. Lamivudine treatment for decompensated cirrhosis resulting from chronic hepatitis B. Hepatology. 2000;31:207–10.
14. Poynard T, McHutchison J, Davis GL et al. Impact of interferon alfa-2b and ribavirin on progression of liver fibrosis in patients with chronic hepatitis C. Hepatology. 2000;32:1131–7.
15. Nakashima E, Kage M, Wanless IR. Idiopathic portal hypertension: Histologic evidence that some cases may be regressed cirrhosis with portal vein thrombosis. Hepatology. 1999;30:218A.
16. Wanless IR, Wong F, Blendis LM, Greig P, Heathcote EJ, Levy G. Hepatic and portal vein thrombosis in cirrhosis: possible role in development of parenchymal extinction and portal hypertension. Hepatology. 1995;21:1238–47.
17. Ward N, Haninec AL, Van Slyke P et al. Angiopoietin-1 causes reversible degradation of the portal microcirculation in mice: implications for treatment of liver disease. Am J Pathol. 2004; in press.
18. Poynard T, Bedossa P, Opolon P. Natural history of liver fibrosis progression in patients with chronic hepatitis C. The OBSVIRC, METAVIR, CLINIVIR, and DOSVIRC groups. Lancet. 1997;349:825–32.
19. Ishak K, Baptista A, Bianchi L et al. Histological grading and staging of chronic hepatitis. J Hepatol. 1995;22:696–9.
20. Scheuer P. Primary biliary cirrhosis. Proc R Soc Med. 1967;60:1257–60.
21. Ludwig J. Etiology of biliary cirrhosis: diagnostic features and a new classification. Zentralbl Allg Pathol. 1988;134:132–41.
22. Wanless IR, Sweeney G, Dhillon AP et al. Lack of progressive hepatic fibrosis during long-term therapy with deferiprone in subjects with transfusion-dependent beta-thalassemia. Blood. 2002;100:1566–9.
23. Wanless IR, Takayama A. Evaluation of regressed cirrhosis on biopsy using the vein/artery ratio. Hepatology. 2004; in press.

# Section III
# Pathophysiology: increased resistance and increased blood flow

# 7
# The paradox: vasoconstriction and vasodilation

YASUKO IWAKIRI and ROBERTO J. GROSZMANN

## INTRODUCTION

One of the most typical characteristics observed in patients with chronic liver diseases is the progressive alteration of the body's homeostatic mechanisms. Electrolyte imbalances, impaired oxygenation and ventilation, as well as abnormalities in vascular tone, are among some of the altered homeostatic functions observed in these patients[1]. Nitric oxide (NO), a key molecule that regulates vascular tone, plays a major role in the pathogenesis of the hyperdynamic circulatory syndrome observed in portal hypertension in liver diseases. NO is paradoxically regulated in portal hypertension (Figure 1).

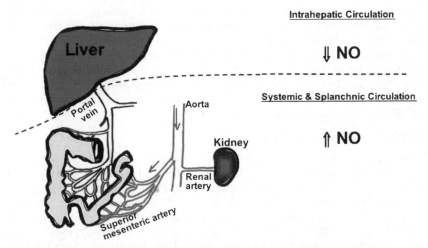

**Figure 1.** Paradoxical regulation of nitric oxide (NO) in portal hypertension. There is a deficit in NO production in the intrahepatic circulation, which increases vascular resistance in the liver. In contrast there is an excessive production of NO in the arteries of the systemic and splanchnic circulation, which is associated with vasodilation

There is excessive production of NO in the splanchnic circulation (thereby leading to vasodilation), while in the intrahepatic microcirculation a deficit of NO production is associated with increased intrahepatic vascular resistance. Both the hyperdynamic splanchnic circulation and increased intrahepatic vascular resistance contribute to the development and progression of portal hypertension[1–3]. This chapter will discuss mechanisms of hemodynamic abnormalities observed in the systemic and splanchnic arterial circulation (vasodilation) and intrahepatic circulation (vasoconstriction) in portal hypertension in liver diseases.

## VASODILATION IN THE SPLANCHNIC AND SYSTEM ARTERIAL CIRCULATION

A hyperdynamic splanchnic and systemic circulatory state is typical of cirrhotic patients and has been observed in all experimental forms of portal hypertension. Its presence is associated with extensive portal–systemic shunting and/or hepatic failure, and contributes to the severity of portal hypertension and to other manifestations of chronic liver disease. The hyperdynamic circulation is most likely initiated by vasodilation, which leads to central hypovolemia, sodium retention and an increased intravascular volume. The combination of vasodilation and an expanded intravascular volume is necessary for the full expression of the hyperdynamic state. The excessive NO production and arterial vasodilation play a central role in the hyperdynamic circulatory state in patients with liver cirrhosis and in animal models of portal hypertension instituted via portal vein ligation. NO is synthesized in mammalian cells, as a by-product of the reaction converting L-arginine to L-citrulline[4], by a family of three NOS: constitutively expressed isoforms, eNOS and neuronal NOS (nNOS), and inducible NOS (iNOS). It has been shown that up-regulation of eNOS in the splanchnic beds is responsible for the overproduction of NO, thus contributing to chronic vasodilation. The initial eNOS activation may be due to the early vasoconstriction (i.e. myogenic response) in the arteries of splanchnic vasculature, which is induced by an increase in portal pressure and the subsequent increase in shear stress[5]. The phosphorylation of eNOS by Akt/protein kinase B activation may play at least in part a role in the early activation of eNOS and subsequent NO production in these vasculatures[6].

### Physiological significance

Systemic and splanchnic arterial vasodilation and chronic elevations in systemic and splanchnic blood flow have been observed in humans and laboratory animals with portal hypertension. Peripheral vasodilation initiates the development of the classic profile of decreased systemic vascular resistance and mean arterial pressure, plasma volume expansion, elevated splanchnic blood flow, and elevated cardiac index. Collectively, these conditions most likely initiate the hyperdynamic circulatory state, which leads to central hypovolemia, sodium retention and an increase in intravascular volume. The combination of vasodilation and an expanded intravascular volume is necessary for the full expression of the hyperdynamic circulatory

58

state. The hyperdynamic circulation manifests in patients with warm, well-perfused extremities, bounding pulses, and rapid heart rate, as well as a high cardiac index and expanded blood volume. Hyperkinetic blood flow is present in the splanchnic as well as systemic circulation with flow to the intestines, stomach, spleen, and pancreas increased by approximately 50% above control values. The well-known increase in blood flow through the splanchnic organs draining into the portal venous system is a major contributing factor for maintenance and aggravation of portal hypertension[1].

## eNOS is the main enzymatic source of vascular NO overproduction

Nitric oxide, an endothelial-derived relaxing factor, is a key player in the etiology of the hyperdynamic circulatory syndrome in portal hypertension. The main enzymatic source of this vascular NO overproduction in the splanchnic arterial circulation has been identified as the endothelial nitric oxide synthase (eNOS). This was evidenced by markedly increased eNOS protein expression[7], enhanced eNOS activity[6,8–10], as well as augmented endothelial NO release in response to flow and shear stress[11] in superior mesenteric arteries of portal hypertensive animals. Normally, NOS present in the vascular endothelium is the constitutive, calcium-dependent eNOS that produces NO transiently in response to physical stimuli, such as an increase in shear stress mediated by blood flow or pressure. The response to shear stress is a unique function of eNOS[12,13]. Knowing that the chronic increases in blood flow induce up-regulation of eNOS, this increase in eNOS-derived NO production could easily be explained as chronic adaptation of the endothelium in response to chronically elevated splanchnic blood flow in portal hypertension.

An important co-factor for eNOS activity is tetrahydrobiopterin ($BH_4$). In cirrhotic rats with bacterial translocation we have observed[14] a significant increase in eNOS activity and eNOS-derived NO overproduction in the mesenteric arterial bed being accompanied by a concomitant increase in $BH_4$. $BH_4$ is an essential and rate-limiting co-factor for NO formation and can directly increase eNOS-derived NO bioavailability[15]. This has been demonstrated in cultured human endothelial cells, isolated rat aortas and human primordial placenta. Furthermore, $BH_4$ has been shown to induce NO-mediated vasorelaxation in various arterial vascular beds and species[15].

## nNOS and iNOS

A recent *in-vivo* study showed that nNOS plays a role in the hyperdynamic circulation in experimental cirrhosis[16]. nNOS was initially found in the neuron and has also been found in skeletal muscle and vascular smooth muscle[17,18], which constitutively produces NO in response to fluid flow[18,19]. This may suggest that nNOS plays a role in vasomotor control. We observed that an nNOS inhibitor normalizes contractile response to methoxamine in endothelium-removed mesenteric arteries isolated from portal hypertensive rats. In contrast, in the presence of endothelial cells there is no effect of the nNOS inhibitor, suggesting that the possible hemodynamic effects induced by nNOS are not seen as long as eNOS is up-regulated, although nNOS may contribute to increased vasodilation observed in portal hypertensive animals to some extent. The iNOS is synthesized *de novo* in macrophages, vascular smooth muscle cells, hepatic stellate cells, hepatocytes, and many others only after induction by endotoxin lipopolysaccharides and inflammatory cytokines[20]. Interestingly, despite the presence of bacterial translocation and endotoxemia in cirrhosis, iNOS is not detected in the splanchnic arterial vasculature in either portal vein ligated or cirrhotic rats[7,9,21]

## The mechanism of the early eNOS induction

What is the mechanism that initiates the splanchnic arterial vasodilation in portal hypertension? A recent study from our group suggests that vasoconstriction in superior mesenteric artery that occurs immediately after an increase in portal pressure may trigger the up-regulation of eNOS enzyme activity[5]. We speculate that this vasoconstriction is probably a myogenic reflex triggered by an increase in portal pressure, resulting in an increase in shear stress and subsequent up-regulation of eNOS activity in superior mesenteric artery. This increase in eNOS activity is sustained along the early course of portal hypertension induced by portal vein constriction and precedes vasodilation, plasma volume expansion, portosystemic shunting and the hyperdynamic circulation. Mesenteric vasoconstriction, the first hemodynamic event after the induction of portal hypertension, may trigger eNOS up-regulation in the superior mesenteric artery of portal hypertensive rats. In a separate study we found that Akt (protein kinase B) is up-regulated in the superior mesenteric artery of early portal hypertension, and that eNOS phosphorylation by activated Akt is involved in early activation of eNOS enzyme activity[6]. Collectively, these observations may suggest that an increase in portal pressure triggers vasoconstriction and a subsequent increase in shear stress in arteries of the splanchnic circulation, which activates Akt and phosphorylation of eNOS. These series of events, at least in part, may contribute to the initial up-regulation of eNOS in portal hypertension.

## Mediators of the splanchnic arterial vasodilation

*Tumor necrosis factor alpha (TNF-α)*

TNF-α, produced by mononuclear cells on activation by bacterial endotoxins, is found in increased levels in portal hypertension[22,23] and is a well-known mediator of NO release[24]. Antagonism of TNF-α with anti-TNF-α antibody, or inhibition of TNF-α synthesis by thalidomide, blunts the development of the hyperdynamic circulation in prehepatic portal hypertensive rats[23,25]. The mechanism of action of TNF-α in portal hypertension in cirrhosis still remains to be studied. However, it is suggested that TNF-α stimulates gene expression and activity of the key enzyme for regulation of $BH_4$ biosynthesis, GTP-cyclohydrolase I, in endothelial cells[15,26], and that enhanced $BH_4$ production directly increases eNOS-derived NO bioavailability[26,27]. Thus, TNF-α can directly increase vascular NO synthesis in absence of any induction of iNOS by up-regulating the production of $BH_4$ (see refs

15 and 27). $BH_4$ was found to be increased in mesenteric vasculature in cirrhotic rats only in conditions of bacterial translocation[14,28].

*Adrenomedullin*

Adrenomedullin is a potent vasodilatory peptide with 52 amino acid residues in the human and 50 amino acid residues in the rat. A growing body of evidence suggests that it plays an important role in regulating the cardiovascular response under various pathophysiological conditions, such as liver cirrhosis[29,30] and sepsis[31]. In liver cirrhotic patients there is an increase in circulating adrenomedullin level[29,30] which was associated with increased plasma nitrite (a stable NO metabolite) and plasma volume expansion[30], and was inversely correlated with peripheral resistance. Furthermore, in a study using rats, the administration of anti-adrenomedullin antibodies prevented the occurrence of the hyperdynamic response[32]. Furthermore, intraportal administration of adrenomedullin leads to the development of a hyperdynamic circulatory state[31]. Collectively the evidence may suggest a role of adrenomedullin in the hyperdynamic circulatory state in portal hypertension.

Adrenomedullin phosphorylates and activates Akt, and increases cGMP production in rat aorta, an indicator of NO production[33]. As mentioned previously, activated Akt directly phosphorylates and activates eNOS in cultured endothelial cells and mesenteric artery isolated from portal hypertensive animals[6], suggesting that adrenomedullin-mediated vasorelaxation is through the production of NO[33]. The evidence implies the possible role of adrenomedullin in the development of the hyperdynamic circulatory state observed in portal hypertension. Currently, the role of adrenomedullin in the development of hyperdynamic circulatory state is not being studied.

*Endocannabinoids*

Endogenous cannabinoids (or endocannabinoids) is a collective term describing a novel class of endogenous lipid ligands, including anandamide (arachidonyl ethanolamide). Cannabinoids, through their binding to the CB1 receptor, have been shown to undergo pronounced cardiovascular effects, including hypotension. It was shown that the endogenous cannabinoid, anandamide, is increased in cirrhotic monocytes and that over-activation of CB1 receptors within the mesenteric vasculature may well contribute to the development of splanchnic vasodilation and portal hypertension. The role of the CB1 receptor in cirrhosis was demonstrated by the work of the laboratory of George Kunos[34]. The blockade of CB1 receptor by the antagonist SR141716A not only increased mean arterial pressure but also reduced mesenteric blood flow in rats with $CCl_4$-induced cirrhosis. Importantly, this reduction in mesenteric flow translated into a reduction in portal pressure in bile duct-ligated rats, another experimental model of cirrhosis[35]. Additional hemodynamic analyses showed a selective loss of anandamide-induced hypotension after an intravenous injection into cirrhotic animals, presumably due to maximal stimulation of the CB1 receptors in portal hypertension. However, in sham rats the hypotensive effect of anandamide was markedly attenuated by the NOS inhibitor, suggesting that a significant component of anandamide-CB1-mediated vasodilation is mediated through downstream NOS activation and NO production. The comparable effects of CB1 receptor blockade and NOS inhibition suggest modulation of upstream and downstream sites within a common signaling pathway. The evidence suggests the possibility that the anandamide/CB1 receptor signaling system may provide a novel target for future treatment of portal hypertensive complications[34].

## VASOCONSTRICTION IN THE INTRAHEPATIC MICROCIRCULATION

Morphological change of liver microcirculation due to fibrosis and nodular regeneration is the most important mechanism for the increased intrahepatic vascular resistance in cirrhosis. Besides this structural alteration in liver cirrhosis, increased vascular tone similar to that observed in arterial hypertension is an important contributor to the increased vascular resistance. This is evidenced by the fact that a pharmacological agent can partially ameliorate intrahepatic vascular resistance, suggesting that non-structural (i.e. functional) abnormalities also play a significant role in the maintenance of intrahepatic vascular resistance[1]. Among other factors, a decrease in NO production seems to play a major role in increased intrahepatic resistance[36,37]. Both structural and non-structural factors are contributing to the development of portal hypertension.

### eNOS dysfunction in liver cirrhosis

Endothelial dysfunction and impaired NO production in cirrhotic livers seems to be evident despite normal eNOS protein expression[38,39]. Interestingly, this reduced NO production is due to the decreased catalytic activity of eNOS, although eNOS protein levels are not altered in cirrhotic liver. A study from our laboratory showed that this reduced eNOS activity was associated with an enhanced interaction with caveolin-1, an inhibitor of eNOS activity, and a diminished interaction with calmodulin, an activator of eNOS[39]. Interestingly, the expression of caveolin-1 markedly increased in sinusoidal endothelial cells of cirrhotic liver. Although the deficit of NO seems to play a major role in the enhanced intrahepatic vascular tone in liver cirrhosis, a decrease in other vasodilators different from NO could also be partly responsible for the increased intrahepatic vascular resistance in chronic liver diseases. By using a NOS inhibitor it has been shown that about 50% of the impairment in agonist-induced vasorelaxation is mediated by NO[39]. What other vasodilators are involved, and to what extent mechanical components participate in increased vascular resistance in cirrhosis, remain to be clarified.

### NO donors and adenovirus delivery of genes to improve hepatic NO production

Nitrovasodilators had been in clinical use as vasorelaxants for years before a mechanism of action was uncovered. NO was identified as endothelium-derived relaxing factor in 1987[40]. Since then it has become well established that NO is a key factor in the hemodynamic abnormalities associated with liver cirrhosis and chronic portal hypertension. Considering the fact that NO overproduction is a serious problem in the splanchnic and systemic arterial circulation, as mentioned earlier, liver-specific delivery of NO would form an important therapeutic approach to reduce resistance in the intrahepatic microcirculation, thereby ameliorating portal hypertension. In this regard, several attempts have been made to reduce resistance in the intrahepatic microcirculation. One of these is delivery of the liver-specific NO donor, NCX1000; the other is an adenovirus delivery of genes (i.e. NOS, nNOS and constitutively active Akt) to the liver to compensate for the lack of eNOS function.

*Liver-specific NO donor (NCX-1000)*

NCX-1000 is a NO-releasing ursodeoxycholic acid (UDCA)-derived compound, being capable of releasing NO selectively into the liver circulation[41-44]. NCX-1000[41] is a stable compound obtained by adding a NO-releasing moiety to UDCA. The fact that UDCA is metabolized only in the liver makes this drug liver-specific. Fiorucci and collaborators[41], using a rat model of $CCl_4$ intoxication, have previously shown that co-administration of NCX-1000 resulted in both prevention of ascites development and maintenance of a normal portal flow/pressure relationship during liver perfusion. In addition, the authors observed a higher liver tissue concentration of nitrite/nitrate in NCX-1000-treated rats. In their study the effects of this NO donor are likely to be related to attenuation in the development of cirrhosis rather than to a regression of this condition. Differently from these previous studies, we used rats that had already developed cirrhosis and portal hypertension to test whether the liver-specific NO donor could reverse, at least in part, the hemodynamic disturbances observed in cirrhosis without inducing systemic hemodynamic side-effects such as the one observed with organic nitrates[41,45,46]. We observed that this liver-specific NO donor improves portal system adaptability to additional increases in portal blood flow, as seen for example in postprandial hyperemia, and decreases the enhanced intrahepatic response to vasoconstrictors in cirrhotic rats without causing systemic arterial hypotension. Furthermore, treatment with NCX-1000 increased cGMP concentration (an effector of NO), suggesting that this improvement is probably secondary to an increase in intrahepatic NO bioavailability[44]. Overall, results suggest that liver-specific NO delivery is an effective approach for reducing intrahepatic vascular resistance in cirrhosis with portal hypertension.

*Targeted gene delivery*

Besides the NO donor molecules, an attempt has been made to introduce a recombinant adenovirus carrying gene encoding eNOS to increase intrahepatic NO production[47]. Delivery of the eNOS gene via tail vein injection significantly increased eNOS protein levels and catalytic activity in the liver. Overexpression of eNOS reduced baseline perfusion pressure and constriction in response to methoxamine, an α-adrenergic agonist and vasoconstric-

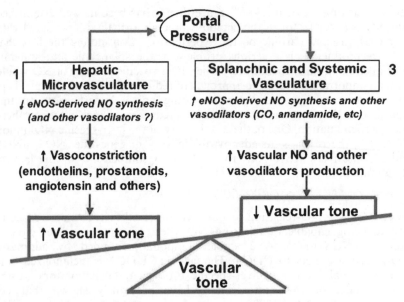

**Figure 2.** Regulation of vascular tone in liver cirrhosis. The sequence of events is depicted by numbers. The modified figure is shown[2]

tor, in perfused liver. Similarly, a study by Yu et al.[48] demonstrated that targeting liver with a recombinant adenovirus-carrying gene encoding nNOS reduces intrahepatic resistance and portal pressure. An interesting observation was also made in a study by Morales-Ruiz et al.[49] which showed that an improvement of eNOS function with adenoviral delivery of myr-Akt (constitutively active form of Akt) is also an effective approach to increase NO production in cirrhotic liver, and more strikingly normalizes portal pressure and increases mean arterial pressure in cirrhotic rats with portal hypertension. Results from these studies may imply the feasibility of using targeted gene delivery approaches to restore vascular tone in the liver. The site-specific control of the eNOS system may be a key to the development of effective treatment of portal hypertension.

## CONCLUSIONS

The regulation of vascular tone in liver disease discussed in this chapter is summarized in Figure 2. The diverse physiological roles of NO and the heterogeneity of liver diseases present a dilemma to the experimental therapist. On the one hand one would like to increase NO production in the liver microcirculation; on the other hand one would like to reduce excessive NO production in the systemic and splanchnic circulations. These are difficult goals to accomplish unless the intrinsic mechanisms leading to decreased hepatic NO and increased splanchnic and systemic production of NO are better understood. The development of liver-specific NO donors will be of great importance for optimizing therapy of liver cirrhosis. Restoring NO bioavailability in the liver microcirculation may not only reverse the direct intrahepatic effects of NO deficiency, but may also prevent the indirect implications that are the result of this deficiency and the associated increase in intrahepatic vascular resistance, vasodilation and the hyperdynamic circulation, thereby ameliorating portal hypertension.

## Acknowledgements

Y. Iwakiri is supported by an American Heart Association Heritage postdoctoral fellowship, and R. J. Groszmann is supported by VA Merit Review and Nicox (Milan, Italy).

## References

1. Groszmann RJ, Loureiro-Silva M, Tsai MH. The Biology of Portal Hypertension, 4th edn. New York: Lippincott Williams & Wilkins; 2001.
2. Wiest R, Groszmann RJ. The paradox of nitric oxide in cirrhosis and portal hypertension: too much, not enough. Hepatology. 2002;35:478–91.
3. Wiest R, Groszmann RJ. Nitric oxide and portal hypertension: its role in the regulation of intrahepatic and splanchnic vascular resistance. Semin Liver Dis. 1999;19:411–26.
4. Moncada S, Higgs A. The L-arginine-nitric oxide pathway. N Engl J Med. 1993;329:2002–12.
5. Tsai MH, Iwakiri Y, Cadelina G, Sessa WC, Groszmann RJ. Mesenteric vasoconstriction triggers nitric oxide overproduction in the superior mesenteric artery of portal hypertensive rats. Gastroenterology. 2003;125:1452–61.
6. Iwakiri Y, Tsai MH, McCabe TJ et al. The phosphorylation of endothelial nitric oxide synthase initiates excessive nitric oxide production in the early phases of portal hypertension. Am J Physiol Heart Circ Physiol. 2002;282:H2084–90.
7. Morales-Ruiz M, Jimenez W, Perez-Sala D et al. Increased nitric oxide synthase expression in arterial vessels of cirrhotic rats with ascites. Hepatology. 1996;24:1481–6.
8. Wiest R, Shah V, Sessa WC, Groszmann RJ. NO overproduction by eNOS precedes hyperdynamic splanchnic circulation in portal hypertensive rats. Am J Physiol. 1999;276: G1043–51.
9. Martin PY, Xu DL, Niederberger M et al. Up-regulation of endothelial constitutive NOS: a major role in the increased NO production in cirrhotic rats. Am J Physiol. 1996;270:F494–9.
10. Cahill PA, Redmond EM, Hodges R, Zhang S, Sitzmann JV. Increased endothelial nitric oxide synthase activity in the hyperemic vessels of portal hypertensive rats. J Hepatol. 1996;25:370–8.
11. Hori N, Wiest R, Groszmann RJ. Enhanced release of nitric oxide in response to changes in flow and shear stress in the superior mesenteric arteries of portal hypertensive rats. Hepatology. 1998;28:1467–73.
12. Buga GM, Gold ME, Fukuto JM, Ignarro LJ. Shear stress-induced release of nitric oxide from endothelial cells grown on beads. Hypertension. 1991;17:187–93.
13. Chaudhuri G, Buga GM, Gold ME, Wood KS, Ignarro LJ. Characterization and actions of human umbilical endothelium derived relaxing factor. Br J Pharmacol. 1991;102:331–6.
14. Wiest R, Cadelina G, Milstien S, McCuskey RS, Garcia-Tsao G, Groszmann RJ. Bacterial translocation up-regulates GTP-cyclohydrolase I in mesenteric vasculature of cirrhotic rats. Hepatology. 2003;38:1508–15.
15. Rosenkranz-Weiss P, Sessa WC, Milstien S, Kaufman S, Watson CA, Pober JS. Regulation of nitric oxide synthesis by proinflammatory cytokines in human umbilical vein endothelial cells. Elevations in tetrahydrobiopterin levels enhance endothelial nitric oxide synthase specific activity. J Clin Invest. 1994;93:2236–43.
16. Xu L, Carter EP, Ohara M et al. Neuronal nitric oxide synthase and systemic vasodilation in rats with cirrhosis. Am J Physiol Renal Physiol. 2000;279:F1110–15.
17. Segal SS, Brett SE, Sessa WC. Codistribution of NOS and caveolin throughout peripheral vasculature and skeletal muscle of hamsters. Am J Physiol. 1999;277:H1167–77.

18. Boulanger CM, Heymes C, Benessiano J, Geske RS, Levy BI, Vanhoutte PM. Neuronal nitric oxide synthase is expressed in rat vascular smooth muscle cells: activation by angiotensin II in hypertension. Circ Res. 1998;83:1271–8.
19. Papadaki M, Tilton RG, Eskin SG, McIntire LV. Nitric oxide production by cultured human aortic smooth muscle cells: stimulation by fluid flow. Am J Physiol. 1998;274:H616–26.
20. Abu-Soud HM, Loftus M, Stuehr DJ. Subunit dissociation and unfolding of macrophage NO synthase: relationship between enzyme structure, prosthetic group binding, and catalytic function. Biochemistry. 1995;34:11167–75.
21. Cahill PA, Foster C, Redmond EM, Gingalewski C, Wu Y, Sitzmann JV. Enhanced nitric oxide synthase activity in portal hypertensive rabbits. Hepatology. 1995;22:598–606.
22. Chu CJ, Lee FY, Wang SS et al. Hyperdynamic circulation of cirrhotic rats with ascites: role of endotoxin, tumour necrosis factor-alpha and nitric oxide. Clin Sci (Lond). 1997;93:219–25.
23. Lopez-Talavera JC, Cadelina G, Olchowski J, Merrill W, Groszmann RJ. Thalidomide inhibits tumor necrosis factor alpha, decreases nitric oxide synthesis, and ameliorates the hyperdynamic circulatory syndrome in portal-hypertensive rats. Hepatology. 1996; 23:1616–21.
24. Kilbourn RG, Belloni P. Endothelial cell production of nitrogen oxides in response to interferon gamma in combination with tumor necrosis factor, interleukin-1, or endotoxin. J Natl Cancer Inst. 1990;82:772–6.
25. Lopez-Talavera JC, Merrill WW, Groszmann RJ. Tumor necrosis factor alpha: a major contributor to the hyperdynamic circulation in prehepatic portal-hypertensive rats. Gastroenterology. 1995;108:761–7.
26. Katusic ZS, Stelter A, Milstien S. Cytokines stimulate GTP cyclohydrolase I gene expression in cultured human umbilical vein endothelial cells. Arterioscler Thromb Vasc Biol. 1998;18:27–32.
27. Wever RM, van Dam T, van Rijn HJ, de Groot F, Rabelink TJ. Tetrahydrobiopterin regulates superoxide and nitric oxide generation by recombinant endothelial nitric oxide synthase. Biochem Biophys Res Commun. 1997;237:340–4.
28. Wiest R, Das S, Cadelina G, Garcia-Tsao G, Milstien S, Groszmann RJ. Bacterial translocation in cirrhotic rats stimulates eNOS-derived NO production and impairs mesenteric vascular contractility. J Clin Invest. 1999;104:1223–33.
29. Fernandez-Rodriguez CM, Prada IR, Prieto J et al. Circulating adrenomedullin in cirrhosis: relationship to hyperdynamic circulation. J Hepatol. 1998;29:250–6.
30. Genesca J, Gonzalez A, Catalan R et al. Adrenomedullin, a vasodilator peptide implicated in hemodynamic alterations of liver cirrhosis: relationship to nitric oxide. Dig Dis Sci. 1999;44:372–6.
31. Zhou M, Chaudry IH, Wang P. The small intestine is an important source of adrenomedullin release during polymicrobial sepsis. Am J Physiol Regul Integr Comp Physiol. 2001;281:R654–60.
32. Wang P, Ba ZF, Cioffi WG, Bland KI, Chaudry IH. The pivotal role of adrenomedullin in producing hyperdynamic circulation during the early stage of sepsis. Arch Surg. 1998;133:1298–304.
33. Nishimatsu H, Suzuki E, Nagata D et al. Adrenomedullin induces endothelium-dependent vasorelaxation via the phosphatidylinositol 3-kinase/Akt-dependent pathway in rat aorta. Circ Res. 2001;89:63–70.
34. Batkai S, Jarai Z, Wagner JA et al. Endocannabinoids acting at vascular CB1 receptors mediate the vasodilated state in advanced liver cirrhosis. Nat Med. 2001;7:827–32.
35. Ros J, Claria J, To-Figueras J et al. Endogenous cannabinoids: a new system involved in the homeostasis of arterial pressure in experimental cirrhosis in the rat. Gastroenterology. 2002;122:85–93.
36. Gupta TK, Toruner M, Chung MK, Groszmann RJ. Endothelial dysfunction and decreased production of nitric oxide in the intrahepatic microcirculation of cirrhotic rats. Hepatology. 1998;28:926–31.
37. Gupta TK, Toruner M, Groszmann RJ. Intrahepatic modulation of portal pressure and its role in portal hypertension. Role of nitric oxide. Digestion. 1998;59:413–15.
38. Rockey DC, Chung JJ. Reduced nitric oxide production by endothelial cells in cirrhotic rat liver: endothelial dysfunction in portal hypertension. Gastroenterology. 1998;114:344–51.

39. Shah V, Haddad FG, Garcia-Cardena G et al. Liver sinusoidal endothelial cells are responsible for nitric oxide modulation of resistance in the hepatic sinusoids. J Clin Invest. 1997;100:2923–30.
40. Ignarro LJ, Buga GM, Wood KS, Byrns RE, Chaudhuri G. Endothelium-derived relaxing factor produced and released from artery and vein is nitric oxide. Proc Natl Acad Sci USA. 1987;84:9265–9.
41. Fiorucci S, Antonelli E, Morelli O et al. NCX-1000, a NO-releasing derivative of ursodeoxycholic acid, selectively delivers NO to the liver and protects against development of portal hypertension. Proc Natl Acad Sci USA. 2001;98:8897–902.
42. Fiorucci S, Mencarelli A, Palazzetti B, Del Soldato P, Morelli A, Ignarro LJ. An NO derivative of ursodeoxycholic acid protects against Fas-mediated liver injury by inhibiting caspase activity. Proc Natl Acad Sci USA. 2001;98:2652–7.
43. Fiorucci S, Antonelli E, Morelli A. Nitric oxide and portal hypertension: a nitric oxide-releasing derivative of ursodeoxycholic acid that selectively releases nitric oxide in the liver. Dig Liver Dis. 2003;35(Suppl. 2):S61–9.
44. Silva M, Iwakiri Y, Cadelina G, Sessa WC, Groszmann RJ. Nitric oxide (NO) delivery by NCX reduced the resistance of hepatic microcirculation of the cirrhotic liver in rats. Hepatology. 2003(AASLD abstract).
45. Garcia-Tsao G. Current management of the complications of cirrhosis and portal hypertension: variceal hemorrhage, ascites, and spontaneous bacterial peritonitis. Gastroenterology. 2001;120:726–48.
46. Kroeger RJ, Groszmann RJ. The effect of the combination of nitroglycerin and propranolol on splanchnic and systemic hemodynamics in a portal hypertensive rat model. Hepatology. 1985;5:425–30.
47. Shah V, Chen AF, Cao S et al. Gene transfer of recombinant endothelial nitric oxide synthase to liver *in vivo* and *in vitro*. Am J Physiol Gastrointest Liver Physiol. 2000; 279:G1023–30.
48. Yu Q, Shao R, Qian HS, George SE, Rockey DC. Gene transfer of the neuronal NO synthase isoform to cirrhotic rat liver ameliorates portal hypertension. J Clin Invest. 2000;105:741–8.
49. Morales-Ruiz M, Cejudo-Martin P, Fernandez-Varo G et al. Transduction of the liver with activated Akt normalizes portal pressure in cirrhotic rats. Gastroenterology. 2003; 125:522–31.

# 8
# Nitric-oxide-mediated vasodilation and portal hypertension

R. WIEST

## PATHOPHYSIOLOGICAL IMPORTANCE OF ARTERIAL VASODILATION

Chronic portal hypertension is associated with reduced splanchnic vascular arteriolar resistance and increased portal venous inflow. This hyperdynamic splanchnic circulatory state is accompanied by a hyperdynamic systemic circulation characterized by a low systemic vascular resistance with decreased arterial pressure and an increased cardiac output/index and regional organ blood flow[1]. Arterial vasodilation represents the initiating mechanism and hence, pathophysiological hallmark, in the development of this hyperdynamic circulation. It occurs early and most predominantly in the splanchnic circulation. Vasodilation can be considered an expression of anatomical (portal–systemic collaterals) or functional (liver cell necrosis/intrahepatic shunts) liver failure, or both. Thus, it is not surprising to find the extent of vasodilation being an excellent prognostic indicator in cirrhotic patients[2].

## NITRIC OXIDE SYNTHESIS AND ITS REGULATION

Three isoforms of nitric oxide synthase (NOS) have been cloned (Figure 1)[3]. All isoforms are dimeric, containing a reductase and an oxidase domain. NO is produced in a complex set of redox reaction steps, using molecular oxygen and the guanidino nitrogen of arginine as the substrates. NADPH is utilized as electron donor, and flavin-adenine dinucleotide (FAD), flavin mononucleotide (FMN), heme, tetrahydrobiopterin ($BH_4$) and $Ca^{2+}$/calmodulin as cofactors[3]. Two distinct but related NOS isoforms, one synthesized by endothelial cells (eNOS) and the other by neuronal cells (nNOS) are expressed constitutively. eNOS releases NO for short periods of time in response to several endogenous and exogenous stimulants including physical stimuli, such as shear stress. eNOS is stimulated further by receptor-dependent agonists that increase intracellular calcium and perturb plasma mem-

# NO – Synthase (NOS): Isoforms and Regulation

| | E(ndothelial) NOS | N(euronal) NOS | I(nducible) NOS |
|---|---|---|---|
| Localisation | Endothelium | Adventitia | Vascular smooth muscle |
| Expression | constitutive | constitutive | constitutive |
| Stimulus | Blood flow, Shear Stress, etc. | Nerval stimulation | LPS, TNF etc. |

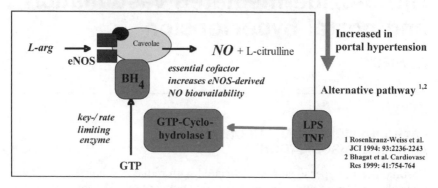

**Figure 1.** Nitric oxide synthase (NOS): isoforms and regulation (Wiest *et al.*)

brane phospholipid asymmetry. Agonists that stimulate eNOS include estrogens, catecholamines, endothelin, angiotensin, thrombin, adenosine-5-diphosphate, bradykinin, substance P, and muscarinic agonists (e.g. acetylcholine), 5-hydroxytryptamine, $Ca^{2+}$-ionophore A23187, arachidonic acid, etc. Depolarization of nerve endings activates nNOS and the presence of such nNOS-containing perivascular nerves has been demonstrated in numerous vascular beds and multiple species[4,5]. Functional studies underline the importance of these adventitial nNOS-immunoreactive fibers for regulation of vascular tone and mediating neurogenic vasodilation by releasing NO[6]. The inducible NOS (iNOS) is synthesized *de novo* in vascular smooth muscle cells, macrophages, hepatic stellate cells (HSC), hepatocytes and many others after induction by lipopolysaccharides (LPS) and inflammatory cytokines, e.g. tumor necrosis factor alpha (TNF-$\alpha$). Once expressed iNOS synthesizes large amounts of NO for extensive periods of time independent of any hemodynamic or mechanical stimuli[3]. Besides this classical pathway LPS and proinflammatory cytokines can enhance vascular NO overproduction via an alternative pathway mediated by tetrahydrobiopterin ($BH_4$) (Figure 1). LPS and/or proinflammatory cytokines have been shown[7,8] to induce GTP-cyclohydrolase I, the key enzyme regulating the *de-novo* synthesis of $BH_4$. $BH_4$ is not only an essential but also rate-limiting co-factor for NO formation[17,18] and can directly increase eNOS-derived NO bioavailability[18,19]. Furthermore, $BH_4$ has been shown to induce NO-mediated vasorelaxation in various arterial vascular beds and species[20,22,23].

The mechanisms by which NO mediates arterial vasodilation are multiple. Reaction with its classical "receptor"-soluble guanylate cyclase, binding at the prosthetic heme moiety, activates the enzyme that catalyzes the conversion of guanosine 5′-triphosphate (GTP) to cyclic guanosine 3′-5′-monophosphate (cGMP). cGMP produces relaxation of the vascular smooth muscle by several mechanisms that basically lead to a reduction of intracellular free $Ca^{2+}$ concentration. Among those mechanisms are discussed: inhibition of $Ca^{2+}$ entry through receptor-operated channels, inhibition of inositol-triphosphate generation, stimulation of intracellular $Ca^{2+}$ sequestration, increase in $K^+$ permeability through $K^+$ channels causing membrane hyperpolarization, stimulation of membrane $Ca^{2+}$-ATPase or cGMP-dependent protein kinase activation that phosphorylates myosin light-chain kinase.

## EVIDENCE FOR NO-MEDIATED VASODILATION IN EXPERIMENTAL PORTAL HYPERTENSION

The importance of NO for arterial vasodilation and associated hemodynamic abnormalities stated above is reflected in the finding of almost complete normalization of splanchnic hemodynamics by acute administration of a non-specific NO synthesis inhibitor[9,10]. Likewise, chronic inactivation of overproduced NO by increasing blood hemoglobin – binding and depleting NO – attenuates splanchnic vasodilation in portal hypertension[11]. Finally, titrating doses of L-NAME to reduce aortic cGMP concentrations to normal, indicating normalization of NO production, in cirrhotic rats with ascites was associated with normalization of arterial pressure, cardiac index and total vascular resistance[12]. A reduced pressor effect of vasoconstrictive substances is a well-documented phenomenon in experimental as well as human portal hypertension. This vascular hyporesponsiveness not only represents a classical expression of arterial vasodilation but is also interpreted as a contributing pathophysiological factor. Impaired vasoconstrictor response has been evidenced for norepinephrine, methoxamine, angiotensin, endothelin and vasopressin in various vascular beds[13–17]. This vascular hyporeactivity was reversed by inhibition of NO synthesis but not by inhibition of cyclooxygenase[13,16,18–20]. Moreover, in cirrhotic rats the pressor effect of inhibition of NO synthesis was significantly greater than in normal animals, suggesting increased activity of endogenous NO[21]. NO also reduces resistance in the collateral portal circulation in animals with portal hypertension[22,23].

## SOURCE OF VASCULAR NO OVERPRODUCTION – WHAT ISOFORM OF NOS IS INVOLVED?

Identification of the type of NOS mediating vascular NO overproduction is of potential therapeutic importance, because of the recent availability of specific or preferential inhibitors of the different NOS isoforms.

### eNOS

A strong line of evidence demonstrates a major role for eNOS involved in vascular NO overproduction in the hyperdynamic circulatory syndrome in chronic portal hypertension. The vascular hyporesponsiveness has been localized to the endothelium, since removal of the endothelium corrects this general vascular defect[24]. Mesenteric arteries as well as aortae of cirrhotic rats contain several-fold more eNOS protein compared with similar vessels from normal rats, and the concentration of mRNA is increased likewise[25-27]. A similar up-regulation of eNOS has also been demonstrated in the rat portal vein ligation (PVL) model, as evidenced by increased eNOS protein levels and enhanced $Ca^{2+}$-dependent NOS activity in aortic and mesenteric arteries from PVL animals[28-31]. This eNOS up-regulation mediates the observed increases in responses to endothelium-dependent vasodilator substances such as acetylcholine, which are prevented by inhibition of NO synthesis[32]. Finally, direct demonstration of enhanced eNOS-derived NO synthesis in the splanchnic vasculature in portal hypertension was shown by monitoring endothelial NO release in *in-vitro* perfused mesenteric arteries. Thereby, NO production in response to vasoconstrictors or increases in flow/shear stress was markedly elevated in portal hypertensive rats[33-35].

## nNOS

Enhanced nerval vasorelaxation has been reported in mesenteric arteries of portal hypertensive rats being partly corrected by inhibition of NO synthesis[36]. In more detail, yet-unpublished personal data demonstrate nNOS up-regulation in the splanchnic circulation in PVL rats. nNOS is localized to the adventitia of the mesenteric arterial tree, showing more intense staining in portal hypertensive as compared to sham rats. Correspondingly, nNOS protein expression is markedly increased in mesenteric arteries in portal hypertensive animals. Finally, the effect of NO inhibition on nNOS-mediated vasorelaxation in *in-vitro* perfused mesenteric vasculature is significantly greater in portal hypertensive than in sham animals, indicating that nNOS-derived vascular NO overproduction contributes to arterial vasodilation in portal hypertension. Indeed, systemic nNOS inhibition in cirrhotic rats *in vivo* for 1 week, using the selective NO-inhibitor 7-NI, resulted in normalization of systemic vascular resistance, mean arterial pressure and cardiac index[37].

## iNOS

Since the hypothesis proposed by Vallance and Moncada, that endotoxemia of cirrhosis induces vascular iNOS expression leading to NO overproduction and arterial vasodilation, multiple independent investigators have failed to prove this hypothesis convincingly. No clear iNOS protein could be demonstrated in different animal models of portal hypertension, even in the presence of bacterial translocation and systemic endotoxinemia[25-27,31]. Moreover, inhibition of iNOS with dexamethasone or aminoguanidine could not prevent the development of the hyperdynamic circulatory syndrome[38,39], arguing against a role of iNOS-dependent NO production in arterial vasodilation in portal hypertension.

## TIME RELATIONSHIP OF VASCULAR NO OVERPRODUCTION WITH EVOLUTION OF HYPERDYNAMIC CIRCULATION

Since we know that chronic increases in blood flow induce up-regulation of eNOS, increased eNOS-derived NO production could easily be explained as a normal adaptation of the endothelium to the splanchnic high-flow state and enhanced shear stress being present in portal hypertension. In accordance with this hypothesis more pronounced vascular NO overproduction is observed in cirrhotic rats with ascites as compared to those without ascites[31,40]. However, eNOS up-regulation in the mesenteric vasculature precedes the development of the hyperdynamic splanchnic circulation in portal hypertension[41]. This has been evidenced by investigating PVL animals early after PVL. The sequence of events after PVL is characterized by vasodilation in non-splanchnic vasculature and vasoconstriction in decreased blood flow in the superior mesenteric vessel bed secondary to a myogenic reflex induced by the acute increase in portal pressure[42]. On day 3 after PVL portal hypertensive animals exhibit superior mesenteric arterial blood flow as well as total portal venous inflow being no different from that in sham rats. Already under such normodynamic conditions increased eNOS-derived NO production by the mesenteric vasculature and higher eNOS protein levels are observed in portal hypertension[41]. A recent elegant investigation could demonstrate enhanced eNOS activity and NO-mediated vascular hyporesponsiveness in mesenteric arteries even as early as 10 h after induction of severe portal hypertension (20 G stenosis of the portal vein)[43]. This eNOS up-regulation appears to be triggered by mesenteric vasoconstriction, since rats with renal artery ligation exhibiting increased mesenteric resistance (but no portal hypertension) also presented with a similar enhancement in eNOS activity and associated vascular hyporesponsiveness. In contrast, portal hypertension *per se*, in the absence of mesenteric vasoconstriction – created by low-level stenosis of the portal vein (18 G diameter) – was not associated with alterations in vascular responsiveness or eNOS activity. Thus, eNOS-mediated vascular NO overproduction is not secondary to chronic increases in flow and shear stress, and may play a primary role in the pathogenesis of the hyperdynamic circulation in portal hypertension.

## STIMULUS FOR VASCULAR NO OVERPRODUCTION AND MECHANISMS INVOLVED

Despite all the evidence stated for vascular NO overproduction, predominantly in the splanchnic circulation, in portal hypertension the mechanism behind this NOS up-regulation remains poorly understood. Particularly the trigger initiating NOS up-regulation is open to speculations, and remains enigmatic due to its apparently vast pathophysiological, and hence clinical, relevance. In the model of PVL, in the very early phase of portal hypertension, cyclic strain (known to up-regulate eNOS) may represent the mechanism by which vasoconstriction increases eNOS activity in mesenteric arteries. Additionally, hypoxia may play a role, since oxygen tension has

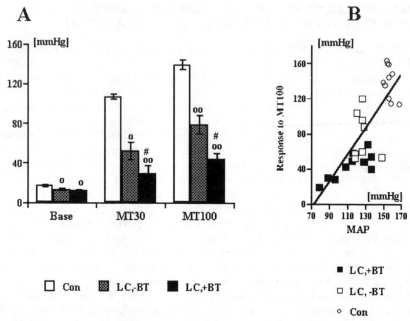

**Figure 2.** **A:** Perfusion pressure under basal conditions (Base) and during the administration of 30 μmol/L and 100 μmol/L of MT (methoxamine) in the *in-vitro*-perfused superior mesenteric vascular bed. $*p < 0.01$ vs. LC, $+ BT$; $°p < 0.01$ vs. control; $°°p < 0.001$ vs. control. **B:** Relationship between *in-vitro* vascular responsiveness and systemic hemodynamic parameter mean arterial pressure (MAP). $r = 0.787$; $p < 0.001$

also been shown to up-regulate eNOS activity. Moreover, receptor-mediated activation of eNOS by circulating mediators may also contribute. Particularly in advanced stages of cirrhosis and portal hypertension increased levels of endotoxins and proinflammatory cytokines have been demonstrated[44–46], and both have been evidenced to enhance endothelial NO synthesis by increasing eNOS activity[47]. TNF has also been implicated in the development of the HCS, since TNF inhibition ameliorated the HCS in PVL rats[46,48]. Endotoxins and TNF are known to be released from the gut in conditions of bacterial translocation (BT); BT is a well-characterized phenomenon in cirrhosis and thought to be responsible for the development of severe spontaneous bacterial infections in cirrhosis. BT has also been demonstrated to increase eNOS-derived NO synthesis in mesenteric arteries in cirrhosis, leading to an additional impairment in vascular contractility (Figure 2A)[49]. Correspondingly, cirrhotic rats with BT presented with lower mean arterial pressure, indicating a more severe arterial vasodilation (Figure 2B). This was found to be associated with increased GTPCH-I activity, the key enzyme for the synthesis of $BH_4$, in the mesenteric vasculature in cirrhotic rats with BT. Both GTPCH-I activity and $BH_4$ content correlated positively with serum NOx levels and mean arterial pressure, indicating a major vasodilatory effect and hemodynamic impact of

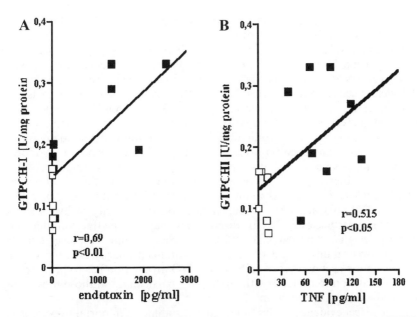

**Figure 3.** Regression analysis of GTPCH-I activity and serum endotoxin (**A**) and TNF (**B**) levels

GTPCH-I up-regulation via enhancement of vascular NO production. Moreover, GTPCH-I activity correlated positively with BT-associated increases in serum endotoxin and TNF (Figure 3). Considering the known stimulatory role of both mediators for GTPCH-I activity these findings support the hypothesis that, in advanced cirrhosis, BT and/or infectious complications aggravate arterial vasodilation via endotoxin-/TNF-stimulated GTPCH-I up-regulation and associated increases in $BH_4$ synthesis, leading to a further increase in eNOS-derived vascular NO overproduction. However, it is difficult to evidence this hypothesis since GTPCH-I is a ubiquitous enzyme and abundantly expressed, and $BH_4$, its product, is involved in other enzymatic reactions independent from NOS; therefore any inhibition of GTPCH-I *in vivo* may lead to multiple various effects completely independent from its impact on NOS. Moreover, inhibitors for GTPCH-I have been criticized for being non-specific and inducing multiple secondary events independent from its effect on $BH_4$. Other candidates that potentially contribute to eNOS up-regulation in portal hypertension include substance P, estrogen and catecholamines, which have been shown to increase eNOS expression and activity and are all known to be increased in chronic portal hypertension[50,51].

## NO AND VASODILATION IN CIRRHOSIS IN HUMANS

Vascular NO overproduction is also observed in patients with cirrhosis who present with increased plasma concentrations of NO and its metabolites

(NOx)[45,52–59]. In decompensated patients with ascites higher NOx plasma levels have been observed as compared to patients without ascites[45,60]. The predominant splanchnic origin of this NO overproduction is reflected in higher plasma NOx concentrations in portal venous plasma than in peripheral venous or arterial plasma[53,58,59]. Moreover, NOS activity in polymorphonuclear cells and monocytes is increased in cirrhotic patients with ascites and correlates with the cardiac index[61,62]. Likewise, multiple studies have observed correlations between NOx plasma levels and hemodynamic parameters reflecting arterial vasodilation[54,55,58]. In addition, increased nocturnal NO production has been reported, and suggested to contribute to hemodynamic changes seen in cirrhotic patients at night-time, indicating a potential role for the increased risk of variceal bleeding at night-time[55]. However, others failed to observe circadian variations in NO production[54] or differences in NOx-plasma levels in dependency on the severity of liver disease or portal hypertension.[53,57] This discrepancy may well be due to differences in study design and patient characterization. Since serum NOx level depends strongly on oral intake of exogenous NOx, and is primarily excreted via the kidney, its use as a marker of endogenous NO production has to be interpreted with caution in patients with cirrhosis[56], particularly in those presenting with reduced kidney function.

More direct evidence for NO-mediated vasodilation in portal hypertensive patients comes from studies investigating forearm blood flow and its response to NO inhibition. The forearm vasoconstrictor response to L-NMMA is greater in cirrhotic patients with ascites than in those without ascites, indicating vascular NO overproduction in the former[63]. Also in comparison with normal subjects, patients with cirrhosis have been reported to present with increased basal forearm blood flow[64]. In addition, cirrhotic patients show a more pronounced increase in forearm blood flow in response to metacholine, which stimulates endothelial NO production, whereas their response to sodium nitroprusside, an endothelium-independent vasodilator, is not different from that of the normal subjects[52]. Finally, enhanced NOS activity has been demonstrated in the splanchnic vasculature of cirrhotic patients undergoing liver transplantation as compared to healthy controls (liver donors)[65]. Highly significant correlations were observed between hepatic artery NOS activity and cardiac output, as well as portal blood flow, supporting the concept of vascular NO overproduction contributing essentially to the hyperdynamic state in those cirrhotic patients.

Acute inhibition of NO synthesis in cirrhotic patients has been demonstrated to increase blood pressure and systemic vascular resistance, as well as reducing cardiac index; hence correcting the hyperdynamic circulation at least partly[66–69]. However, no change in portal venous pressure could be detected[66,68] which may reflect a simultaneous reduction in splanchnic arterial blood flow and increase in intrahepatic portal venous resistance[70,71]. Moreover, results of acute NO blockade on renal function in cirrhotic patients are controversial[67–69]. This may well relate to differences in the severity of liver disease and renal function in patients studied at basal conditions, but also to duration and continuity of drug administration. Most likely, acute inhibition of NO-synthesis (< 3 h) is not long enough to induce sustained changes in the circulatory system reversing the enhanced release of vasoconstrictor mediating renal vasoconstriction and sodium and water retention. Therefore, further studies evaluating the role of chronic NO inhibition are clearly needed in humans, in order to develop a new approach to the management of circulatory and renal dysfunction in patients with cirrhosis.

## References

1. Groszmann RJ. Hyperdynamic circulation of liver disease 40 years later: pathophysiology and clinical consequences. Hepatology. 1994;20:1359–63.
2. Llach J, Gines P, Arroyo V et al. Prognostic value of arterial pressure, endogenous vasoactive systems, and renal function in cirrhotic patients admitted to the hospital for the treatment of ascites. Gastroenterology. 1988;94:482–7.
3. Sessa WC. The nitric oxide synthase family of proteins. J Vasc Res. 1994;31:131–43.
4. Ignacio CS, Curling PE, Childres WF, Bryan RM Jr. Nitric oxide-synthesizing perivascular nerves in the rat middle cerebral artery. Am J Physiol. 1997;273:R661–8.
5. Toda N, Ayajiki K, Uchiyama M, Okamura T. Nitric oxide-mediated neurogenic vasodilation in isolated monkey lingual arteries. Am J Physiol. 1997;272:H1582–8.
6. Toda N, Okamura T. Regulation of arterial tone by nitroxidergic nerves. News in Physiol Sci. 1991;7:148–52.
7. Hattori Y, Oka M, Kasai K, Nakanishi N, Shimoda S. Lipopolysaccharide treatment *in vivo* induces tissue expression of GTP cyclohydrolase I mRNA. FEBS Lett. 1995;368:336–8.
8. Katusic ZS, Stelter A, Milstien S. Cytokines stimulate GTP cyclohydrolase I gene expression in cultured human umbilical vein endothelial cells. Arterioscler Thromb Vasc Biol. 1998; 18:27–32.
9. Pizcueta P, Pique JM, Fernandez M et al. Modulation of the hyperdynamic circulation of cirrhotic rats by nitric oxide inhibition. Gastroenterology. 1992;103:1909–15.
10. Pizcueta MP, Pique JM, Bosch J, Whittle BJ, Moncada S. Effects of inhibiting nitric oxide biosynthesis on the systemic and splanchnic circulation of rats with portal hypertension. Br J Pharmacol. 1992;105:184–90.
11. Casadevall M, Pique JM, Cirera I et al. Increased blood hemoglobin attenuates splanchnic vasodilation in portal-hypertensive rats by nitric oxide inactivation. Gastroenterology. 1996;110:1156–65.
12. Niederberger M, Martin PY, Gines P et al. Normalization of nitric oxide production corrects arterial vasodilation and hyperdynamic circulation in cirrhotic rats. Gastroenterology. 1995;109:1624–30.
13. Sieber CC, Groszmann RJ. *In vitro* hyporeactivity to methoxamine in portal hypertensive rats: reversal by nitric oxide blockade. Am J Physiol. 1992;262:G996–1001.
14. Kiel JW, Pitts V, Benoit JN, Granger DN, Shepherd AP. Reduced vascular sensitivity to norepinephrine in portal-hypertensive rats. Am J Physiol. 1985;248:G192–5.
15. Hartleb M, Moreau R, Cailmail S, Gaudin C, Lebrec D. Vascular hyporesponsiveness to endothelin 1 in rats with cirrhosis [see comments]. Gastroenterology. 1994;107:1085–93.
16. Sieber CC, Groszmann RJ. Nitric oxide mediates hyporeactivity to vasopressors in mesenteric vessels of portal hypertensive rats. Gastroenterology. 1992;103:235–9.
17. Sieber CC, Sumanovski LT, Moll-Kaufmann C, Stalder GA. Hyposensitivity to nerve stimulation in portal hypertensive rats: role of nitric oxide. Eur J Clin Invest. 1997;27:902–7.
18. Weigert AL, Martin PY, Niederberger M et al. Endothelium-dependent vascular hyporesponsiveness without detection of nitric oxide synthase induction in aortas of cirrhotic rats. Hepatology. 1995;22:1856–62.
19. Sieber CC, Lopez-Talavera JC, Groszmann RJ. Role of nitric oxide in the *in vitro* splanchnic vascular hyporeactivity in ascitic cirrhotic rats. Gastroenterology. 1993;104:1750–4.
20. Castro A, Jimenez W, Claria J et al. Impaired responsiveness to angiotensin II in experimental cirrhosis: role of nitric oxide [see comments]. Hepatology. 1993;18:367–72.
21. Claria J, Jimenez W, Ros J et al. Pathogenesis of arterial hypotension in cirrhotic rats with ascites: role of endogenous nitric oxide. Hepatology. 1992;15:343–9.

22. Lee FY, Colombato LA, Albillos A, Groszmann RJ. Administration of $N$ omega-nitro-L-arginine ameliorates portal-systemic shunting in portal-hypertensive rats. Gastroenterology. 1993;105:1464–70.
23. Mosca P, Lee FY, Kaumann AJ, Groszmann RJ. Pharmacology of portal–systemic collaterals in portal hypertensive rats: role of endothelium. Am J Physiol. 1992;263:G544–50.
24. Atucha NM, Shah V, Garcia-Cardena G, Sessa WE, Groszmann RJ. Role of endothelium in the abnormal response of mesenteric vessels in rats with portal hypertension and liver cirrhosis. Gastroenterology. 1996;111:1627–32.
25. Martin PY, Xu DL, Niederberger M et al. Up-regulation of endothelial constitutive NOS: a major role in the increased NO production in cirrhotic rats. Am J Physiol. 1996;270:F494–9.
26. Morales-Ruiz M, Jimenez W, Perez-Sala D et al. Increased nitric oxide synthase expression in arterial vessels of cirrhotic rats with ascites. Hepatology. 1996;24:1481–6.
27. Wiest R, Garcia-Tsao G, Cadelina G, Das S, Shah V, Groszmann RJ. Bacterial translocation to mesenteric lymph nodes enhances eNOS-derived NO overproduction in mesenteric vasculature of cirrhotic rats: role for impairment in vascular contractility. J Clin Invest. 1999;104:1223–33.
28. Cahill PA, Foster C, Redmond EM, Gingalewski C, Wu Y, Sitzmann JV. Enhanced nitric oxide synthase activity in portal hypertensive rabbits. Hepatology. 1995;22:598–606.
29. Cahill PA, Redmond EM, Hodges R, Zhang S, Sitzmann JV. Increased endothelial nitric oxide synthase activity in the hyperemic vessels of portal hypertensive rats. J Hepatol. 1996;25:370–8.
30. Gadano AC, Sogni P, Yang S et al. Endothelial calcium-calmodulin dependent nitric oxide synthase in the *in vitro* vascular hyporeactivity of portal hypertensive rats. J Hepatol. 1997;26:678–86.
31. Niederberger M, Gines P, Martin PY et al. Comparison of vascular nitric oxide production and systemic hemodynamics in cirrhosis versus prehepatic portal hypertension in rats. Hepatology. 1996;24:947–51.
32. Claria J, Jimenez W, Ros J et al. Increased nitric oxide-dependent vasorelaxation in aortic rings of cirrhotic rats with ascites [see comments]. Hepatology. 1994;20:1615–21.
33. Hori N, Groszmann RJ. Direct evidence for increased functional activity of eNOS in superior mesenteric arterial beds of portal hypertensive rats. Hepatology. 1996;24:A749.
34. Shah V, Wiest R, Garcia-Cardena G, Sessa WC, Groszmann R. HSP 90 regulation of endothelial nitric oxide synthase contributes to vascular control in portal hypertension. Am J Physiol. 1999;277:G463–8.
35. Wiest R, Hori N, Cadelina G, Das S, Groszmann RJ. Increased nitric oxide release in response to vasoconstrictors in the superior mesenteric arterial bed of cirrhotic rats. Hepatology. 1997;26:A390.
36. Moll-Kaufmann C, Sumanovski LT, Sieber CC. Neurally-mediated vasodilation in normal and portal hypertensive rats: role of nitric oxide and calcitonin gene-related peptide. J Hepatol. 1998;28:1031–6.
37. Xu L, Carter EP, Ohara M et al. Neuronal nitric oxide synthase and systemic vasodilation in rats with cirrhosis. Am J Physiol. 2000;279:F1110–15.
38. Fernandez M, Garcia-Pagan JC, Casadevall M et al. Evidence against a role for inducible nitric oxide synthase in the hyperdynamic circulation of portal-hypertensive rats. Gastroenterology. 1995;108:1487–95.
39. Heinemann A, Stauber RE. The role of inducible nitric oxide synthase in vascular hyporeactivity of endotoxin-treated and portal hypertensive rats. Eur J Pharmacol. 1995;278:87–90.
40. Niederberger M, Gines P, Tsai P et al. Increased aortic cyclic guanosine monophosphate concentration in experimental cirrhosis in rats: evidence for a role of nitric oxide in the pathogenesis of arterial vasodilation in cirrhosis. Hepatology. 1995;21:1625–31.
41. Wiest R, Shah V, Sessa WC, Groszmann RJ. NO overproduction by eNOS precedes hyperdynamic splanchnic circulation in portal hypertensive rats. Am J Physiol. 1999;276:G1043–51.
42. Colombato LA, Albillos A, Groszmann RJ. Temporal relationship of peripheral vasodilation, plasma volume expansion and the hyperdynamic circulatory state in portal-hypertensive rats. Hepatology. 1992;15:323–8.
43. Tsai MH, Iwakiri Y, Cadelina G, Sessa WC, Groszmann R. Mesenteric vasoconstriction triggers nitric oxide overproduction in the superior mesenteric artery of portal hypertensive rats. Gastroenterology. 2003;125:1452–61.

44. Chu CJ, Lee FY, Wang SS et al. Splanchnic endotoxin levels in cirrhotic rats induced by carbon tetrachloride. Chung Hua I Hsueh Tsa Chih. 2000;63:196–204.
45. Guarner C, Soriano G, Tomas A et al. Increased serum nitrite and nitrate levels in patients with cirrhosis: relationship to endotoxemia. Hepatology. 1993;18:1139–43.
46. Lopez-Talavera JC, Merrill WW, Groszmann RJ. Tumor necrosis factor alpha: a major contributor to the hyperdynamic circulation in prehepatic portal-hypertensive rats. Gastroenterology. 1995;108:761–7.
47. Bhagat K, Hingorani AD, Palacios M, Charles IG, Vallance P. Cytokine-induced venodilation in humans in vivo: eNOS masquerading as iNOS. Cardiovasc Res. 1999;41:754–64.
48. Lopez-Talavera JC, Cadelina G, Olchowski J, Merrill W, Groszmann RJ. Thalidomide inhibits tumor necrosis factor alpha, decreases nitric oxide synthesis, and ameliorates the hyperdynamic circulatory syndrome in portal-hypertensive rats. Hepatology. 1996; 23:1616–21.
49. Wiest R, Das S, Cadelina G, Garcia-Tsao G, Milstien S, Groszmann RJ. Bacterial translocation in cirrhotic rats stimulates eNOS-derived NO production and impairs mesenteric vascular contractility. J Clin Invest. 1999;104:1223–33.
50. Fernandez-Rodriguez CM, Prieto J, Quiroga J et al. Plasma levels of substance P in liver cirrhosis: relationship to the activation of vasopressor systems and urinary sodium excretion. Hepatology. 1995;21:35–40.
51. John Judy S, Ding-Liu X. Effect of circulating substances known to be increased in cirrhosis on endothelial nitric oxide synthase (eNOS) mRNA. J Am Soc Nephrol. 1996;7:A1619.
52. Albillos A, Rossi I, Cacho G et al. Enhanced endothelium-dependent vasodilation in patients with cirrhosis. Am J Physiol. 1995;268:G459–64.
53. Battista S, Bar F, Mengozzo G, Zanon E, Grosso M, Molino G. Hyperdynamic circulation in patients with cirrhosis: direct measurement of nitric oxide levels in hepatic and portal veins. J Hepatol. 1997;26:75–80.
54. Arkenau HT, Stichtenoth DO, Frolich JC, Manns MP, Boker KH. Elevated nitric oxide levels in patients with chronic liver disease and cirrhosis correlate with disease stage and parameters of hyperdynamic circulation. Z Gastroenterol. 2002;40:907–13.
55. Genesca J, Segura R, Gonzalez A et al. Nitric oxide may contribute to nocturnal hemodynamic changes in cirrhotic patients. Am J Gastroenterol. 2000;95:1539–44.
56. Heller J, Kristeleit H, Brensing KA, Woitas R, Spengler U, Sauerbruch T. Nitrite and nitrate levels in patients with cirrhosis of the liver: influence of kidney function and fasting state. Scand J Gastroenterol. 1999;34:297–302.
57. Sansoe G, Silvano S, Mengozzo G et al. Systemic nitric oxide production and renal function in nonazotemic human cirrhosis: a reappraisal. Am J Gastroenterol. 2002;97:2383–90.
58. Shijo H, Yokoyama M, Ota K et al. Nitrate kinetics in patients with compensated cirrhosis: correlation with hemodynamics. Am J Gastroenterol. 1996;91:2190–4.
59. Sarela AI, Mihaimeed FMA, Batten JJ, Davidson BR, Mathie RT. Hepatic and splanchnic nitric oxide activity in patients with cirrhosis. Gut. 1999;44:749–53.
60. Campillo B, Bories PN, Benvenuti C, Dupeyron C. Serum and urinary nitrate levels in liver cirrhosis: endotoxemia, renal function and hyperdynamic circulation. J Hepatol. 1996; 25:707–14.
61. Criado-Jimenez M, Rivas-Cabanero L, Martin-Oterino JA, Lopez-Novoa JM, Sanchez-Rodriguez A. Nitric oxide production by mononuclear leukocytes in alcoholic cirrhosis. J Mol Med. 1995;73:31–3.
62. Laffi G, Foschi M, Masini E et al. Increased production of nitric oxide by neutrophils and monocytes from cirrhotic patients with ascites and hyperdynamic circulation. Hepatology. 1995;22:1666–73.
63. Campillo B, Chabrier PE, Pelle G et al. Inhibition of nitric oxide synthesis in the forearm arterial bed of patients with advanced cirrhosis. Hepatology. 1995;22:1423–9.
64. Calver A, Harris A, Maxwell JD, Vallance P. Effect of local inhibition of nitric oxide synthesis on forearm blood flow and dorsal hand vein size in patients with alcoholic cirrhosis. Clin Sci (Colch.). 1994;86:203–8.
65. Albornoz L, Motta M, Alvarez E et al. Nitric oxide synthase activity in the splanchnic vasculature of patients with cirrhosis: relationship with hemodynamic disturbances. J Hepatol. 2001;35:452–6.
66. Forrest EH, Jones AL, Dillon JF, Walker J, Hayes PC. The effect of nitric oxide synthase inhibition on portal pressure and azygos blood flow in patients with cirrhosis. J Hepatol. 1995;23:254–8.

67. La Villa G, Barletta G, Pantaleo P et al. Hemodynamic, renal and endocrine effects of acute inhibition of nitric oxide synthase in compensated cirrhosis. Hepatol. 2001;34:19–27.
68. Spahr L, Martin P, Niederberger M, Lang U, Capponi A, Hadengue A. Acute effects of nitric oxide synthase inhibition on systemic, hepatic, and renal hemodynamics in patients with cirrhosis and ascites. J Invest Med. 2002;50:116–24.
69. Thiesson HC, Skott O, Jespersen B, Schaffalitzky de Muckadell OB. Nitric oxide synthase inhibition does not improve renal function in cirrhotic patients with ascites. Am J Gastroenterol. 2003;98:180–6.
70. Pilette C, Moreau R, Sogni P et al. Haemodynamic and hormonal responses to long-term inhibition of nitric oxide synthesis in rats with portal hypertension. Eur J Pharmacol. 1996;312:63–8.
71. Wiest R, Groszmann RJ. The paradox of nitric oxide in cirrhosis and portal hypertension: too much, not enough. Hepatology. 2001;35:478–91.

# 9
# Impaired vasodilation in cirrhotic livers

MAURICIO R. LOUREIRO-SILVA
and ROBERTO J. GROSZMANN

## INTRODUCTION

Similarly to other vascular systems, the intrahepatic circulation has an intrinsic mechanism of vascular tone control. In addition to humoral and neural factors intrahepatic vascular tone is modulated by local production of vasoactive substances with autocrine and paracrine effects. Although different liver cells are able to produce vasoactive substances that can modulate intrahepatic vascular tone, endothelial cells play a central role in this function. Interposed between the lumen and the contractile elements of the vessel wall, endothelial cells react to different intraluminal stimuli releasing vasoconstrictor and vasodilator substances to adjust vascular tone to a particular situation[1].

Although anatomical abnormalities are the main cause of increased vascular resistance in cirrhotic livers, an enhanced intrahepatic vascular tone has been demonstrated in cirrhotic patients[2,3] and cirrhotic rats[4]. Decreased availability of vasodilators[5-9], increased production of vasoconstrictors[10,11], and increased endothelin receptor density[12] are major functional intrinsic mechanisms that generate an imbalance between vasoconstrictor and vasodilator forces, causing the increased intrahepatic vascular tone observed in cirrhosis. Although the liver produces different vasodilator substances, only nitric oxide (NO) production was shown to be impaired in cirrhotic livers.

## NITRIC OXIDE (NO) MODULATES INTRAHEPATIC VASCULAR TONE

Among the endothelial-derived vasodilators, NO plays a central role in the intrinsic vascular tone control in different vascular beds[13-15] including the intrahepatic circulation[16,17]. Because of its importance in health and disease the regulation of NO synthesis has been studied extensively[18]. Most of the information regarding the role of NO on intrinsic intrahepatic vascular tone

81

control came from studies using rat liver perfusion as an experimental model. The availability of specific NO synthase inhibitors and NO donor compounds was essential to uncover the hemodynamic effect of this vasodilator in the liver circulation.

Using rat liver perfusion as an experimental model, Mittal and collaborators showed that the presence of the NO synthase blocker $N\omega$-nitro-L-arginine (NNA) in the perfusate increased the vasoconstrictive response of the intrahepatic circulation to norepinephrine[16], suggesting that NO modulates vascular tone in normal livers. Later, this result was confirmed using different vasoconstrictors such as angiotensin II, endothelin-1 (authors' unpublished data), and methoxamine (specific $\alpha_1$-adrenergic agonist)[19] or vasoconstrictive doses of bradykinin[17].

Additional studies reinforced the conclusion that NO modulates intrahepatic vascular tone control. Acetylcholine caused vasodilation of preconstricted (methoxamine) perfused livers, an effect that was significantly decreased by the presence of NNA[5]. Liver perfusion performed in a recirculating mode was shown to cause accumulation of the NO end-products in the perfusate, indicating the presence of intrahepatic NO production stimulated by shear stress, one of the most potent stimuli of endothelial NO production. As expected, this NO production was significantly reduced by preincubation in the presence of NNA[5]. Liver endothelial cells in culture were also shown to produce NO in response to shear stress[20].

## NITRIC OXIDE PRODUCTION IS DECREASED IN CIRRHOTIC LIVERS

As mentioned above, an increased vascular tone is a significant component of the increased intrahepatic vascular resistance in cirrhosis. In studies performed in isolated perfused cirrhotic livers the greatest reduction in portal pressure by vasodilator compounds was observed after infusion of the NO donor sodium nitroprusside[4]. Shear stress-induced NO production and acetylcholine-induced vasodilation were shown to be severely impaired in cirrhotic livers[5].

Shah and collaborators have shown that, although the expression of endothelial NO synthase in cirrhotic livers was similar to the expression in normal livers, the activity of this enzyme was significantly reduced in cirrhotic livers previously treated with carbon tetrachloride. This deficient activity was associated with increased protein levels of caveolin-1 and an increased binding of eNOS to caveolin-1, probably preventing the binding of the enzyme to calmodulin and its consequent activation[7]. Later, this mechanism of NO production impairment was also observed in bile duct-ligated rats, a model of liver fibrosis with cholestasis[21].

## LOCALIZATION OF THE NO HEMODYNAMIC EFFECTS IN THE LIVER

Recently we have developed a modified rat liver perfusion model in which not only the perfusion pressure but also the sinusoidal pressure is measured

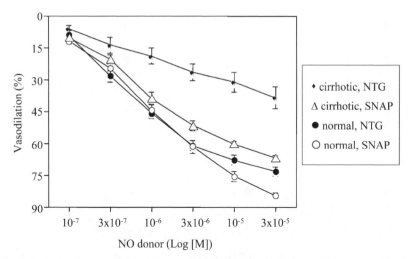

**Figure 1.** Vasorelaxation induced by nitroglycerin (NTG) and $S$-nitroso-$N$-acetylpenicillamine (SNAP) in normal and cirrhotic rat livers after preconstriction with methoxamine ($10^{-4}$ M) during liver perfusion. SNAP and NTG promoted similar vasorelaxant responses in normal livers ($p = 0.435$); in cirrhotic livers, SNAP produced a greater relaxation than NTG ($p < 0.001$). Both SNAP ($p < 0.001$) and NTG ($p = 0.002$) induced a greater vasorelaxation in normal livers than in cirrhotic livers[23]. Comparison: repeated measures ANOVA (from Dudenhoefer et al., 2002[23], with permission)

during the experiment[19]. Using this innovative experimental model we observed that, normally, NO modulates the vascular tone in the presinu-soidal, sinusoidal, and postsinusoidal segments of the intrahepatic circula-tion. In addition we observed that, in cirrhotic livers, NO production is preserved in the presinusoidal area but severely impaired in the sinusoidal and postsinusoidal areas[19].

## DELIVERING NO TO THE LIVER

Nitrates have been used with success for treating different cardiovascular conditions. However, for different reasons, nitrates are not so efficient in treating portal hypertension in cirrhotic patients[22]. We studied the vasodila-tion induced by nitroglycerin (NTG, a nitrate) and $S$-nitroso-$N$-acetylpenicil-lamine (SNAP) in normal and cirrhotic rat livers (Figure 1)[23]. Differently from the spontaneous NO donor SNAP, NTG requires bioactivation to cause its vasodilatory effect[24,25]. We observed that NTG caused less vasodila-tion in cirrhotic livers than in normal livers, indicating that its bioactivation is impaired in this condition. This may explain, at least in part, the poor response to nitrates among cirrhotic patients.

In cirrhotic livers SNAP caused more vasodilation than NTG. However, the vasodilation induced by SNAP was still less in cirrhotic livers than in normal livers. This indicates that, in addition to a decreased NO production, a decreased response to NO is also involved in the development of the increased vascular tone observed in cirrhotic livers. A decreased vascular

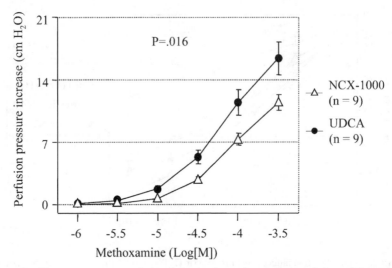

**Figure 2.** Dose–response curve induced by methoxamine during perfusion of livers from cirrhotic rats previously treated with NCX-1000 or ursodeoxycholic acid (UDCA; control)[32]. Comparison: repeated measures ANOVA (from Loureiro-Silva *et al.*, 2003[32], with permission)

response to NO in cirrhotic livers could be caused by: (a) increased NO inactivation by superoxide anion, a product of oxidative stress; (b) dysfunction of the cGMP cascade, an enzymatic system that mediates NO-induced vasorelaxation; and (c) dysfunction of cGMP-independent mechanisms of NO-induced vasorelaxation.

Physical impairment of NO diffusion through structurally changed vessel walls could also be involved in the impaired vascular response to NO in cirrhotic livers. The intrahepatic vascular permeability, particularly to high molecular-weight molecules such as albumin (FW 66 000), is decreased in cirrhotic livers[26,27]. However, small molecules such as water and sucrose (FW 342.3) have a normal diffusion from the intravascular to the extravascular space in CCl$_4$-induced cirrhotic livers[27], practically ruling out a physical impairment to NO (FW 30) diffusion in this condition. An altered redox status, however, may impose an important spatial range constraint to NO because of its high reactivity[28].

Portal hypertension in cirrhosis is frequently associated with the development of splanchnic and systemic vasodilation, which is, at least in part, mediated by an overproduction of NO[29–31]. The use of liver-specific NO donors would replenish the intrahepatic circulation with NO, reducing intrahepatic vascular resistance without causing arterial hypotension. NCX-1000, an ursodeoxycholic derivative, was designed to deliver NO exclusively to the liver.

We observed that, during liver perfusion, this compound was able to significantly reduce the hyper-responsiveness of cirrhotic rat livers to methoxamine (Figure 2). *In vivo*, NCX-1000 abolished the portal pressure increase induced by increase in portal blood flow observed in cirrhotic rats (Figure 3).

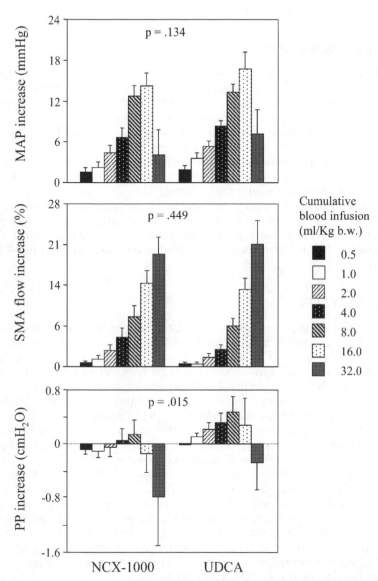

**Figure 3.** Mean arterial pressure (MAP), superior mesenteric artery (SMA) blood flow, and portal pressure (PP) *in-vivo* measurements during blood infusion in cirrhotic rats previously treated with NCX-1000 or ursodeoxycholic acid (UDCA)[32]; b.w.: body weight. Comparison: two-way ANOVA (from Loureiro-Silva *et al.*, 2003[32], with permission)

These beneficial hemodynamic effects of NCX-1000 were associated with an increased cGMP concentration in cirrhotic liver tissue[32].

## CARBON MONOXIDE

Carbon monoxide (CO) is a co-product of the degradation of protoheme IX to biliverdin by heme oxygenases. Similarly to NO, it activates guanylyl cyclase, increasing the production of cGMP[33]. Inhibition of heme oxygenase activity by protoporphyrin IX was shown to increase perfusion pressure during rat liver perfusion, an effect that was further reversed by addition of CO to the perfusate[34]. In addition, CO overproduction by induced heme oxygenase-1 caused a reduction in intrahepatic vascular resistance during liver perfusion[35]. Taken together, these observations indicate that CO participates in intrahepatic vascular tone control.

Heme oxygenase-1 activity in liver tissue from cirrhotic patients was shown to be higher than in normal liver tissue[36], suggesting that CO production in cirrhotic livers is not impaired. It has been suggested that increased CO production could be involved in decreased production of NO in cirrhotic livers[36].

## PROSTACYCLIN

Prostacyclin ($PGE_1$) is a potent vasodilator derived from arachidonic acid metabolism. It is produced not only by endothelial cells but also by vascular smooth muscle cells. $PGE_1$ causes relaxation by activating adenyl cyclase and increasing cAMP production. The same humoral and physical factors that are involved in endothelial NO production stimulate the release of $PGE_1$ (see ref. 37). Using rat liver perfusion, Mittal and collaborators have shown that indomethacin (an inhibitor of $PGE_1$ production) increases the intrahepatic vascular response to norepinephrine only in the presence of the NO synthase inhibitor NNA, indicating that $PGE_1$ plays a role in intrahepatic vascular tone control that is secondary to the role of NO[16].

Using liver perfusion, Graupera and collaborators have studied the production of prostanoids in normal and cirrhotic livers. They observed[11] that, after vasoconstriction induced by methoxamine ($\alpha_1$-adrenergic agonist), normal and cirrhotic livers produced similar amounts of 6-keto prostaglandin $F_1$, the end metabolite of $PGE_1$. This finding indicates that normal livers produce $PGE_1$ in response to a hemodynamic challenge, and that this production is preserved in cirrhotic livers. However, it does not seem enough to compensate for the decreased NO production.

## CONCLUSION

Among different vasodilator substances involved in intrinsic vascular tone control in the intrahepatic circulation, only NO seems to be depleted in cirrhotic livers. NO is an important component of intrinsic vascular tone control in the intrahepatic circulation. Endothelial dysfunction and a consequent deficit in NO production play a major role in the development of an increased intrahepatic vascular tone in cirrhotic livers. This deficit in NO production is located in both the sinusoidal and postsinusoidal areas. Although the cirrhotic liver has an impaired response to NO, the use of liver-specific NO donors is effective in improving the intrahepatic hemodynamic abnormalities observed in cirrhosis.

## References

1. Vane JR, Botting RM. Endothelium-derived vasoactive factors and the control of circulation. Semin Perinatol. 1991;15:4–10.
2. Groszmann RJ, Kravetz D, Bosch J et al. Nitroglycerin improves the hemodynamic response to vasopressin in portal hypertension. Hepatology. 1982;2:757–62.
3. Albillos A, Llebo JL, Banares R et al. Hemodynamic effects of α-adrenergic blockade with prazosin in cirrhotic patients with portal hypertension. Hepatology. 1994;20:611–17.
4. Bhathal PS, Grossman HJ. Reduction of the increased portal vascular resistance of the isolated perfused cirrhotic rat liver by vasodilators. J Hepatol. 1985;1:325–37.
5. Gupta TK, Toruner M, Chung MK, Groszmann RJ. Endothelial dysfunction and decreased production of nitric oxide in the intrahepatic microcirculation of cirrhotic rats. Hepatology. 1998;28:926–31.
6. Rockey DC, Chung JJ. Reduced nitric oxide production by endothelial cells in cirrhotic rat liver: endothelial dysfunction in portal hypertension. Gastroenterology. 1998;114:344–51.
7. Shah V, Toruner M, Haddad F et al. Impaired endothelial nitric oxide synthase activity associated with enhanced caveolin binding in experimental cirrhosis in the rat. Gastroenterology. 1999;117:1222–8.
8. Moralez-Ruiz M, Cajudo-Martin P, Fernandes-Varo G et al. Transduction of the liver with activated Akt normalizes portal pressure in cirrhotic rats. Gastroenterology. 2003;125:522–31.
9. Van de Casteele M, van Pelt JF, Nevens F, Fevery J, Reichein J. Low NO bioavailability in $CCl_4$ cirrhotic rat livers might result from low NO synthesis combined with decreased superoxide dismutase activity allowing superoxide-mediated NO breakdown: a comparison of two portal hypertensive models with healthy controls. Comp Hepatol. 2003;2:2.
10. Pinzani M, Milani S, De Franco R et al. Endothelin 1 is overexpressed in human cirrhotic liver and exerts multiple effect on activated hepatic stellate cells. Gastroenterology. 1996;110:534–48.
11. Graupera M, Garcia-Pagan JC, Abraldes JG et al. Cyclooxygenase-derived products modulate the increased intrahepatic resistance of cirrhotic rat livers. Hepatology. 2003;37:172–81.
12. Gandhi CR, Sproat LA, Subbotin VM. Increased hepatic endothelin-1 levels and endothelin receptors density in cirrhotic rat livers. Life Sci. 1996;58:55–62.
13. Furchgott RF, Zawadski JV. The obligatory role of endothelial cells in the relaxation of arterial smooth muscle by acetylcholine. Nature. 1980;288:373–6.
14. Lowenstein CJ, Dinerman JL, Snyder SH. Nitric oxide: a physiological messenger. Ann Intern Med. 1994;120:227–37.
15. Moncada S, Higgs A. The L-arginine-nitric oxide pathway. N Engl J Med. 1993;329:2002–12.
16. Mittal MK, Gupta TK, Lee FY, Sieber CC, Groszmann RJ. Nitric oxide modulates hepatic vascular tone in normal rat liver. Am J Physiol. 1994;267:416–22.
17. Loureiro-Silva MR, Molina HM, Borges DR. The portal hypertensive response to bradykinin is mediated by the B2-type receptor and modulated by nitric oxide. Intern Hepatol Commun. 1995;4:175–80.
18. Bellamy TC, Wood J, Garthwaite J. On the activation of soluble guanylyl cyclase by nitric oxide. Proc Natl Acad Sci USA. 2002;99:507–10.
19. Loureiro-Silva MR, Cadelina GW, Groszmann RJ. Deficit in nitric oxide production in cirrhotic livers is located in the sinusoidal and pre-sinusoidal areas. Am J Physiol. 2003;284:G567–74.
20. Shah V, Haddad FG, Garcia-Gardena G et al. Liver sinusoidal endothelial cells are responsible for nitric oxide modulation of resistance in hepatic sinusoids. J Clin Invest. 1997;100:2923–30.

21. Shah V, Cao S, Hendrickson H, Yao J, Katusic Z. Regulation of hepatic eNOS by caveolin and calmodulin after bile duct ligation in rats. Am J Physiol Gastrointest Liver Physiol. 2001;280:G1209–16.
22. Garcia-Tsao G. Current management of the complications of cirrhosis and portal hypertension: variceal hemorrhage, ascites, and spontaneous bacterial peritonitis. Gastroenterology. 2001;120:726–48.
23. Dudenhoefer AA, Loureiro-Silva MR, Cadelina GW, Gupta T, Groszmann RJ. Bioactivation of nitroglycerin and vasomotor response to nitric oxide are impaired in cirrhotic rat livers. Hepatology. 2002;36:381–5.
24. Brien JF, McLaughlin BE, Kobus SA, Kawamoto LH, Nakatsu JK, Marks GS. Mechanisms of glyceril trinitrate-induced vasodilation. I. Relationship between drug biotransformation, tissue cyclic GMP elevation and relaxation of rabbit aorta. J Pharmacol Exp Ther. 1988;244:322–7.
25. Feelish M. The use of nitric oxide donors in pharmacological studies. Naunyn Schmiedebergs Arch Pharmacol. 1998;358:113–22.
26. Villeneuve J-P, Dagenais M, Huet P-M, Roy A, Lapoint R, Marleua D. The hepatic microcirculation in the isolated perfused human liver. Hepatology. 1996;23:24–31.
27. Hung DY, Chang P, Cheung K, Winterford C, Roberts MS. Quantitative evaluation of altered hepatic spaces and membrane transport in fibrotic rat liver. Hepatology. 2002;36:1180–9.
28. Stamler JS. Redox signaling: nitrosylation and related target interactions of nitric oxide. Cell. 1994;78:931–6.
29. Sieber CC, Lopez-Talavera JC, Groszmann RJ. Role of nitric oxide in the *in vivo* splanchnic hyporeactivity in ascitic cirrhotic rats. Gastroenterology. 1993;104:1750–4.
30. Ros J, Jimenez W, Lamas S et al. Nitric oxide production in arterial vessels of cirrhotic rats. Hepatology. 1995;21:554–60
31. Niederberger M, Gines P, Tsai P et al. Increased aortic cyclic guanosine monophosphate concentration in experimental cirrhosis in rats: evidence for a role of nitric oxide in the pathogenesis of arterial vasodilation in cirrhosis. Hepatology. 1995;21:1625–31.
32. Loureiro-Silva MR, Cadelina GW, Iwakiri Y, Groszmann RJ. A liver-specific nitric oxide donor improves the intra-hepatic vascular response to portal blood flow increase and methoxamine in cirrhotic rats. J Hepatol. 2003;39:940–6.
33. Maines MD. Heme oxygenase: function, multiplicity, regulatory mechanisms, and clinical applications. FASEB J. 1988;2:2557–68.
34. Suematsu M, Kashiwagi S, Sano T, Goda N, Shinoda Y, Ishimura Y. Carbon monoxide as an endogenous modulator of hepatic vascular perfusion. Biochem Biophys Res Commun. 1994;205:1333–7.
35. Wakabayashi Y, Takamiya R, Mizuki A et al. Carbon monoxide overproduced by heme oxygenase-1 causes a reduction of vascular resistance in perfused rat liver. Am J Physiol. 1999;277:G1088–96.
36. Makino N, Suematsu M, Sugiura Y et al. Altered expression of heme oxygenase-1 in the livers of patients with portal hypertensive diseases. Hepatology. 2001;33:32–42.
37. Cahill PA, Redmond EM, Sitzmann JV. Endothelial dysfunction in cirrhosis and portal hypertension. Pharmacol Ther. 2001;89:273–93.

# 10
# Enhanced release of vasoconstrictors

JUAN CARLOS GARCÍA-PAGÁN

## INCREASED INTRAHEPATIC VASCULAR RESISTANCE

Increased resistance to portal blood flow is the primary factor in the pathophysiology of portal hypertension, and may occur at any site within the portal venous system. In cirrhosis, increased intrahepatic vascular resistance is the consequence of the distortion of the liver vascular architecture caused by fibrosis, scarring and nodule formation. Careful pathological studies have suggested that thrombosis of medium and small portal and hepatic veins occurs frequently in cirrhosis, and that these events may be important in causing further progression of cirrhosis and worsening portal hypertension[1]. In addition, the active contraction, in response to several agonists, of different contractile cell types in the liver promotes a further increase in intrahepatic resistance[2]. It has been claimed that this dynamic and reversible component may represent up to 40% of the increased intrahepatic vascular resistance in cirrhosis.

Contractile elements influencing the hepatic vascular bed can be located at sinusoidal as well as at extrasinusoidal levels[3,4]. These elements include vascular smooth muscle cells of the intrahepatic vasculature (i.e. small portal venules in portal areas)[5] and activated hepatic stellate cells (HSC), that are pericyte cells located in the perisinusoidal space of Disse with extensions that wrap around the sinusoids, and reduce its caliber after contraction[3,4]. Contraction of hepatic myofibroblasts, either derived from activated HSC or from other cellular sources, by compression of venous shuntings that have been shown to be located in the fibrous septa, may also contribute to the dynamic increase in intrahepatic vascular resistance. Whatever the location in which they act, it is now clear that vasoactive mediators, either vasoconstrictors or vasodilators, may modulate intrahepatic vascular resistance either in health or liver disease.

An increased production of vasoconstrictors and an exaggerated response of the hepatic vascular bed to some of them are one of the mechanisms that have been implicated in the pathogenesis of the dynamic component of

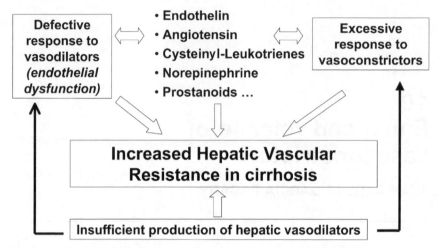

**Figure 1.** Mechanisms involved in the increased hepatic vascular resistance of the cirrhotic liver

increased intrahepatic resistance of the cirrhotic liver. In addition, the defective response of the hepatic vascular bed to endothelium-dependent vasodilators, what has been called endothelial dysfunction, is also increasing the intrahepatic resistance of the cirrhotic liver. Endothelial dysfunction has been empirically attributed to an insufficient release of hepatic vasodilators. However, as will be shown later in this chapter, endothelial dysfunction is, at least in part, also due to an increased production of hepatic vasoconstrictors (Figure 1).

## INCREASED PRODUCTION/EXAGGERATED RESPONSE OF THE HEPATIC VASCULAR BED TO VASOCONSTRICTORS

An increased activity of several endogenous vasoconstrictors such as endothelin, norepinephrine, angiotensin II, vasopressin and more recently leukotrienes and thromboxane A2, has been demonstrated in cirrhosis. Additionally, an increased vasoconstrictive response of the hepatic vascular bed to some of these vasoconstrictors magnifies its role. The next section will discuss more deeply the role of this pathophysiological mechanism increasing hepatic vascular tone.

### Endothelin

Endothelin comprises a family of homologous 21-amino acid peptides (ET-1, ET-2, and ET-3). Biological properties of endothelins are mediated essentially by two major endothelin receptors, endothelin A ($ET_A$) and endothelin B ($ET_B$)[6]. The role of a presumed type C endothelin receptor ($ET_C$) has not yet been clarified. While the $ET_A$ receptor shows a high affinity for ET-1, but not ET-3, and mediates constriction, the $ET_B$ receptor has equal affinity for ET-1 and ET-3 and is considered to mediate dilation and constriction[7]. In base to this different effect they have been designated as $ET_{B1}$ and $ET_{B2}$

respectively[7]. Many patients with liver cirrhosis have increased circulating plasma levels of ET-1 and ET-3[8–12]. Although the increase is greater and more consistently found in cirrhotic patients with ascites[8,11,12] it is also observed in pre-ascitic cirrhotic patients[12]. A net release of ET-1 and ET-3 during splanchnic passage has been observed in cirrhotic patients, but not in control subjects, suggesting an increased production of ET-1 and ET-3 in the splanchnic territory in liver cirrhosis[10]. Recently, immunostaining and *in-situ* hybridization studies have detected an increased expression of ET-1 in cirrhotic human livers[13]. Endothelial cells, HSC in their activated phenotype, as well as bile duct epithelial cells, were the major intrahepatic sources of ET-1[13]. The exact mechanism promoting such increases is not well known; however, cultured HSC stimulated with angiotensin II and transforming growth factor beta (TGF-$\beta$) have been shown to increase its production of ET-1[13]. Therefore, it is conceivable that in liver cirrhosis these and other factors, that are usually increased, may stimulate the production of endothelins[13]. A decreased clearance of ET-1 by the liver has also been demonstrated in cirrhotic rats[14].

ET-1 increases portal pressure in isolated and perfused normal livers. This effect is associated with a reduction in sinusoidal diameter, promoted by HSC contraction, causing a marked redistribution of sinusoidal blood flow[15–17]. ET-3 and Safarotoxin S6C, a specific $ET_B$ receptor agonist, also increase portal pressure but fail to induce any significant change in sinusoidal diameter because of a concomitant increase in NO production due to the activation of endothelial $ET_B$ receptors[18].

ET-1[16,17] and Safarotoxin S6C[17] administration has also been shown to increase portal pressure in isolated and perfused $CCl_4$ cirrhotic livers. A slightly increased[17] or blunted[16] portohepatic response to ET-1 has been reported in cirrhotic in comparison with normal livers. Safarotoxin S6C has been suggested to promote a much greater increase in portal pressure in cirrhotic than in normal rats, suggesting a major action of $ET_B$ receptors in cirrhosis[16]. The role played by HSC in the portohepatic response to vasoconstrictors in cirrhosis is unknown. *In-vitro* studies show that the progressive activation and phenotypical modulation of human HSC in culture is associated with a progressive transformation from a relative dominion of $ET_A$ receptors to a relative dominion of $ET_B$ receptors[13]. In addition, HSC isolated from rats pretreated with $CCl_4$ for 10 weeks (histologically proven cirrhotic rats) exhibited a marked contraction to $ET_B$ agonists[16]. It is therefore possible that the marked phenotypical transformation of HSC observed in cirrhosis may promote marked changes in the response of these cells to different vasoactive agents. In addition one of the postulated origins of the myofibroblast located in the fibrous septa of the cirrhotic livers is the phenotypical transformation of HSC. It is therefore possible that the contraction of such cells in response to endothelin or other vasoconstrictors may play a role in modulating the vascular resistance of cirrhotic livers.

Endothelin has also been shown to promote the closing of endothelium fenestrae in normal rat liver[19]. This may be relevant since the capillarization process and occlusion of fenestrae are thought to play a role in increasing resistance in cirrhosis.

The role of endothelin modulating the increase in sinusoidal resistance in cirrhosis is further emphasized by a study in isolated livers showing that administration of the $ET_A$ and $ET_B$ antagonist bosentan produces a slight but significant reduction in portal pressure in cirrhotic but not in normal livers[16,19]. This, however, is controversial, since no reduction in portal pressure after endothelin blockade has been shown in other studies[20]. There is also controversy regarding the role of each different endothelin receptor subtype in the regulation of the increased intrahepatic vascular resistance of cirrhotic livers. Different experimental studies have suggested a major role of $ET_A$ or $ET_B$ activation, respectively. However, most studies using endothelin antagonists suggest that both types of receptor need to be blocked to significantly reduce portal pressure.

Other vasoconstrictive factors have also been involved in the regulation of hepatic vascular tone. Indeed, studies in perfused cirrhotic livers have shown that norepinephrine, angiotensin II and vasopressin, three circulating vasoactive factors which are usually found to be increased in cirrhosis, are also able to increase intrahepatic vascular resistance[21]. The increased resistance promoted by norepinephrine is completely blunted by the administration of α-adrenergic antagonists such as prazosin. This agent by itself markedly reduces hepatic resistance and portal pressure in patients with cirrhosis. On the other hand, administration of α-adrenergic antagonists, such as prazosin, reduces intrahepatic vascular resistance in the perfused cirrhotic liver. These data suggest that adrenergic receptors may be involved in the regulation of intrahepatic resistance in cirrhosis, and that α-adrenergic receptor blockers may have a potential for decreasing portal pressure in cirrhosis.

In addition, the hepatic vascular bed of cirrhotic livers exhibits a vasoconstrictor hyperresponse to the α-adrenergic agonist methoxamine. This hyperresponse is associated with an overproduction of thromboxane A2 (TxA2) by the COX-1 isoenzyme and completely corrected by pretreating the livers either with COX non-selective blockers, with COX-1, but not with COX-2, selective blockers or with TxA2 antagonists. Thus, the coupling of an increased production of TxA2 markedly enhances the vasoconstrictive response of the cirrhotic hepatic vascular bed to methoxamine[22]. Whether this effect is also shared by other vasoconstrictors has not been investigated so far; however, it is known that the coupling of different agonists to its membrane G-coupled receptors promotes the release of arachidonic acid from the plasma membrane, facilitating its metabolization to different prostanoids[23,24].

Angiotensin II is a powerful vasoconstrictor that may increase hepatic resistance. Angiotensin II blockade may reduce portal pressure, but causes systemic hypotension[25-27].

Cysteinyl-leukotrienes are a group of biologically highly potent vasoactive substances derived from arachidonic acid after its oxygenation and dehydratation by 5-lipoxygenase[28,29]. These substances have also been shown to increase intrahepatic vascular resistance in normal and $CCl_4$ cirrhotic rat livers[28]. This response is significantly greater in cirrhotic livers that also exhibit an increased cysteinyl-leukotriene production and 5-lipoxygenase mRNA expression[28,30]. In addition, 5-lipoxygenase inhibition produces a significant and marked reduction in PP in cirrhotic livers, suggesting that 5-lipoxygenase-derived eicosanoids contribute to increase hepatic vascular resistance in cirrhosis[28].

It is clear than an increase in the production, as well as an enhanced response to several vasoconstrictors, is involved in the increased vascular resistance of cirrhotic livers. This overactivation of vasoconstrictors is not counterbalanced by a compensatory activation of the hepatic vasodilatory systems, which are even reduced.

## ENDOTHELIAL DYSFUNCTION AND INCREASED PRODUCTION OF VASOCONSTRICTOR PROSTANOIDS IN CIRRHOTIC LIVERS

In normal conditions the endothelium of the hepatic vascular bed, similar to what happens in other vascular territories, is able to generate vasodilator stimuli in response to increases in blood volume, blood pressure or vasoconstrictor agents in an attempt to prevent or attenuate the consequent increase in pressure. In several pathological conditions there is an impairment in this endothelium-dependent vasodilation that has been named endothelial dysfunction[31-33]. Endothelial dysfunction is considered one of the main pathological mechanisms involved in the increased vascular tone observed in several vascular disorders such as arterial hypertension, diabetes and atherosclerosis, and has been attributed to a diminished NO bioavailability[32,34], to an increased production of endothelial-derived contracting factors (EDCF), such as, $PGH_2/TXA_2$ (see refs 33, 35–37), endothelin[38] or anion superoxide[39].

The hepatic vascular bed of cirrhotic livers also exhibits endothelial dysfunction[40]; indeed, studies performed either in patients with cirrhosis or in experimental models of cirrhosis have shown that, contrary to what happens in normal livers, the cirrhotic liver cannot accommodate the increase in portal blood flow caused by the postprandial hyperemia, which determines an abrupt postprandial increase in portal pressure[41]. This is important because such repeated brisk increases in portal pressure and portal–collateral blood flow, in response to meals and other physiological stimuli, is thought to be a major determinant of the progressive dilation of the varices in patients with cirrhosis[42]. In addition, endothelial dysfunction has been further characterized by showing that the vascular bed of the cirrhotic liver exhibits an impaired response to the endothelium-dependent vasodilator acetylcholine[40,43]. This impaired response to acetylcholine was shown to be associated with an increased production of TxA2, and completely prevented by COX-1 selective blockers and by TxA2 antagonists. These results suggest that an increased production of a COX-1-derived vasoconstrictor prostanoid, probably TxA2, is, at least in part, responsible for endothelial dysfunction[43]. Acetylcholine coupling to the endothelial muscarinic $M_3$ receptor has been shown to promote the stimulation of NO synthase as well as COX-1, with the subsequent release of NO and vasoconstrictor endoperoxides, respectively[31]. In physiological states a vasodilating response is the final balance between the interaction of these endothelial vasoactive mediators.

However, in cirrhosis – but also in other different pathophysiological situations, such as hypertension, diabetes, and arteriosclerosis – there is a perturbation of this balance, resulting in endothelial dysfunction with the consequent impaired response to acetylcholine. All these findings suggest that in cirrhotic livers there is over-activation of the COX-1 pathway with increased production of their vasoconstrictor-derived compounds.

## Acknowledgements

These studies were supported by grants from the Fondo de Investigaciones Sanitarias (FIS 02/0692 and FIS 02/0739) and a grant from the Instituto de Salud Carlos III (C03/02).

## References

1. Wanless IR, Wong F, Blendis LM, Greig P, Heathcote EJ, Levy G. Hepatic and portal vein thrombosis in cirrhosis: possible role in development of parenchymal extinction and portal hypertension. Hepatology. 1995;21:1238–47.
2. Bathal PS, Grossmann HJ. Reduction of the increased portal vascular resistance of the isolated perfused cirrhotic rat liver by vasodilators. J Hepatol. 1985;1:325–9.
3. Zhang JX, Pegoli W, Clemens MG. Endothelin-1 induces direct constriction of hepatic sinusoids. Am J Physiol. 1994; 266:G624–32.
4. Kawada N, Tran-Thi TA, Klein H, Decker K. The contraction of hepatic stellate (Ito) cells stimulated with vasoactive substances. Possible involvement of endothelin 1 and nitric oxide in the regulation of the sinusoidal tonus. Eur J Biochem. 1993;213:815–23.
5. Kaneda K, Ekataksin W, Sogawa M, Matsumura A, Cho A, Kawada N. Endothelin-1-induced vasoconstriction causes a significant increase in portal pressure of rat liver: localized constrictive effect on the distal segment of preterminal portal venules as revealed by light and electron microscopy and serial reconstruction. Hepatology. 1998;27:735–47.
6. Rubanyi GM, Botelho LH. Endothelins. FASEB J. 1991;5:2713–20.
7. Clozel M, Gray GA, Breu V, Loffler BM, Osterwalder R. The endothelin $ET_B$ receptor mediates both vasodilation and vasoconstriction in vivo. Biochem Biophys Res Commun. 1992;186:867–73.
8. Asbert M, Gines A, Gines P et al. Circulating levels of endothelin in cirrhosis. Gastroenterology. 1993;104:1485–91.
9. Moller S, Gulberg V, Henriksen JH, Gerbes AL. Endothelin-1 and endothelin-3 in cirrhosis: relations to systemic and splanchnic haemodynamics. J Hepatol. 1995;23:135–44.
10. Gerbes AL, Moller S, Gulberg V, Henriksen JH. Endothelin-1 and -3 plasma concentrations in patients with cirrhosis: role of splanchnic and renal passage and liver function. Hepatology. 1995;21:735–9.
11. Bernardi M, Gulberg V, Colantoni A, Trevisani F, Gasbarrini A, Gerbes AL. Plasma endothelin-1 and -3 in cirrhosis: relationship with systemic hemodynamics, renal function and neurohumoral systems. J Hepatol. 1996;24:161–8.
12. Trevisani F, Colantoni A, Gerbes AL et al. Daily profile of plasma endothelin-1 and -3 in pre-ascitic cirrhosis: relationships with the arterial pressure and renal function. J Hepatol. 1997;26:808–15.
13. Pinzani M, Milani S, De Franco R et al. Endothelin 1 is overexpressed in human cirrhotic liver and exerts multiple effects on activated hepatic stellate cells. Gastroenterology. 1996;110:534–48.
14. Gandhi CR, Sproat LA, Subbotin VM. Increased hepatic endothelin-1 levels and endothelin receptor density in cirrhotic rats. Life Sci. 1996;58:55–62.
15. Zhang JX, Pegoli Jr W, Clemens MG. Endothelin-1 induces direct constriction of hepatic sinusoids. Am J Physiol (Gastrointest Liver Physiol). 1994;29:G264–632.
16. Rockey DC, Weisiger RA. Endothelin induced contractility of stellate cells from normal and cirrhotic rat liver: implications for regulation of portal pressure and resistance. Hepatology. 1996;24:233–40.

17. Elliot AJ, Vo LT, Grossman VL, Bhathal PS, Grossman HJ. Endothelin-induced vasoconstriction in isolated perfused liver preparations from normal and cirrhotic rats. J Gastroenterol Hepatol. 1997;12:314–18.
18. Zhang JX, Bauer M, Clemens MG. Vessel- and target cell-specific actions of endothelin-1 and endothelin-3 in rat liver. Am J Physiol. 1995;269:G269–77.
19. Reichen J, Gerbes AL, Steiner MJ, Sagesser H, Clozel M. The effect of endothelin and its antagonist Bosentan on hemodynamics and microvascular exchange in cirrhotic rat liver. J Hepatol. 1998;28:1020–30.
20. Poo JL, Jimenez W, Maria MR et al. Chronic blockade of endothelin receptors in cirrhotic rats: hepatic and hemodynamic effects. Gastroenterology. 1999;116:161–7.
21. Ballet F, Chretien Y, Rey C, Poupon R. Differential response of normal and cirrhotic liver to vasoactive agents. A study in the isolated perfused rat liver. J Pharmacol Exp Ther. 1988;244:283–9.
22. Graupera M, Garcia-Pagan JC, Abraldes JG et al. Cyclooxygenase-derived products modulate the increased intrahepatic resistance of cirrhotic rat livers. Hepatology. 2003;37:172–81.
23. Xing M, Insel PA. Protein kinase C-dependent activation of cytosolic phospholipase A2 and mitogen-activated protein kinase by alpha 1-adrenergic receptors in Madin–Darby canine kidney cells. J Clin Invest. 1996;97:1302–10.
24. Athari A, Hanecke K, Jungermann K. Prostaglandin F2 alpha and D2 release from primary Ito cell cultures after stimulation with noradrenaline and ATP but not adenosine. Hepatology. 1994;20:142–8.
25. Schneider AW, Kalk JF, Klein CP. Effect of losartan, an angiotensin II receptor antagonist, on portal pressure in cirrhosis. Hepatology. 1999;29:334–9.
26. Gonzalez-Abraldes J, Albillos A, Banares R et al. Randomized comparison of long-term losartan versus propranolol in lowering portal pressure in cirrhosis. Gastroenterology. 2001;121:382–8.
27. Debernardi-Venon W, Barletti C, Alessandria C et al. Efficacy of irbesartan, a receptor selective antagonist of angiotensin II, in reducing portal hypertension. Dig Dis Sci. 2002;47:401–4.
28. Graupera M, Garcia-Pagan JC, Titos E et al. 5-Lipoxygenase inhibition reduces intrahepatic vascular resistance of cirrhotic rat livers: a possible role of cysteinyl-leukotrienes. Gastroenterology. 2002;122:387–93.
29. Back M, Norel X, Walch L et al. Prostacyclin modulation of contractions of the human pulmonary artery by cysteinyl-leukotrienes. Eur J Pharmacol. 2000;401:389–95.
30. Titos E, Claria J, Bataller R et al. Hepatocyte-derived cysteinyl leukotrienes modulate vascular tone in experimental cirrhosis. Gastroenterology. 2000;119:794–805.
31. Aleixandre de Artiñano A, Lopez-Miranda Gonzalez V. Endothelial dysfunction and hypertensive vasoconstriction. Pharmacol Res. 1999;40:113–24.
32. Harrison DG. Cellular and molecular mechanisms of endothelial cell dysfunction. J Clin Invest. 1997;100:2153–7.
33. Fu-Xiang D, Jameson M, Skopec J, Diederich A, Diederich D. Endothelial dysfunction of resistance arteries of spontaneously hypertensive rats. J Cardiovasc Pharmacol. 1992;20(Suppl. 12):S190–2.
34. Wilcox JN, Subramanian RR, Sundell CL et al. Expression of multiple isoforms of nitric oxide synthase in normal and atherosclerotic vessels. Arterioscler Thromb Vasc Biol. 1997;17:2479–88.
35. Ge T, Hughes H, Junquero DC, Wu KK, Vanhoutte PM, Boulanger CM. Endothelium-dependent contractions are associated with both augmented expression of prostaglandin H synthase-1 and hypersensitivity to prostaglandin H2 in the SHR aorta. Circ Res. 1995;76:1003–10.
36. Mayhan WG. Role of prostaglandin H2-thromboxane A2 in responses of cerebral arterioles during chronic hypertension. Am J Physiol. 1992;262:H539–43.
37. Mayhan WG, Simmons LK, Sharpe GM. Mechanism of impaired responses of cerebral arterioles during diabetes mellitus. Am J Physiol. 1991;260:H319–26.
38. Lerman A, Holmes DR Jr, Bell MR, Garratt KN, Nishimura RA, Burnett JC Jr. Endothelin in coronary endothelial dysfunction and early atherosclerosis in humans. Circulation. 1995;92:2426–31.
39. Tagawa H, Tomoike H, Nakamura M. Putative mechanisms of the impairment of endothelium-dependent relaxation of the aorta with atheromatous plaque in heritable hyperlipidemic rabbits. Circ Res. 1991;68:330–7.

40. Gupta TK, Toruner M, Chung MK, Groszmann RJ. Endothelial dysfunction and decreased production of nitric oxide in the intrahepatic microcirculation of cirrhotic rats. Hepatology. 1998;28:926–31.
41. Bellis L, Berzigotti A, Abraldes JG et al. Low doses of isosorbide mononitrate attenuate the postprandial increase in portal pressure in patients with cirrhosis. Hepatology. 2003;37:378–84.
42. Bosch J, Garcia-Pagan JC. Complications of cirrhosis. I. Portal hypertension. J Hepatol. 2000;32(Suppl. 1):141–56.
43. Graupera M, Garcia-Pagan JC, Pares M, Abraldes JG et al. Cyclooxyenase-1 inhibition corrects endothelial dysfunction in cirrhotic rat livers. J Hepatol. 2003;39:521.

# 11
# Endogenous cannabinoids and circulatory dysfunction in cirrhosis

WLADIMIRO JIMÉNEZ and JOSEFA ROS

## INTRODUCTION

Cirrhosis of the liver is among the most prevalent diseases in Western countries. The prognostic expectations for these patients are grim, except for those who may benefit from liver transplantation. This is due to the multiple organic derangement, including renal failure, variceal bleeding or bacterial peritonitis, developed by these individuals[1]. Several clinical and experimental studies have demonstrated that the trigger for these disturbances is the existence of an important and progressively accentuated cardiocirculatory dysfunction of which portal hypertension, arterial hypotension, high cardiac output and diminished systemic vascular resistance are the most relevant features[2]. Thus, during the past decade the mechanisms leading to decreased arterial pressure and concomitant arterial vasodilation in cirrhosis have been a subject of great interest. Moreover, vasodilation seems to be localized in the splanchnic circulation because direct blood flow and/or resistive index measurements in skin, skeletal muscle or extremities have found normal or even elevated values of these parameters in cirrhotic patients[3,4]. Although it is generally believed that increased endothelial production of nitric oxide (NO) by the splanchnic vasculature is of major importance in the pathogenesis of this phenomenon[5], other mechanisms are probably implicated.

Cloning and characterization of central and peripheral specific receptors for plant-derived cannabinoids have suggested the existence of endogenously produced cannabinoid substances mimicking the properties of these natural compounds[6,7]. Several endocannabinoids have been described including anandamide, 2-arachydonylglycerol, noladin ether and palmitoylethanolamide, the former being the most extensively investigated[8]. In addition to displaying analgesic, hypothermic and locomotor inhibitory properties, endocannabinoids may also deeply affect systemic hemodynamics[9]. Exogenous administration of anandamide to anesthetized rats results in a transient hypertension followed by a long-lasting hypotension[10]. This vasodepressor effect is mediated by the interaction of anandamide with a central and peripherally located G-protein coupled receptor, namely the CB1 receptor[11]. CB1 receptor blockade prevents the hypotensive effect of anandamide[12], and this substance loses its long-lasting hypotensive effect when given to CB1 receptor knockout mice[13]. The CB1 receptor is peripherally located in endothelial[14,15] and smooth muscle cells[15,16] and in perivascular nerves[16]. Anandamide promotes vasodilation in some particular territories such as the lungs and the splanchnic and renal vascular bed[17–19], and may also inhibit contraction, proliferation and migration in human hepatic stellate cells[20]. In addition, several investigations have demonstrated that the induction of a hemorrhagic shock or the intravenous administration of bacterial lipopolysaccharide (LPS) in rats stimulates anandamide production by circulating blood cells which, in turn, promotes a marked hypotensive effect in recipient euvolemic animals[21,22].

Anandamide is thought to be produced on demand from the enzymatic cleavage of $N$-arachydonyl phosphatidylethanolamine by a $Ca^{2+}$-dependent $N$-acetyltransferase in several cell types including neurons, human umbilical vein endothelial cells, neuroblastoma cells, leukocytes, monocytes and macrophages[6,23]. It is important to note, however, that endogenous cannabinoids do not exert tonic control on arterial pressure in normal conditions, since genetically engineered mice lacking the CB1 receptor gene do not show alterations in blood pressure[13].

Several investigations have recently demonstrated that endocannabinoids are involved in the pathogenesis of the cardiovascular dysfunction occurring in cirrhosis[24,25]. Systemic administration of a selective CB1 receptor antagonist, SR141716A, increased arterial pressure and total peripheral resistance and decreased mesenteric blood flow and portal pressure in cirrhotic rats, but not in control rats. These effects were peripherally mediated because injection of the antagonist in the fourth cerebral ventricle of both control and cirrhotic rats, failed to alter blood pressure. Furthermore, a significant reduction in mean arterial pressure was observed in recipient animals in response to circulating blood cells of cirrhotic rats, a phenomenon not observed when cells were collected from control rats. A remarkably similar pattern of cardiovascular behavior was observed in recipient animals in response to isolated circulating monocytes of cirrhotic rats with ascites. This hypotensive effect induced by isolated monocytes of cirrhotic rats was prevented by the prior administration of the CB1-specific receptor antagonist. The endocannabinoid system operates in cirrhotic animals not only in resting conditions but also after experimentally induced stimulation. Infusion of monocytes from hemorrhaged cirrhotic rats resulted in a sharp, long-lasting diminution of blood pressure in recipient animals, which was of markedly higher intensity than that produced by isolated monocytes of hemorrhaged healthy rats. Monocytes of control rats did not contain anandamide, whereas detectable amounts of this compound were found in monocytes of cirrhotic rats. Since it has been shown that anandamide can elicit arterial hypotension through CB1 receptors, it is likely that anandamide mediates, at least in part, the hypotension induced by monocytes of cirrhotic rats. Moreover, Bátkai et al.[24] assessed mRNA expression and protein abundance of CB1 receptors in endothelial cells isolated from hepatic arteries of normal subjects and cirrhotic patients. CB1 receptor mRNA was markedly overexpressed in samples from cirrhotic patients. Likewise, binding experiments showed increased CB1 receptor abundance in hepatic arteries of cirrhotic patients. As to whether this system operates independently from the NO-metabolic pathway has not been fully established. Whereas in the study by Bátkai et al.[24], NO inhibition with L-NAME prevented the hypotensive effect of anandamide in bile duct-ligated cirrhotic rats, in the investigation by Ros et al[25]. prior L-NAME treatment did not prevent the decrease in arterial pressure produced by the administration of monocytes of cirrhotic rats with ascites to recipient control rats.

More recently, experiments in isolated third-order mesenteric arteries of cirrhotic rats[26] with ascites have shown that these vessels display an altered and differential response to anandamide. The endocannabinoid induced a greater relaxation in mesenteric resistance arteries of cirrhotic rats with ascites than in mesenteric arteries of control rats. Since increased circulating levels of anandamide have been found in cirrhotic patients[27], these results suggest that the endocannabinoid system may have a greater local vasodilator activity in the splanchnic circulation under this condition. This distinct pattern response was not modified by preincubating the vessels with the NO synthase inhibitor, L-NAME, or when the vascular reactivity assays were performed in endothelium-denuded vessels, indicating that the effect of anandamide in resistance mesenteric arteries is not dependent on functional endothelium integrity, and suggesting that endothelium-derived NO does not play a major role in this response. The effect of anandamide was selective for the mesenteric vessels since no effects were seen when vascular reactivity experiments were performed in distal femoral arteries of cirrhotic and control rats.

The presence of CB1 receptor messenger and protein in rat resistance mesenteric arteries has recently been demonstrated in our laboratory[28]. Indeed, RT-PCR experiments showed higher transcript expression in cirrhotic than in control vessels. Furthermore, no messenger expression was detected in femoral arteries, irrespective of whether they were obtained from cirrhotic or control rats. The CB1 gene was not only transcribed, but also translated, in the mesenteric arteries. Western blot experiments yielded parallel results to those found in the RT-PCR. In mesenteric arteries the CB1-specific antibody recognized the CB1 protein, while in femoral arteries CB1 protein expression was absent. Moreover, receptor signal intensity was higher in protein extracts obtained from mesenteric vessels of cirrhotic animals than in those of control animals. CB1 cellular distribution within cirrhotic and control mesenteric arteries was also assessed by immunohistochemistry. Specific CB1 staining was detectable in endothelial and adventitial cells. In addition, CB1 receptor immunoreactivity was more intense in the adventitial cells of the cirrhotic vessels than in those of controls. This pattern of staining is consistent with the increased CB1 mRNA and protein expression observed in the cirrhotic arteries, and coincides with those obtained in the vascular reactivity assays, thus suggesting a major involvement of the

CB1 receptor in the increased vascular responsiveness to anandamide detected in the resistance mesenteric arteries of cirrhotic rats.

Overall, these results indicate that anandamide is an important specific splanchnic vasodilator acting predominantly in a non-endothelium-, non-NO-dependent manner, a phenomenon not observed in the peripheral vasculature and mediated by interaction with CB1 receptors. These findings point to the endocannabinoid system as a potentially significant pathogenic mediator of the splanchnic arteriolar vasodilation in advanced liver disease.

## References

1. Arroyo V, Jimenez W. Complications of cirrhosis. II. Renal and circulatory dysfunction. Lights and shadows in an important clinical problem. J Hepatol. 2000;32:157–70.
2. Arroyo V, Ginés P, Jiménez W, Rodes J. Renal dysfunction in cirrhosis. In: Bircher J, Benhamou JP, McIntyre N, Rizzetto M, Rodés J, editors. Oxford Textbook of Clinical Hepatology, 2nd edn. Oxford: Oxford Medical Publications, 1999:733–61.
3. Maroto A, Ginès A, Saló J et al. Diagnosis of functional renal failure of cirrhosis by doppler sonography. Prognostic value of resistive index. Hepatology. 1994;20:839–44.
4. Maroto A, Ginès P, Arroyo V et al. Brachial and femoral artery blood flow in cirrhosis. Relationship with renal dysfunction. Hepatology. 1993;17:788–93.
5. Martin PY, Ginès P, Schrier RW. Nitric oxide as a mediator of hemodynamic abnormalities and sodium and water retention in cirrhosis. N Engl J Med. 1998;339:533–41.
6. Di Marzo V. Endocannabinoids and other fatty acid derivatives with cannabimimetic properties: biochemistry and possible physiopathological relevance. Biochim Biophys Acta. 1998;1392:153–75.
7. Martin BR, Mechoulam R, Razdan RK. Discovery and characterization of endogenous cannabinoids. Life Sci. 1999;65:573–95.
8. Di Marzo V, Bisogno T, De Petrocellis L, Melck D. Martin BR. Cannabimimetic fatty acid derivatives: the anandamide family and other "endocannabinoids". Curr Med Chem. 1999;6:721–44.
9. Randall MD, Kendall DA. Endocannabinoids: a new class of vasoactive substances. TIPS. 1998;19:55–8.
10. Dewey WL. Cannabinoid pharmacology. Pharmacol Rev. 1986;38:151–78.
11. Felder CC, Glass M. Cannabinoid receptors and their endogenous agonists. Annu Rev Pharmacol Toxicol. 1998;38:179–200.
12. Varga K, Lake K, Martin BR, Kunos G. Novel antagonist implicates the CB1 cannabinoid receptor in the hypotensive effect of anandamide. Eur J Pharmacol. 1995;278:279–83.
13. Ledent C, Valverde O, Cossu G et al. Unresponsiveness to cannabinoids and reduced addictive effects of opiates in CB1 receptor knockout mice. Science. 1999;283:401–4.
14. Högestätt ED, Zygmunt PM. Cardiovascular pharmacology of anandamide. Prostagland Essent Fatty Acids. 2002;66:343–51.
15. Begg M, Baydoun A, Person ME, Molleman A. Signal transduction of cannabinoid CB1 receptors in a smooth muscle cell line. J Physiol. 2001;531:95–104.
16. Ralevic V, Kendall DA, Randall MD, Smart D. Cannabinoid modulation of sensory neurotransmission via cannabinoid and vanilloid receptor: roles in regulation of cardiovascular system. Life Sci. 2002;71:2577–94.
17. Calignano A, Kátona I, Désarnaud F et al. Bidirectional control of airway responsiveness by endogenous cannabinoids. Nature. 2000;408:96–101.
18. Garcia N, Járai Z, Faridoddin M, Kunos G, Sanyal AJ. Systemic and portal hemodynamic effects of anandamide. Am J Physiol Gastrointest Liver Physiol. 2001;280:G14–20.
19. Deutsch DJ, Goligorsky MS, Schmid PC et al. Production and physiological actions of anandamide in the vasculature of the rat kidney. J Clin Invest. 1997;100:1538–46.
20. Bataller R, Ros J, Jimenez W, Brenner DA. Anandamide, an endogenous cannabinoid, inhibits contraction, proliferation and migration of human hepatic stellate cells. J Hepatol. 2004;40:94.
21. Wagner JA, Varga K, Ellis EF, Rzigalinski BA, Martin BR, Kunos G. Activation of peripheral CB1 receptors in hemorrhagic shock. Nature. 1997;390:518–21.

22. Varga K, Wagner JA, Bridgen DT, Kunos G. Platelet- and macrophage-derived endogenous cannabinoids are involved in endotoxin-induced hypotension. FASEB J. 1998;12:1035–44.
23. Hillard CJ, Jarrahian A. The movement of $N$-arachidonoyethanolamine (anandamide) across cellular membranes. Chem Phys Lipids. 2000;108:123–34.
24. Bátkai S, Járai Z, Wagner JA et al. Endocannabinoids acting at vascular CB1 receptors mediate the vasodilated state in advanced liver cirrhosis. Nature Med. 2001;7:827–32.
25. Ros J, Clària J, To-Figueras J et al. Endogenous cannabinoids: a new system involved in the homeostasis of arterial pressure in experimental cirrhosis in rats. Gastroenterology. 2002;122:85–93.
26. Domenicali M, Ros J, Crespo M et al. The endogenous cannabinoid, anandamide, produces a specific and high vasodilator effect in mesenteric vessels of cirrhotic rats. J Hepatol. 2003;38(Suppl. 2):28.
27. Fernandez-Rodriguez CM, Romero J, Petros TJ et al. Circulating levels of the endogenous cannabinoid anandamide and portal, systemic, renal hemodynamics and activation of neurohormonal systems in cirrhosis. J Hepatol. 2004;40(Suppl. 1):59.
28. Ros J, Domenicali M, Cejudo-Martin P et al. Cannabinoid CB1 receptors are overexpressed in resistance mesenteric arteries of cirrhotic rats with ascites. J Hepatol. 2004;40(Suppl. 1):63.

# Section IV
# Mini-symposium: Possibilities of manipulating NO biosynthesis in the treatment of portal hypertension

# 12
# NCX-1000: a liver-specific NO donor

STEFANO FIORUCCI, ELISABETTA ANTONELLI
and ANTONIO MORELLI

## INTRODUCTION

Recent advances in the knowledge of the pathophysiology of portal hypertension show that cirrhotic liver exhibits endothelial dysfunction of sinusoidal endothelial cells. This alteration results in a defective or absent vasodilatory response to acetylcholine and in insufficient nitric oxide (NO) production by endothelial NO synthase in the intrahepatic vascular bed. Such deficient NO production increases hepatic vascular tone, and may decrease the intrahepatic vasodilatory adaptive response to sudden increases in blood flow[1-3]. Therefore, drugs that deliver NO to the intrahepatic circulation, such as nitrates, should be able to compensate for reduced NO generation and reduce portal pressure gradient. For this reason vasodilators have been studied in recent years as a possible alternative to β-blockers in the pharmacologic treatment of portal hypertension.

## NO-BASED THERAPY FOR THE TREATMENT OF PORTAL HYPERTENSION

Nitrovasodilators were used to treat portal hypertension long before the discovery of NO, on account of their capacity to lower portal pressure[4-6]. In studies performed in the isolated perfused cirrhotic rat liver, nitroprusside was found to cause a significant reduction of perfusion resistance (20–30% of the increased resistance)[7]. These drugs reduce portal pressure by decreasing the vascular resistance to portal–collateral blood flow. In some cases an additional fall in portal pressure may be promoted because of reflex splanchnic vasoconstriction in response to reduced mean arterial and cardiac filling pressures. Long-acting nitrovasodilators, such as isosorbide dinitrate or ISMN, have been shown to reduce hepatic venous pressure gradient (HVPG) and esophageal variceal pressure[6]. Unfortunately it has recently been demonstrated that ISMN does not have any beneficial effect in preventing first variceal bleeding in patients with cirrhosis that cannot be treated with β-blockers. Indeed, it can even promote a slight increase in the risk of bleeding[8]. Moreover, a direct correlation exists between the decrease in mean arterial pressure and HVPG, suggesting that NO vasodilators lower portal pressure mainly through a baroreflex-mediated splanchnic arterial vasoconstriction that occurs in response to arterial hypotension[6]. Organic nitrates such as nitroglycerin and isosorbide-5-mononitrate are non-liver-specific NO donors and cause vasodilation in both arterial and venous vascular beds and cause systemic hypotension which, in cirrhotic patients, might result in progression of the vasodilatory syndrome, aggravating renal dysfunction and sodium retention. Thus, the ideal drug for the treatment of portal hypertension should act by decreasing intrahepatic vascular resistance, without worsening splanchnic/systemic vasodilation.

## NO-RELEASING URSODEOXYCHOLIC ACID DERIVATIVES (NCX-1000)

### Chemistry and metabolism

As NCX-1000 consists of two active moieties, ursodeoxycholic acid (UDCA) and the NO-releasing moiety, its liver metabolism can be tracked by measuring the appearance of UDCA in supernatants of cell culture and in bile of NCX-1000-treated animals[9]. Preclinical studies have shown that NCX-1000 is rapidly and completely metabolized in rat, dog and human liver S9 fraction with half-lives of 1.31–2.31 min, 1.24–2.47 min and 3.92–4.24 min in rats, dogs and humans, respectively. The data obtained *in vitro* are confirmed *in vivo*, with tauroursodeoxycholic acid (TUDCA) being the main conjugation pathway for both UDCA and NCX-1000, as assessed by the quantitative analysis of bile acids in bile of BDL rats chronically treated with NCX-1000[10]. Preliminary data on the human safety of NCX-1000, derived from studies in healthy volunteers treated with four dose levels (500, 1000, 2000 or 3000 mg) of NCX-1000 oral powder, were available. No acute or subchronic toxicity was observed. No clinically significant trend or dose-dependent relationship was observed in the evolution of sitting systolic and diastolic blood pressure values or heart rate during treatment, indicating that NCX-1000 does not reduce systemic blood pressure.

## NCX-1000: EFFECTS ON PORTAL PRESSURE

Preclinical studies have demonstrated that NCX-1000 is exclusively metabolized in the liver, it delivers NO directly to HSC and selectively releases NO into the liver microcirculation with no detectable effect on systemic circulation[9]. Long-term administration of NCX-1000 to rats with chronic liver injury induced by $CCl_4$ intoxication lowers intrahepatic resistance, resulting in both prevention of ascites development and maintenance of a normal portal flow/pressure relationship during liver perfusion[9]. Moreover, while, similar to UDCA, NCX-1000 exerts antifibrotic effects, only the NO-releasing derivative protects against portal hypertension. In addition,

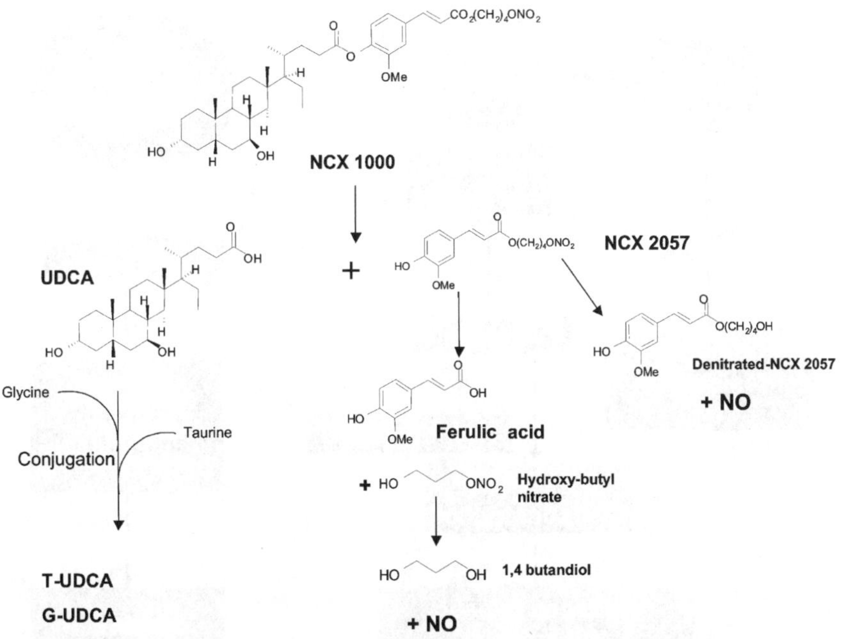

**Figure 1.** Structure and metabolic pathway of NCX-1000, 2-(acetyloxy) benzoic acid 3-(nitroxymethyl) phenyl ester. NCX-1000 is a NO-releasing derivative of ursodeoxycholic acid (UDCA), a stable compound obtained by adding a nitroxybutyl moiety to UDCA. Proposed metabolism

NCX-1000 has no effect on liver eNOS expression and activity, but significantly increases liver content of nitrite/nitrate, demonstrating that liver cells are able to use NCX-1000, *in vivo*, as a source of NO despite a defect in post-translational handling of eNOS. As a further index of its ability to protect against development of portal hypertension, NCX-1000 reduces the nitrite/nitrate content in the ascitic fluid, suggesting a beneficial effect of this compound on the hyperdynamic circulation. To exclude the possibility that the hemodynamic effect observed after this treatment is likely to be related to attenuation of the development of cirrhosis, rather than to a regression of this condition, more recently two additional studies have examined the effect of NCX-1000 on rats with established liver cirrhosis[10,11]. The studies used identical doses of NCX-1000 (28 mg/kg) and equimolar amounts of UDCA as control therapy (although the length of therapy was longer in the CCl$_4$ study). Both studies documented an increase of cGMP levels in liver homogenates from rats receiving NCX-1000 which, together with the findings of increased liver nitrite/nitrate content and increased biliary levels of total bile acids and TUDCA, indicate that NCX-1000 was absorbed, metabolized by the liver and resulted in increased hepatic levels of biologically active NO. Since there were no differences in arterial pressure between animals receiving NCX-1000 or UDCA, both studies conclude that NCX-1000 indeed behaves as a liver-selective NO donor. The two studies further coincided in

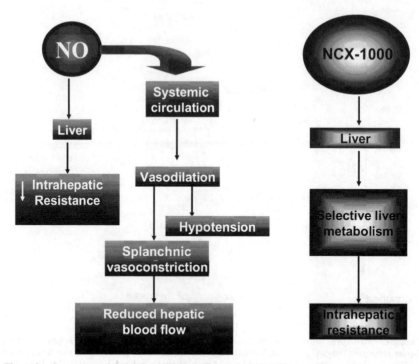

**Figure 2.** Systemic and local vasodilatory effects of NCX-1000 in comparison with conventional nitrates

showing that NCX-1000, but not UDCA, resulted in a significant attenuation of the hyper-response to α-adrenergic stimulation in liver perfusion experiments, supporting the view that NCX-1000 reduces portal hypertension, reversing the dynamic component of portal hypertension. These data are obtained 16 h after the administration of the last dose of NCX-1000, suggesting that hepatic cells can store and/or metabolize NCX-1000 at a low rate, resulting in a long-lasting release of NO. On the other hand, it cannot be excluded that the storage of NO in vessels may play a role in controlling vascular tone. In addition, after NCX-1000 administration, Loureiro-Silva et al.[11] observed an improved adaptability of the cirrhotic intrahepatic circulation to increase in portal blood flow induced by blood volume expansion. This finding suggests that this nitro-compound could be useful to prevent further increases in portal pressure secondary to the increase in portal blood flow and, consequently, could reduce the risk of bleeding in cirrhotic patients. Moreover, both studies used an empirical dose, which may have sub-optimal effects in cirrhotic animals, known to have a decreased sensitivity to nitrovasodilators. It is obvious that additional studies are required, testing a wide range of NCX-1000 doses in cirrhotic rats or, even better, in portal hypertensive cirrhotic patients.

## SYSTEMIC EFFECT OF NCX-1000

Preclinical data show that NCX-1000 does not affect systemic hemodynamics in healthy animals. In all the animal models tested the treatment of cirrhotic rats with NCX-1000 did not change the basal mean arterial pressure (MAP) or basal heart rate measured after the last dose of the NO donor, suggesting that NCX-1000 releases a low amount of NO in the blood stream[9].

## A SECOND-GENERATION NO-UDCA

A second-generation NO-UDCA has been developed (NCX-999). This nitro-UDCA derivative has a better hydrosolubility than NCX-1000, which would confer to the compound a high capability of circulating into the sinusoids and delivering NO into the hepatic microcirculation, instead of being stored into the hepatocytes. Preliminary studies performed in freshly isolated rat hepatocytes and hepatic stellate cells have demonstrated that NCX-999 releases nitrite and nitrate *in vitro* at the same level as NCX-1000, suggesting that this compound, as well as NCX-1000, is metabolized by liver cells to produce NO. Moreover, as well as NCX-1000, NCX-999 can affect HSC function, as demonstrated by its capability in reducing MCP-1 release. Thus, it seemed reasonable that this compound could have modulated intrahepatic circulation. Preliminary data obtained using the isolated perfused rat liver system demonstrated that NCX-999 can significantly reduce the vasoconstriction induced by norepinephrine in normal rat liver, suggesting a potential role of this second-generation NO compound for the treatment of portal hypertension.

## NITRATE VERSUS NCX-1000 FOR THE TREATMENT OF PORTAL HYPERTENSION

The obvious potential pharmacological treatment of portal hypertension in cirrhosis is replenishment of the intrahepatic vasculature with NO by using stable NO-donating compounds. However, it should be underlined that the liver metabolic impairment observed in cirrhosis can be responsible for the blunted vasorelaxant response to nitroglycerin administration in cirrhotic animals[12]. On the other hand our results demonstrated that hepatic biotransformation of NCX-1000 is not significantly altered in injured liver: (1) being capable of increasing the concentration of the tauro-conjugate of UDCA in bile of cirrhotic rats and increasing hepatic nitrite/nitrate content in NCX-1000 treated animals and (2) causing a similar reduction of vasoconstriction induced by the maximally effective concentration of norepinephrine in sham-operated and cirrhotic animals[10]. It is of relevance that, in cirrhosis, the liver metabolic impairment and its inability to release NO after nitrate administration presumably account for the observation that the use of nitrates frequently shows more pronounced systemic side-effects than therapeutic advantage. Conversely, NCX-1000 is devoid of hypotensive systemic effect. Moreover, nitrite therapy is frequently associated with the well-known tolerance phenomenon (tachyphylaxia) that is more pronounced for the venous than for the arterial vascular bed. This effect is not observed after NCX-1000, which is capable of producing the same antihypertensive effect in the liver after short treatment (5 days) and long treatment (7 weeks).

## CONCLUSIONS

Preclinical data suggest that, by selectively delivering therapeutic quantities of NO to the liver microcirculation without apparent effect on systemic and splanchnic circulation, NCX-1000 may provide a novel therapy for the treatment of patients with portal hypertension, without affecting systemic pressure.

## References

1. Rockey D.C, Chung J.J, Reduced nitric oxide production by endothelial cells in cirrhotic rat liver: endothelial dysfunction in portal hypertension. Gastroenterology. 1998;114:344–51.
2. Gupta T, Toruner M, Chung M, Groszmann R. Endothelial dysfunction and decreased production of nitric oxide in the intrahepatic microcirculation of cirrhotic rats. Hepatology. 1998;28:926–31.
3. Shah V, Cao S, Hendrickson H, Yao J, Katusic ZS. Regulation of hepatic eNOS by caveolin and calmodulin after bile duct ligation in rats. Am J Physiol Gastrointest Liver Physiol. 2001;280:G1209–16.
4. Merkel C, Finucci G, Zuin R et al. Effects of isosorbide dinitrate on portal hypertension in alcoholic cirrhosis. J Hepatol. 1987;4:174–80.
5. Mols P, Hallemans R, Melot C, Lejeune P, Naeije R. Systemic and regional hemodynamic effects of isosorbide dinitrate in patients with liver cirrhosis and portal hypertension. J Hepatol. 1989;8:316–24.
6. Escorsell A, Feu F, Bordas JM et al. Effects of isosorbide-5-mononitrate on variceal pressure and systemic and splanchnic haemodynamics in patients with cirrhosis. J Hepatol. 1996;24:423–9.
7. Bhathal P, Grossman H. Reduction of the increased portal vascular resistance of the isolated perfused cirrhotic rat liver by vasodilators. J Hepatol. 1985;1:325–37.
8. Garcia-Pagan JC, Villanueva C, Vila MC et al. MOVE Group. Mononitrato Varices Esofagicas. Isosorbide mononitrate in the prevention of first variceal bleed in patients who cannot receive beta-blockers. Gastroenterology. 2001;121:908–14.
9. Fiorucci S, Antonelli E, Morelli O et al. NCX-1000, a NO-releasing derivative of ursodeoxy-cholic acid, selectively delivers NO to the liver and protects against development of portal hypertension. Proc Natl Acad Sci USA. 2001;98:8897–902.
10. Fiorucci S, Antonelli E, Brancaleone V et al. NCX-1000, a nitric oxide-releasing derivative of ursodeoxycholic acid, ameliorates portal hypertension and lowers norepinephrine-induced intrahepatic resistance in the isolated and perfused rat liver. J Hepatol. 2003; 39:932–9.
11. Loureiro-Silva MR, Cadelina GW, Iwakiri Y, Groszmann RJ. A liver-specific nitric oxide donor improves the intra-hepatic vascular response to both portal blood flow increase and methoxamine in cirrhotic rats. J Hepatol. 2003;39:940–6.
12. Dudenhoefer AA, Loureiro-Silva MR, Cadelina GW, Gupta T, Groszmann RJ. Bioactivation of nitroglycerin and vasomotor response to nitric oxide are impaired in cirrhotic rat livers. Hepatology. 2002;36:381–5.

# 13
# Possibilities of manipulating nitric oxide biosynthesis in the treatment of portal hypertension: statins

JUAN G. ABRALDES, CARMEN ZAFRA and JAIME BOSCH

---

## THE PLEIOTROPIC EFFECTS OF STATINS

Statins are lipid-lowering agents that act by inhibiting the activity of the rate-limiting enzyme for cholesterol synthesis, the 3-hydroxyl-3-methylglutaryl coenzyme A (HMG-CoA) reductase. Statins are among the most widely prescribed drug class in Western countries, and have been consistently shown to decrease the incidence of cardiovascular events and to improve survival in patients with ischemic heart disease[1]. Although the beneficial effects of statins were initially entirely attributed to their lipid-lowering effects, detailed analysis of randomized controlled trials suggested that some of their benefits were independent of their cholesterol-lowering capacity[2,3]. This prompted further investigations that showed a variety of effects of statins beyond cholesterol reduction, which have been called the pleiotropic effects of statins[4]. Statins reduce oxidant stress and inflammation at the vessel wall, have antithrombotic and antiproliferative properties and improve endothelial function, increasing nitric oxide (NO) production in endothelial cells[5-11]. Statins' effects on angiogenesis are more controversial, but it seems that at clinically relevant doses statins are proangiogenic agents[7,12,13]. Many of these effects have been demonstrated to occur as early as within 24 hours of statin administration, further reinforcing their independence from plasma cholesterol changes[14-16].

## STATINS INCREASE NO PRODUCTION IN ENDOTHELIAL CELLS

In the past few years it has been shown that much of the cholesterol-independent vascular protection achieved by statins is the result of an up-regulation of endothelial NO production[7,17-19]. This has recently been emphasized by showing that vascular protection by statins is abolished in

**Table 1.** Mechanisms by which HMG-CoA reductase inhibitors may increase NO production

---

Increase in eNOS activity
    Activation of PI3K/Akt pathway $\Rightarrow$ eNOS phosphorylation
    Decrease in caveolin expression
    Increase in Hsp90–eNOS interaction
    Increase in $BH_4$

Increase in eNOS expression
    Decrease in LDL-cholesterol $\Rightarrow$ increase in eNOS mRNA stability
    Decrease in Rho activity $\Rightarrow$ increase in eNOS mRNA stability

Increase in NO availability
    Decrease in NADPH oxidase $\Rightarrow$ decrease in superoxide

---

endothelial NO synthase (eNOS) knockout mice or after eNOS block-ade[20,21]. Statins may increase NO production by at least three mechanisms (Table 1): by increasing eNOS expression, by increasing eNOS activity at the post-translational level, and by increasing NO bioavailability.

The most immediate effect of statins on endothelial NO production is an increase in eNOS phosphorylation at ser 1177/1179, with subsequent increased activity[7]. This is mediated by the activation of the phosphatidyl inositol 3 kinase (PI3K)/Akt pathway[7,22] that leads to an increase in Akt phosphorylation (present as early as 15 min after exposure to simvastatin) with ensuing eNOS phosphorylation[23] (Figure 1). The mechanism of PI3K/Akt pathway activation seems related to a decrease in the levels of an endogenous endothelial cholesterol pool[24].

Statins can also modify eNOS activity at the post-translational level by other mechanisms. Statins reduce the expression of the eNOS inhibitory protein caveolin-1[25], an effect that seems to depend in part on cholesterol synthesis inhibition[26], and increases the interaction of eNOS with its stimula-tory protein Hsp90[25]. These effects occur more slowly than PI3K/Akt path-way activation. Statins also increase the expression of GTP cyclohydrolase I (GTPCH), the rate-limiting enzyme for *de-novo* tetrahydrobiopterin ($BH_4$) synthesis[27]. This is mediated by the inhibition of the isoprenoid intermediate geranylgeranylpyrophosphate (GGPP), which is required for Rho activation (Figure 1). Rho decreases the expression of GTPCH; the result is that statins increase the production of $BH_4$, a cofactor that increases eNOS activity by preventing eNOS uncoupling and, thus, superoxide generation.

Statins also up-regulate eNOS expression. This occurs at the translational level, by increasing eNOS mRNA stability[17], and is mediated by the inhibi-tion of Rho, since Rho negatively regulates eNOS expression[28]. Additionally, this effect might also be mediated by a decrease in low density lipoprotein (LDL) cholesterol, since LDL also down-regulates eNOS mRNA[29].

Finally, statins may increase NO bioavailability by a reduction of oxida-tive stress through a decrease in the expression of NADPH oxidase. A decrease in the isoprenoid GGPP that leads to a decrease in the activity of Rac1 protein (Figure 1) seems to mediate this effect[30].

The ability of statins to increase NO production and vasomotor response has been confirmed *in vivo* both in experimental animals and in humans[19],

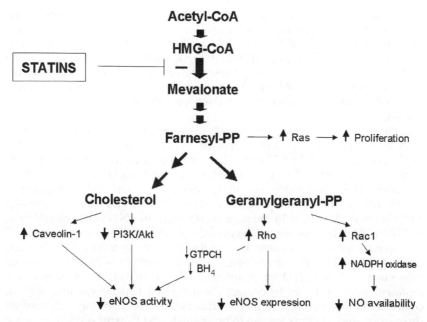

**Figure 1.** Cholesterol synthesis pathway, with biological actions of isoprenoid intermediates and cholesterol. Cholesterol increases caveolin-1 and inhibits the PI3K/Akt signaling pathway. Both effects contribute to a decrease in eNOS activity. Farnesyl-PP activates Ras, a protein implicated in cell proliferation. Geranylgeranyl-PP activates among others Rho and Rac1. Rho down-regulates eNOS and GTP cyclohydrolase I (GTPCH). Rac up-regulates NADPH oxidase. Statins block the rate-limiting step in the synthesis of cholesterol. In this way statins decrease the levels of cholesterol and isoprenoid intermediates, increasing eNOS expression, eNOS activity and NO bioavailability

and it has been shown to occur within 24 h[14,15]. Whether this effect is due to a direct action of statins on endothelial cells, or whether it is the result of a decrease in liver synthesis and circulating levels of the cholesterol precursor mevalonate, has not been yet clarified[19].

## TARGETS FOR STATINS IN PORTAL HYPERTENSION

Increased hepatic resistance is the first pathophysiological phenomenon causing portal hypertension in cirrhosis[31]. This occurs predominantly through mechanical factors, but there is also a vasculogenic component which is clearly reversible[32]. This concept was first demonstrated by Bathal and Grossmann in the isolated perfused cirrhotic rat liver[33]. Insufficient NO production by endothelial cells in liver microvasculature seems to be the major factor involved in increased hepatic resistance in cirrhosis[32,34–37]. In addition, such an insufficient availability of NO may explain the incapacity of the intrahepatic vasculature to relax in response to acute increases in portal blood flow, such as those induced by meals[38]. As a result, in cirrhotic patients marked postprandial increases in portal pressure occur[38–44].

It is implicit that delivering NO to the liver circulation should result in a decrease in hepatic resistance. A straightforward way to achieve this goal is to generate bioavailable NO that diffuses directly to the effector contractile cells by means of NO donors. Although these agents are effective in reducing portal pressure[45,46], their systemic vasodilatory effects could exacerbate the systemic hypotension of cirrhotic patients with adverse effects on renal function[47]. Thus, new strategies to selectively deliver NO to the liver are needed.

Both unaltered[35,36] and decreased[48,49] protein levels of NO eNOS have been found in cirrhosis, but decreased hepatic eNOS activity has been uniformly reported[34-37,50]. This has been attributed to complex post-translational modifications of eNOS; indeed, in the cirrhotic liver eNOS activity has been shown to be down-regulated due to an increased interaction of eNOS with the inhibitory protein caveolin-1[36,50-52], and also to decreased Akt phosphorylation, with subsequent decrease in eNOS phosphorylation at 1779/1799[53]. In addition, an increased scavenging of NO by superoxide[49] has been proposed to account for the decreased response to NO observed in the cirrhotic liver. Pharmacological up-regulation of eNOS activity and/or expression and/or reduction in intracellular superoxide anion levels may represent new strategies to correct the increased hepatic vascular tone in cirrhosis. As discussed previously, statins are able to favorably influence all these steps, since they are known to up-regulate eNOS expression, to increase eNOS activity at a post-translational level, and to decrease superoxide production. Therefore, statins have a good potential to increase intrahepatic NO bioavailability in the cirrhotic liver.

## STATINS IN LIVER CIRRHOSIS

Only one study has so far evaluated the effects of statins on hepatic hemodynamics and NO levels in patients with cirrhosis of the liver[54]. This study investigated the effects of simvastatin administration on resting and meal-stimulated hepatic hemodynamics and NO output in a series of cirrhotic patients, most of them with varices, and with a mean Child–Pugh score of 6.9. A first protocol showed that single-dose oral administration of 40 mg of simvastatin decreased hepatic resistance by 14% at 30 min ($p = 0.03$) and by 11% at 60 min (n.s.). This was followed by a significant increase in total hepatic blood flow, which did not cause an increase in the portal pressure gradient (evaluated by measuring the hepatic venous pressure gradient (HVPG)) because of the decrease in hepatic resistance (Figure 2). Since there were no changes in systemic hemodynamics (cardiac output and mean arterial pressure), the increase in hepatic blood flow was probably due to a redistribution of collateral flow to the liver. This would be consistent with the concept that simvastatin promoted a selective decrease in intrahepatic resistance through enhanced hepatic NO production, while the collateral resistance was not modified. Of note, a redistribution of flow from the collaterals to the liver after decreasing portal resistance has been previously demonstrated experimentally in the partial portal vein ligation model after removal of the ligature[55].

114

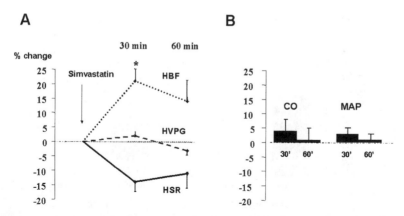

**Figure 2.** Acute hemodynamic changes after a single dose of 40 mg of simvastatin. Simvastatin administration decreased hepatic sinusoidal resistance (HSR), which allowed an increase in hepatic blood flow (HBF), without changes in hepatic venous pressure gradient (HVPG). Mean arterial pressure (MAP) and cardiac output (CO) were not significantly modified

Since direct, NO-independent vasoactive effects of simvastatin have not been described, the hemodynamic changes observed in that study were most likely mediated by the up-regulation of NO production. This is supported by the observed significant increase in plasma NOx products selectively at the hepatic vein[54], which suggests an up-regulation in NO production localized at the hepatosplanchnic territory. Both the hepatic hemodynamic effects and the increase in NO induced by simvastatin were observed as early as 30 min after drug administration, a finding that fits with an effect on post-translational regulation of eNOS.

A second protocol of this study[54] demonstrated that hepatic vein NOx levels increased further after stimulating the splanchnic circulation with a meal in patients pre-treated with simvastatin, but not with placebo. This indicates that simvastatin not only increased basal NO production, but also restored a vasorelaxing response after the volume load caused by postprandial hyperemia (Figure 3). As a consequence the brisk postprandial increase in HVPG observed in patients pretreated with placebo was markedly attenuated in those receiving simvastatin (Figure 4) despite a similar increase in hepatic blood flow in the simvastatin and placebo groups.

These results demonstrate that, in patients with cirrhosis and portal hypertension, simvastatin administration increases hepatosplanchnic output of NOx, decreases hepatic resistance and attenuates the postprandial increase in portal pressure, without deleterious effects on the systemic circulation. This suggests that statins might represent an effective strategy to selectively increase intrahepatic NO in patients with cirrhosis of the liver, without worsening the systemic vasodilation observed in this condition. The apparent selectivity of statins increasing NO levels in the hepatic circulation, but not in the systemic circulation, is intriguing and calls for further investigation in experimental studies. The beneficial effects on hepatic hemodynamics and NO levels observed in patients with cirrhosis[53] should also be confirmed

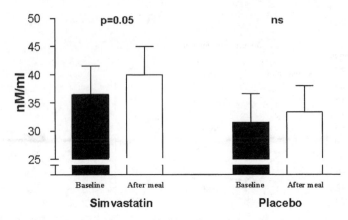

**Figure 3.** Hepatic vein NOx levels increased significantly after the test meal in patients pretreated with simvastatin, but not with placebo (error bars represent SEM)

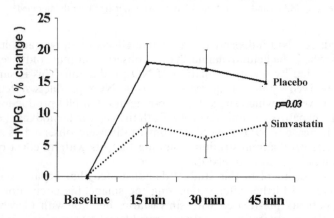

**Figure 4.** Postprandial changes in HVPG in patients treated with simvastatin or placebo. Simvastatin significantly attenuated the increase in portal pressure induced by the meal (error bars represent SEM)

after continuous administration of the drug. It is of note that studies in experimental animals have shown that statins are able to decrease arterial pressure in spontaneously hypertensive rats, which show diffuse endothelial dysfunction, but do not modify arterial pressure in normal animals[56]. Thus, it is possible that, in liver cirrhosis, the selective effect of statins on hepatic NO production might be explained by the fact that simvastatin targeted to the dysfunctioning hepatic endothelium, while it did not further increase the already-enhanced NO production in the systemic circulation.

## FUTURE PERSPECTIVES

These preliminary studies set the rationale to explore further the potential of statins in the treatment of patients with cirrhosis and portal hypertension.

Studies in experimental animals are under way to clarify the mechanism of simvastatin effects in liver cirrhosis. Preliminary results suggest that $CCl_4$-cirrhotic rats also exhibit an improved flow-mediated vasorelaxation after simvastatin pretreatment. In patients the next step would be to examine the hemodynamic effects of simvastatin after continuous administration. Although acute administration of simvastatin resulted in no changes in portal pressure, it is possible that a sustained reduction in hepatic resistance and an increase in liver NO availability could lead to a decrease in portal pressure. In that regard it has recently been shown, in an experimental model of cirrhosis, that a steady increase in Akt signaling (by transfecting the liver with adenovirus encoding a constitutively active form of Akt), leads to a marked decrease in portal pressure[53]. On the other hand, the observed attenuation of the brisk postprandial increases in portal pressure may by itself represent a clinically relevant beneficial effect of statins, since it has been proposed that the portal hypertension flares related to meals play an important role contributing to the development and progressive dilation of gastroesophageal varices that leads to their eventual rupture[38,57].

Statins may also influence other pathophysiological aspects of liver disease. A potential antifibrotic effect has been suggested, since simvastatin has been shown to decrease hepatic stellate cell proliferation[58,59] and collagen synthesis[59], probably by reducing the levels of active Ras (Figure 1)[59]. In relation to its anti-inflammatory properties, trials are under way to evaluate the effects of atorvastatin on liver function in patients with primary biliary cirrhosis.

Lastly, an important concern with statins that must be addressed is the potential liver toxicity of these drugs. Simvastatin increases liver transaminases in up to 2% of patients, but serious liver injury is exceedingly rare, if it ever occurs[1]. Furthermore, a very recent large study concluded that the risk of statins-related hepatotoxicity is not increased in patients with elevated baseline liver enzymes[60]. Simvastatin has also proved safe in patients in early stages of primary biliary cirrhosis[61]. However, if a relevant benefit of these drugs in cirrhotic patients is confirmed, the safety of statins in these particular patients after continued administration should be carefully evaluated.

In summary, statins are drugs that might act on several mechanisms that lead to cirrhosis progression and to the development of complications derived from portal hypertension. Since these drugs are readily available, and appear to have a good safety profile, they deserve priority in the search for new agents for the treatment of patients with cirrhosis.

## Acknowledgements

This work was supported in part by grants from Fundación Ramón Areces and Asociación Española para el Estudio del Hígado (to J.G.A.) and from the Instituto de Salud Carlos III (CO3-02) and Fondo de Investigación Sanitaria (PI 020739).

# References

1. Pasternak RC, Smith SC Jr, Bairey-Merz CN, Grundy SM, Cleeman JI, Lenfant C. ACC/AHA/NHLBI Clinical Advisory on the Use and Safety of Statins. Stroke. 2002;33:2337–41.
2. Influence of pravastatin and plasma lipids on clinical events in the West of Scotland Coronary Prevention Study (WOSCOPS). Circulation. 1998;97:1440–5.
3. Baseline serum cholesterol and treatment effect in the Scandinavian Simvastatin Survival Study (4S). Lancet. 1995;20:1274–5.
4. Takemoto M, Liao JK. Pleiotropic effects of 3-hydroxy-3-methylglutaryl coenzyme a reductase inhibitors. Arterioscler Thromb Vasc Biol. 2001;21:1712–19.
5. Dangas G, Smith DA, Unger AH et al. Pravastatin: an antithrombotic effect independent of the cholesterol-lowering effect. Thromb Haemost. 2000;83:688–92.
6. Lefer DJ. Statins as potent antiinflammatory drugs. Circulation. 2002;106:2041–2.
7. Kureishi Y, Luo Z, Shiojima I et al. The HMG-CoA reductase inhibitor simvastatin activates the protein kinase Akt and promotes angiogenesis in normocholesterolemic animals. Nat Med. 2000;6:1004–10.
8. McGirt MJ, Lynch JR, Parra A et al. Simvastatin increases endothelial nitric oxide synthase and ameliorates cerebral vasospasm resulting from subarachnoid hemorrhage. Stroke. 2002;33:2950–6.
9. Bates K, Ruggeroli CE, Goldman S, Gaballa MA. Simvastatin restores endothelial NO-mediated vasorelaxation in large arteries after myocardial infarction. Am J Physiol Heart Circ Physiol. 2002;283:H768–75.
10. Laufs U, Gertz K, Dirnagl U, Bohm M, Nickenig G, Endres M. Rosuvastatin, a new HMG-CoA reductase inhibitor, upregulates endothelial nitric oxide synthase and protects from ischemic stroke in mice. Brain Res. 2002;942:23–30.
11. Kalinowski L, Dobrucki LW, Brovkovych V, Malinski T. Increased nitric oxide bioavailability in endothelial cells contributes to the pleiotropic effect of cerivastatin. Circulation. 2002;105:933–8.
12. Weis M, Heeschen C, Glassford AJ, Cooke JP. Statins have biphasic effects on angiogenesis. Circulation. 2002;105:739–45.
13. Dimmeler S, Aicher A, Vasa M et al. HMG-CoA reductase inhibitors (statins) increase endothelial progenitor cells via the PI 3-kinase/Akt pathway. J Clin Invest. 2001;108:391–7.
14. Omori H, Nagashima H, Tsurumi Y et al. Direct *in vivo* evidence of a vascular statin: a single dose of cerivastatin rapidly increases vascular endothelial responsiveness in healthy normocholesterolaemic subjects. Br J Clin Pharmacol. 2002;54:395–9.
15. Laufs U, Wassmann S, Hilgers S, Ribaudo N, Bohm M, Nickenig G. Rapid effects on vascular function after initiation and withdrawal of atorvastatin in healthy, normocholesterolemic men. Am J Cardiol. 2001;88:1306–7.
16. Sironi L, Cimino M, Guerrini U et al. Treatment with statins after induction of focal ischemia in rats reduces the extent of brain damage. Arterioscler Thromb Vasc Biol. 2003;23:322–7.
17. Laufs U, La F, V, Plutzky J, Liao JK. Up-regulation of endothelial nitric oxide synthase by HMG CoA reductase inhibitors. Circulation. 1998;97:1129–35.
18. Sessa WC. Can modulation of endothelial nitric oxide synthase explain the vasculoprotective actions of statins? Trends Mol Med. 2001;7:189–91.
19. Laufs U. Beyond lipid-lowering: effects of statins on endothelial nitric oxide. Eur J Clin Pharmacol. 2003;58:719–31.
20. Endres M, Laufs U, Huang Z et al. Stroke protection by 3-hydroxy-3-methylglutaryl (HMG)-CoA reductase inhibitors mediated by endothelial nitric oxide synthase. Proc Natl Acad Sci USA. 1998;95:8880–5.
21. Wolfrum S, Grimm M, Heidbreder M et al. Acute reduction of myocardial infarct size by a hydroxymethyl glutaryl coenzyme A reductase inhibitor is mediated by endothelial nitric oxide synthase. J Cardiovasc Pharmacol. 2003;41:474–80.
22. Mukai Y, Shimokawa H, Matoba T et al. Acute vasodilator effects of HMG-CoA reductase inhibitors: involvement of PI3-kinase/Akt pathway and Kv channels. J Cardiovasc Pharmacol. 2003;42:118–24.
23. Fulton D, Gratton JP, McCabe TJ et al. Regulation of endothelium-derived nitric oxide production by the protein kinase Akt. Nature. 1999;399:597–601.

24. Skaletz-Rorowski A, Lutchman M, Kureishi Y, Lefer DJ, Faust JR, Walsh K. HMG-CoA reductase inhibitors promote cholesterol-dependent Akt/PKB translocation to membrane domains in endothelial cells. Cardiovasc Res. 2003;57:253–64.
25. Feron O, Dessy C, Desager JP, Balligand JL. Hydroxy-methylglutaryl-coenzyme A reductase inhibition promotes endothelial nitric oxide synthase activation through a decrease in caveolin abundance. Circulation. 2001;103:113–18.
26. Pelat M, Dessy C, Massion P, Desager JP, Feron O, Balligand JL. Rosuvastatin decreases caveolin-1 and improves nitric oxide-dependent heart rate and blood pressure variability in apolipoprotein E-/- mice in vivo. Circulation. 2003;20:2480–6.
27. Hattori Y, Nakanishi N, Akimoto K, Yoshida M, Kasai K. HMG-CoA reductase inhibitor increases GTP cyclohydrolase I mRNA and tetrahydrobiopterin in vascular endothelial cells. Arterioscler Thromb Vasc Biol. 2003;23:176–82.
28. Laufs U, Liao JK. Targeting Rho in cardiovascular disease. Circ Res. 2000;87:526–8.
29. Vidal F, Colome C, Martinez-Gonzalez J, Badimon L. Atherogenic concentrations of native low-density lipoproteins down-regulate nitric-oxide-synthase mRNA and protein levels in endothelial cells. Eur J Biochem. 1998;252:378–84.
30. Wassmann S, Laufs U, Muller K et al. Cellular antioxidant effects of atorvastatin in vitro and in vivo. Arterioscler Thromb Vasc Biol. 2002;22:300–5.
31. Bosch J, D'Amico G, Garcia-Pagan JC. Portal hypertension. In: Schiff ER, Sorrell MF, Maddrey WC, editors. Diseases of the Liver, 9th edn. Philadelphia: Lippincott Williams & Wilkins, 2003:429–86.
32. Wiest R, Groszmann RJ. The paradox of nitric oxide in cirrhosis and portal hypertension: too much, not enough. Hepatology. 2002;35:478–91.
33. Bathal PS, Grossmann HJ. Reduction of the increased portal vascular resistance of the isolated perfused cirrhotic rat liver by vasodilators. J Hepatol. 1985;1:325–9.
34. Gupta TK, Toruner M, Chung MK, Groszmann RJ. Endothelial dysfunction and decreased production of nitric oxide in the intrahepatic microcirculation of cirrhotic rats. Hepatology. 1998;28:926–31.
35. Rockey DC, Chung JJ. Reduced nitric oxide production by endothelial cells in cirrhotic rat liver: endothelial dysfunction in portal hypertension. Gastroenterology. 1998;114:344–51.
36. Shah V, Toruner M, Haddad F et al. Impaired endothelial nitric oxide synthase activity associated with enhanced caveolin binding in experimental cirrhosis in the rat. Gastroenterology. 1999;117:1222–8.
37. Sarela AI, Mihaimeed FM, Batten JJ, Davidson BR, Mathie RT. Hepatic and splanchnic nitric oxide activity in patients with cirrhosis. Gut. 1999;44:749–53.
38. Bellis L, Berzigotti A, Abraldes JG et al. Low doses of isosorbide mononitrate attenuate the postprandial increase in portal pressure in patients with cirrhosis. Hepatology. 2003; 37:378–84.
39. Lee SS, Hadengue A, Moreau R, Sayegh R, Hillon P, Lebrec D. Postprandial hemodynamic responses in patients with cirrhosis. Hepatology. 1988;8:647–51.
40. Tsunoda T, Ohnishi K, Tanaka H. Portal hemodynamic responses after oral intake of glucose in patients with cirrhosis. Am J Gastroenterol. 1988;83:398–403.
41. O'Brien S, Keogan M, Patchett S, McCormick PA, Afdhal N, Hegarty JE. Postprandial changes in portal haemodynamics in patients with cirrhosis. Gut. 1992;33:364–7.
42. Albillos A, Rossi I, Iborra J et al. Octreotide prevents postprandial splanchnic hyperemia in patients with portal hypertension. J Hepatol. 1994;21:88–94.
43. Bendtsen F, Simonsen L, Henriksen JH. Effect on hemodynamics of a liquid meal alone and in combination with propranolol in cirrhosis. Gastroenterology. 1992;102:1017–23.
44. Vorobioff JD, Gamen M, Kravetz D et al. Effects of long-term propranolol and octreotide on postprandial hemodynamics in cirrhosis: a randomized, controlled trial. Gastroenterology. 2002;122:916–22.
45. Navasa M, Chesta J, Bosch J, Rodes J. Reduction of portal pressure by isosorbide-5-mononitrate in patients with cirrhosis. Effects on splanchnic and systemic hemodynamics and liver function. Gastroenterology. 1989;96:1110–18.
46. Garcia-Pagan JC, Feu F, Navasa M et al. Long-term haemodynamic effects of isosorbide 5-mononitrate in patients with cirrhosis and portal hypertension. J Hepatol. 1990;11:189–95.
47. Salmeron JM, Ruiz dA, Gines A et al. Renal effects of acute isosorbide-5-mononitrate administration in cirrhosis. Hepatology. 1993;17:800–6.

48. Van de CM, Omasta A, Janssens S et al. *In vivo* gene transfer of endothelial nitric oxide synthase decreases portal pressure in anaesthetised carbon tetrachloride cirrhotic rats. Gut. 2002;51:440–5.
49. Van De CM, Van Pelt JF, Nevens F, Fevery J, Reichen J. Low NO bioavailability in CCl4 cirrhotic rat livers might result from low NO synthesis combined with decreased superoxide dismutase activity allowing superoxide-mediated NO breakdown: a comparison of two portal hypertensive rat models with healthy controls. Comp Hepatol. 2003;2:2.
50. Shah V, Cao S, Hendrickson H, Yao J, Katusic ZS. Regulation of hepatic eNOS by caveolin and calmodulin after bile duct ligation in rats. Am J Physiol Gastrointest Liver Physiol. 2001;280:G1209–16.
51. Chatila R, Theise N, Shah V, West AB, Sessa RJ, Groszmann RJ. Caveolin-1 in normal and cirrhotic human liver. Gastroenterology. 2000;118:A979.
52. Yokomori H, Oda M, Ogi M, Sakai K, Ishii H. Enhanced expression of endothelial nitric oxide synthase and caveolin-1 in human cirrhosis. Liver. 2002;22:150–8.
53. Morales-Ruiz M, Cejudo-Martin P, Fernandez-Varo G et al. Transduction of the liver with activated Akt normalizes portal pressure in cirrhotic rats. Gastroenterology. 2003; 125:522–31.
54. Zafra C, Abraldes JG, Turnes J et al. Simvastatin enhances hepatic nitric oxide production and decreases the hepatic vascular tone in patients with cirrhosis. Gastroenterology. 2004;126:749–55.
55. Sikuler E, Groszmann RJ. Interaction of flow and resistance in maintenance of portal hypertension in a rat model. Am J Physiol. 1986;250:G205–12.
56. Susic D, Varagic J, Ahn J, Slama M, Frohlich ED. Beneficial pleiotropic vascular effects of rosuvastatin in two hypertensive models. J Am Coll Cardiol. 2003;42:1091–7.
57. Polio J, Groszmann RJ. Hemodynamic factors involved in the development and rupture of esophageal varices: a pathophysiologic approach to treatment. Semin Liver Dis. 1986; 6:318–31.
58. Mallat A, Preaux AM, Blazejewski S, Dhumeaux D, Rosenbaum J, Mavier P. Effect of simvastatin, an inhibitor of hydroxy-methylglutaryl coenzyme A reductase, on the growth of human Ito cells. Hepatology. 1994;20:1589–94.
59. Rombouts K, Kisanga E, Hellemans K, Wielant A, Schuppan D, Geerts A. Effect of HMG-CoA reductase inhibitors on proliferation and protein synthesis by rat hepatic stellate cells. J Hepatol. 2003;38:564–72.
60. Chalasani N, Aljadhey H, Kesteron J, Murray MD, Hall SD. Patients with elevated liver enzymes may not be at higher risk for statin hepatotoxicity than those with normal enzymes. Gastroenterology. 2004;126:1287–92.
61. Ritzel U, Leonhardt U, Nather M, Schafer G, Armstrong VW, Ramadori G. Simvastatin in primary biliary cirrhosis: effects on serum lipids and distinct disease markers. J Hepatol. 2002;36:454–8.

# 14
# Pathophysiological role of Akt and endothelial nitric oxide synthase in cirrhosis

MANUEL MORALES-RUIZ

## INTRODUCTION

Due to the fact that nitric oxide (NO) is a component of air pollution, produced in lightning and also a by-product of microbial metabolism, this substance has been the focus of environmental and microbiological research for many years. However the original clues for a biological role of NO came from studies suggesting the implication of this gas as the active component of nitroglycerin[1], which has long been used in the treatment of angina pectoris because of its vasoactive properties. In 1980 Furchgott et al. described a labile and diffusible substance produced by endothelial cells responsible for acetylcholine-dependent blood vessel relaxation[2]. It was not until a few years later when the two discoveries were connected by Palmer et al.[3] and Ignarro et al.[4]. They published the first evidence that the biological activity of NO was indistinguishable from that of endothelium-derived relaxing factor described by Furchgott et al. These first observations awakened great interest among the scientific community, and generated an enormous amount of literature that culminated in 1992 with the nomination of "Molecule of the Year" by *Science* journal[5]. In addition, in 1998 the investigators Robert Furchgott, Ferid Murad, and Louis Ignarro were awarded the Nobel Prize for their research on the effects of NO on blood vessels.

Due to the properties of NO as an important regulator of vascular tone, it was not surprising that in 1991 Vallance and Moncada proposed an association between the altered systemic hemodynamics in cirrhosis and the vasoactive properties of NO[6]. This first publication stimulated an important scientific effort in experimental models of cirrhosis (induced by carbon tetrachloride ($CCl_4$) or bile duct ligation (BDL)) and prehepatic portal hypertension (in mice, rats or rabbits by partial portal vein ligation) and in cirrhotic patients, that contributed to the current knowledge of the role of NO in cirrhosis.

## ROLE OF THE PI3-KINASE/Akt/eNOS SIGNALING PATHWAY IN CIRRHOTIC LIVERS

Increased resistance to portal blood flow is the primary factor in the pathophysiology of portal hypertension, and is the main cause of morbidity and mortality of patients with cirrhosis. This increased intrahepatic vascular resistance is the consequence of anatomic abnormalities caused by fibrosis and the formation of regenerating nodules[7]. It is well established that this is not a purely mechanical phenomenon, and different vasoactive agents such as NO play an important role in the development of the intrahepatic resistance associated with cirrhosis. In this regard there are studies showing that NO production and endothelial nitric oxide synthase (eNOS) protein activity are decreased in perfused cirrhotic livers from $CCl_4$-treated rats and isolated endothelial cells from $CCl_4$-treated rats and BDL rats, respectively[8,9]. In the study performed by Rockey et al.[9], equal levels of mRNA and protein of eNOS were associated with a significant decrease in sinusoidal eNOS activation in cirrhotic animals, suggesting a post-translational control of eNOS activity. In this context it has recently been shown that enhanced expression and interaction of caveolin-1 with eNOS may contribute to impaired NO production and reduced NOS activity in livers from $CCl_4$-treated and BDL rats[10–12]. Similar to these findings, Yokomory and colleagues demonstrated, by immunohistochemistry and Western blot, that liver specimens from cirrhotic patients presented an over-expression of caveolin-1[13]. However, although the authors presented data of eNOS and caveolin-1 colocalization, the *in-vivo* interaction of these two proteins still needs to be demonstrated in human cirrhosis.

The serine/threonine kinase Akt (or protein kinase B) is an important regulator of various cellular processes including metabolism, cell survival and migration[14–18]. This enzyme is activated by phosphoinositide 3-kinase (PI3-kinase) which catalyzes the phosphorylation of the inositol ring of phosphatidylinositol (PtdIns) lipids at the D-3 position producing PtdIns(3,4)P2 and PtdIns(3,4,5)P3. Direct binding of Akt to the membrane phosphoinositide products of the PI3-kinase reaction (through its pleckstrin homology domain) permits its phosphorylation by a phosphoinositide-dependent kinase (PDK1). PDK1 is also activated by phosphoinositol lipids and phosphorylates Akt at Thr-308, resulting in autophosphorylation of Ser-473 (Figure 1), thus increasing Akt catalytic activity toward a variety of diverse substrates[19,20].

Recently it has been shown that Akt can phosphorylate eNOS on serine 1179 (bovine sequence)/1177 (human sequence) resulting in eNOS activation and an increase in NO production of several-fold in comparison to basal levels[21,22]. In addition, there are several articles linking the activation of the PI3-kinase/Akt signaling pathway to the release of NO in endothelial cells and, therefore, the regulation of vascular tone[23,24]. It can be predicted, therefore, that Akt-dependent eNOS phosphorylation may be an important mechanism in the control of vascular function.

So far, only two papers have assessed the role of the Akt/eNOS signaling pathway in portal hypertension[25,26]. The results published by Iwakiri et al. suggest that the activation of eNOS by Akt may be the first step leading to an initial increase in NO production in mesenteric arterial beds, leading to splanchnic vasodilation. By contrast, in the intrahepatic circulation there is an impaired activation of Akt in livers of cirrhotic rats treated with $CCl_4$ and a subsequent decrease in the incorporation of phosphate groups into

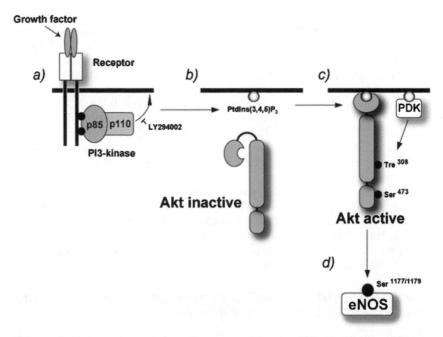

**Figure 1.** Schematic overview of eNOS activation through the PI3-kinase/Akt signaling pathway. (**a**) Activation of growth factor receptor protein tyrosine kinase results in autophosphorylation on tyrosine residues. PI3-kinase is recruited to the membrane by directly binding to phosphotyrosine consensus residues of growth factor receptors or adaptors through one or both SH2 domains in the adaptor subunit (p85). This leads to allosteric activation of the catalytic subunit (p110). (**b**) Activation results in production of the second messenger phosphatidylinositol-3,4,5-triphosphate (PtdIns(3,4,5)P3). (**c**) The lipid product of PI3-kinase recruits a subset of signaling proteins with pleckstrin homology domains to the membrane, including PDKs and Akt. (**d**) Once activated, Akt phosphorylates eNOS on serine 1179 (bovine sequence)/1177 (human sequence) resulting in eNOS activation and increase in NO production

serine 1176 in the rat eNOS sequence[26]. On the basis of these results, Morales-Ruiz et al. used a gene transfer approach to restore the intrahepatic eNOS activity in cirrhosis using a recombinant replication-deficient adenovirus vector carrying a constitutively active mutant of Akt (myr-Akt). The *in vivo* experiments performed in the same study showed that the intravenous administration of myr-Akt adenovirus to cirrhotic rats at a dose of $5 \times 10^{10}$ p.f.u., resulted in transgene expression, increased eNOS phosphorylation and enhanced intrahepatic release of NO, as estimated by the hepatic content of cGMP. Furthermore, restoring eNOS activity by myr-Akt gene delivery normalizes portal pressure, decreases superior mesenteric blood flow and ameliorates arterial hypotension in cirrhotic rats. Related to these findings, detailed histologic examination of the animals used in this study, which underwent a cirrhosis induction protocol for 17–19 weeks, revealed that cirrhotic livers have predominantly thin and often incomplete fibrous septa. Therefore, these results strongly suggest that, in this cirrhotic stage, vascular liver tone is still highly modulated by the vasculogenic component, and probably this therapy would not have been as effective in a late scenario, in which abundant collagen deposition and concomitant mechanical obstruction would have been the most important contributors to the intrahepatic resistance.

Although it had been shown that myr-Akt liver transduction correlates with an increase in phosphorylated eNOS, it is difficult to discount the possibility that other upstream regulators such as AMP-activated kinase, protein kinase A and protein kinase G, which *in vitro* phosphorylate eNOS on serine 1177/1179[27], may affect intrahepatic NO production in cirrhosis. An important question that also remains unanswered is the underlying mechanism that promotes a differential activation of Akt in the setting of portal hypertension.

Due to the fact that splanchnic arterial vasodilation and intrahepatic resistance contribute to the increase in portal pressure, we can conclude that these results, obtained in the experimental model of portal hypertension and in $CCl_4$-treated rats, point to Akt activity as a major modulator of portal blood flow in cirrhosis. Thus, pharmacological modulation of Akt activity remains an area of further investigation in cirrhosis.

## NEW THERAPEUTIC STRATEGIES FOR CIRRHOSIS BASED ON TISSUE SPECIFIC NITRIC OXIDE AVAILABILITY

Without any doubt, experimental models of cirrhosis and portal hypertension have improved our understanding of the pathophysiological role of NO. There is now a strong body of evidence supporting the concept of increased NOS activity in the systemic and splanchnic areas of both cirrhotic patients and rats with experimental cirrhosis and/or portal hypertension[28–30]. These results raise the possibility that the use of specific NOS inhibitors could be explored as treatment for the hyperdynamic state in cirrhosis.

This situation differs substantially from the defective eNOS activation described in cirrhotic livers, where the restoration of intrahepatic eNOS activity may be associated with undesirable side-effects such as the aggravation of systemic vasodilation, as observed with the use of conventional NO donors[28]. Several pharmacological and gene therapy approaches have been followed to specifically deliver NO to this organ. These new therapies include the use of liver-targeted NO donors, such as the NO-releasing derivative of ursodeoxycholic acid NCX-1000[31,32], and the hepatic gene transfer of nNOS[33], eNOS[34] or a constitutively active mutant of Akt[26]. Although all these methods have successfully reduced portal pressure in experimental models of cirrhosis, the relevance of these new therapeutic approaches in cirrhotic patients remains to be determined. Moreover, some conflicting issues should be solved before the promising translation of these treatments to patients. For example, in contrast to the results obtained in the transduction of a wild-type form of eNOS, BDL rats transduced with a mutant form of eNOS, that mimics phosphorylated eNOS, did not display reduced portal pressure[10]. These findings raise the need for a deeper study of the precise molecular mechanisms involved in the impaired intrahepatic eNOS activity found in experimental models of cirrhosis.

Further research should provide a solid basis for therapeutic approaches to specifically supplement NO or activate eNOS in cirrhotic livers and suppress splanchnic and systemic NO overproduction without affecting the immunological response to bacterial infection. We predict that the combination of all these theoretical concepts in the design of new therapeutic approaches for the treatment of cirrhosis will produce results superior to those obtainable with the consideration of only a single pathophysiological role of NO in cirrhosis.

## Acknowledgements

This work was supported by the Ministerio de Ciencia y Tecnología (SAF 2001-2585). M.M.-R. is an established investigator of the Programa Ramón y Cajal (Ministerio de Ciencia y Tecnología).

## References

1. Arnold WP, Mittal CK, Katsuki S, Murad F. Nitric oxide activates guanylate cyclase and increases guanosine $3':5'$-cyclic monophosphate levels in various tissue preparations. Proc Natl Acad Sci USA. 1977;74:3203–7.
2. Furchgott RF, Zawadzki JV. The obligatory role of endothelial cells in the relaxation of arterial smooth muscle by acetylcholine. Nature. 1980;288:373–6.
3. Palmer RM, Ferrige AG, Moncada S. Nitric oxide release accounts for the biological activity of endothelium-derived relaxing factor. Nature. 1987;327:524–6.
4. Ignarro LJ, Buga GM, Wood KS, Byrns RE, Chaudhuri G. Endothelium-derived relaxing factor produced and released from artery and vein is nitric oxide. Proc Natl Acad Sci USA. 1987;84:9265–9.
5. Culotta E, Koshland DE Jr. NO news is good news. Science. 1992;258:1862–5.
6. Vallance P, Moncada S. Hyperdynamic circulation in cirrhosis: a role for nitric oxide? Lancet. 1991;337:776–8.
7. Bosch J, Garcia-Pagan JC. Complications of cirrhosis. I. Portal hypertension. J Hepatol. 2000;32(Suppl. 1):141–56.
8. Gupta TK, Toruner M, Chung MK, Groszmann RJ. Endothelial dysfunction and decreased production of nitric oxide in the intrahepatic microcirculation of cirrhotic rats. Hepatology. 1998;28:926–31.
9. Rockey DC, Chung JJ. Reduced nitric oxide production by endothelial cells in cirrhotic rat liver: endothelial dysfunction in portal hypertension. Gastroenterology. 1998;114:344–51.
10. Hendrickson H, Chatterjee S, Cao S, Morales-Ruiz M, Sessa WC, Shah V. Influence of caveolin on constitutively activated recombinant eNOS: insights into eNOS dysfunction in BDL rat liver. Am J Physiol Gastrointest Liver Physiol. 2003;285:G652–60.
11. Shah V, Toruner M, Haddad F et al. Impaired endothelial nitric oxide synthase activity associated with enhanced caveolin binding in experimental cirrhosis in the rat. Gastroenterology. 1999;117:1222–8.
12. Shah V, Cao S, Hendrickson H, Yao J, Katusic ZS. Regulation of hepatic eNOS by caveolin and calmodulin after bile duct ligation in rats. Am J Physiol Gastrointest Liver Physiol. 2001;280:G1209–16.
13. Yokomori H, Oda M, Ogi M, Sakai K, Ishii H. Enhanced expression of endothelial nitric oxide synthase and caveolin-1 in human cirrhosis. Liver. 2002;22:150–8.
14. Franke TF, Hornik CP, Segev L, Shostak GA, Sugimoto C. PI3K/Akt and apoptosis: size matters. Oncogene. 2003;22:8983–98.
15. Lee MJ, Thangada S, Paik JH et al. Akt-mediated phosphorylation of the G protein-coupled receptor EDG-1 is required for endothelial cell chemotaxis. Mol Cell. 2001;8:693–704.
16. Gratton JP, Morales-Ruiz M, Kureishi Y, Fulton D, Walsh K, Sessa WC. Akt down-regulation of p38 signaling provides a novel mechanism of vascular endothelial growth factor-mediated cytoprotection in endothelial cells. J Biol Chem. 2001;276:30359–65.

17. Morales-Ruiz M, Lee MJ, Zollner S et al. Sphingosine 1-phosphate activates Akt, nitric oxide production, and chemotaxis through a Gi protein/phosphoinositide 3-kinase pathway in endothelial cells. J Biol Chem. 2001;276:19672–7.
18. Morales-Ruiz M, Fulton D, Sowa G et al. Vascular endothelial growth factor-stimulated actin reorganization and migration of endothelial cells is regulated via the serine/threonine kinase Akt. Circ Res. 2000;86:892–6.
19. Toker A, Newton AC. Akt/protein kinase B is regulated by autophosphorylation at the hypothetical PDK-2 site. J Biol Chem. 2000;275:8271–4.
20. Downward J. Mechanisms and consequences of activation of protein kinase B/Akt. Curr Opin Cell Biol. 1998;10:262–7.
21. Dimmeler S, Fleming I, Fisslthaler B, Hermann C, Busse R, Zeiher AM. Activation of nitric oxide synthase in endothelial cells by Akt-dependent phosphorylation. Nature. 1999; 399:601–5.
22. Fulton D, Gratton JP, McCabe TJ et al. Regulation of endothelium-derived nitric oxide production by the protein kinase Akt. Nature. 1999;399:597–601.
23. Luo Z, Fujio Y, Kureishi Y et al. Acute modulation of endothelial Akt/PKB activity alters nitric oxide-dependent vasomotor activity *in vivo*. J Clin Invest. 2000;106:493–9.
24. Scotland RS, Morales-Ruiz M, Chen Y et al. Functional reconstitution of endothelial nitric oxide synthase reveals the importance of serine 1179 in endothelium-dependent vasomotion. Circ Res. 2002;90:904–10.
25. Iwakiri Y, Tsai MH, McCabe TJ et al. Phosphorylation of eNOS initiates excessive NO production in early phases of portal hypertension. Am J Physiol Heart Circ Physiol. 2002;282:H2084–90.
26. Morales-Ruiz M, Cejudo-Martin P, Fernandez-Varo G et al. Transduction of the liver with activated Akt normalizes portal pressure in cirrhotic rats. Gastroenterology. 2003; 125:522–31.
27. Fulton D, Gratton JP, Sessa WC. Post-translational control of endothelial nitric oxide synthase: why isn't calcium/calmodulin enough? J Pharmacol Exp Ther. 2001;299:818–24.
28. Groszmann RJ. Beta-adrenergic blockers and nitrovasodilators for the treatment of portal hypertension: the good, the bad, the ugly. Gastroenterology. 1997;113:1794–7.
29. Martin PY, Gines P, Schrier RW. Nitric oxide as a mediator of hemodynamic abnormalities and sodium and water retention in cirrhosis. N Engl J Med. 1998;339:533–41.
30. Shah V. Cellular and molecular basis of portal hypertension. Clin Liver Dis. 2001;5:629–44.
31. Fiorucci S, Antonelli E, Morelli O et al. NCX-1000, a NO-releasing derivative of ursodeoxycholic acid, selectively delivers NO to the liver and protects against development of portal hypertension. Proc Natl Acad Sci USA. 2001;98:8897–902.
32. Loureiro-Silva MR, Cadelina GW, Iwakiri Y, Groszmann RJ. A liver-specific nitric oxide donor improves the intra-hepatic vascular response to both portal blood flow increase and methoxamine in cirrhotic rats. J Hepatol. 2003;39:940–6.
33. Yu Q, Shao R, Qian HS, George SE, Rockey DC. Gene transfer of the neuronal NO synthase isoform to cirrhotic rat liver ameliorates portal hypertension. J Clin Invest. 2000;105:741–8.
34. Van de CM, Omasta A, Janssens S et al. *In vivo* gene transfer of endothelial nitric oxide synthase decreases portal pressure in anaesthetised carbon tetrachloride cirrhotic rats. Gut. 2002;51:440–5.

# 15
# Nitric oxide synthase gene transfer

**JUNE SUNG LEE and VIJAY SHAH**

## INTRODUCTION

Chronic liver diseases are often characterized by portal hypertension, an important component of which is increased intrahepatic vascular resistance. Portal hypertension in turn has profound clinical consequences, many of which are associated with substantial morbidity and mortality[1]. Nitric oxide (NO) modulates numerous physiological processes in the liver circulation[2]. The basal production of NO in the hepatic circulation is generated through the catalytic activity of the endothelial NO synthase (eNOS) isoform, localized within liver endothelial cells (LEC) and regulated through physiological stimuli including shear stress[3,4]. Several recent studies suggest that the biological activity of hepatic eNOS is diminished in portal hypertension[3,5,6]. Thus, NO supplementation is a rational therapeutic approach in portal hypertension. While NO donor therapy in portal hypertension may be beneficial under specific clinical circumstances, its benefits are limited by several factors including short half-life, high reactivity, tolerance and, most importantly, the unwanted systemic delivery of these compounds that tends to exacerbate an existing hyperdynamic circulatory state and create untoward side-effects and limit effectiveness of clinical application[7,8].

Gene therapy refers to the transfer of functional genes to the host tissue to correct the malfunction of a specific gene or to replace a missing gene[9]. Owing to the liver homing predilection of systemically delivered adenoviral vectors, recent studies have examined the potential efficacy of gene transfer of eNOS and neuronal NOS (nNOS) isoforms in preclinical experimental models of portal hypertension, and are reviewed here[10-13] (Table 1).

## eNOS GENE TRANSFER AND PORTAL HYPERTENSION

One recent study examined whether delivery of an adenoviral vector encoding eNOS gene to liver influenced vasomotor regulation *in vivo* and possible mechanisms of NO production *in vitro*[13]. In these studies, rats were administered adenoviruses encoding β-galactosidase (AdLacZ) or eNOS (AdeNOS) via tail vein injection. One week later, β-galactosidase activity was increased

**Table 1.** NOS activation in liver by gene transfer

| Reference | NOS isoform | Ameliorates portal hypertension |
|---|---|---|
| Van de Casteele et al.[10] | eNOS | Yes |
| Yu et al.[11] | nNOS | Yes |
| Hendrickson et al.[12] | Constitutive active eNOS | No |
| Shah et al.[13] | eNOS | n.a. |
| Morales-Ruiz et al.[18] | AKT (upstream kinase) | Yes |

in the liver of animals transduced with AdLacZ, most prominently in hepatocytes. In AdeNOS-transduced animals the eNOS protein levels and catalytic activity were significantly increased. eNOS gene delivery diminished baseline perfusion pressure and constriction in response to the $\alpha_1$-agonist methoxamine in the perfused liver. In complementary *in-vitro* studies, transduction of cultured hepatocytes with AdeNOS resulted in the binding of recombinant eNOS with the NOS-activating protein heat-shock protein 90 and targeting of NOS to a perinuclear distribution, reminiscent of Golgi membranes. These processing events were associated with increased stimulated NO release from the cells. Therefore, this proof-of-concept study demonstrated that recombinant eNOS gene could be delivered to liver *in vivo* and *in vitro* with ensuing NO production[13].

Further publications have examined for a potential beneficial effect of NOS gene delivery in portal hypertension models[10-12]. In one of these studies Casteele and colleagues showed that *in-vivo* eNOS gene transfer decreased portal pressure in $CCl_4$ cirrhotic rats[10]. They injected the recombinant adenovirus, carrying cDNA encoding human eNOS into the portal vein of $CCl_4$ cirrhotic rats. The result of Casteele and colleagues' study showed that, in liver parenchyma, eNOS immunoreactivity was observed in sinusoidal and hepatic vein endothelium but hepatocytes were negative. In specimens of $CCl_4$ cirrhotic rats treated with placebo or transfected with Ad$\beta$Gal, or with empty vectors, the intensity of the eNOS immunoreactivity was markedly reduced compared with normal livers. Cirrhotic rats transfected with AdeNOS showed enhanced eNOS immunoreactivity in the sinusoidal lining cells compared with placebo-treated animals. The amount of immunoreactive hepatic eNOS protein, measured by Western blotting, was lower in $CCl_4$ cirrhotic rats than in normal control rats. Following eNOS gene transfer, deficient eNOS protein levels in cirrhotic rats were partially restored and portal pressure was significantly improved by about 35%. This study indicates that eNOS gene transfer to cirrhotic rat liver may lead to a marked decrease in portal hypertension without systemic effects[12].

Another recent study, in the bile duct ligation (BDL) model of portal hypertension, examined the effect of a constitutively active form of eNOS (Sl179DeNOS)[14] in both liver cells *in vitro* and in the sham and BDL rat liver *in vivo*, using an adenoviral vector encoding green fluorescent protein (AdGFP) and S1179DeNOS (AdS1179DeNOS)[12]. Transduction of S1179DeNOS increased both basal and agonist-stimulated NO generation in non-parenchymal liver cells and in hepatocytes. Sham rats transduced *in vivo* with AdS1179DeNOS evidenced a decreased pressor response to incremental doses of the vasoconstrictor methoxamine compared with sham rats transduced with AdGFP consistent with prior studies demonstrating an increase in hepatic vasodilatory responses in response to eNOS gene transfer. However, BDL rats transduced with AdS1179DeNOS did not display improved vasodilatory responses. This was evidenced by similar flow-dependent pressure increases to that observed in BDL rats transduced with AdGFP, and was not due to inadequate levels of viral transduction in the injured liver as evidenced by similar levels of viral transgene expression. Thus, S1179DeNOS gene delivery did not appear to improve portal hypertension in the BDL model. Additional studies were performed *in vitro* to better examine the influence of the eNOS inhibitory protein caveolin on S1179DeNOS dysfunction in cirrhotic liver. Caveolin-1 in BDL liver was prominently detected, not only in liver endothelial cells but also in hepatic stellate cells, as assayed by immunogold electron microscopic analysis. *In vitro* studies in the LX2 hepatic stellate cell line demonstrated that caveolin and S1179DeNOS coprecipitated[15]. Furthermore, adenoviral-based overexpression of caveolin-1 in these cells, used to mimic caveolin overexpression in cirrhosis, was associated with enhanced S1179DeNOS-caveolin-1 binding and diminished recombinant S1179DeNOS activity. In sum these studies indicate that recombinant S1179DeNOS protein functions in normal liver cells and tissue, but evidences dysfunction in the cirrhotic rat liver, similar to the endogenous hepatic eNOS protein, and that caveolin expression and inhibition in BDL non-parenchymal cells, including hepatic stellate cells, may be the cause of this dysfunction[12]. These events preclude efficacy of eNOS gene transfer in this pre-clinical model.

## nNOS GENE TRANSFER AND PORTAL HYPERTENSION

In endothelial cells eNOS must undergo extensive post-translational processing, including myristolation and dissociation from caveolin, to be functionally active[16]. Because of the potential of a post-translational handling defect in eNOS after liver injury[5,17], Yu and colleagues transduced a heterologous NOS isoform, nNOS, to cirrhotic liver[11]. After demonstrating that hepatic stellate cells are efficiently transduced with adenoviral vectors *in vitro* and *in vivo*, they next determined the effectiveness of *in-vivo* gene transfer of AdnNOS after liver injury (BDL and $CCl_4$). Although transduction efficiency was reduced after liver injury, nitrite production did increase in all cell types after liver injury and nNOS gene transfer inhibited endothelin-1-induced contractility of perisinusoidal stellate cells. *In vivo*, transduction of portal hypertensive liver with recombinant AdnNOS significantly reduced intrahepatic resistance and portal pressure. In sum, these studies made several meaningful advances by: (a) establishing a "vasorelaxing" effect with a non-endothelial NOS isoform in the liver (which has important therapeutic implications for endothelial disorders in which eNOS may be dysfunctional); (b) suggesting that liver injury and caveolin overexpression do not impair, in endothelial or other cell types, the function of nNOS in liver; and (c) providing a proof-in-concept of the portal hypertension-improving effect of NOS gene transfer[11].

## FUTURE DIRECTIONS AND LIMITATIONS OF GENE TRANSFER FOR PORTAL HYPERTENSION

It is important to note that the adenoviral vectors utilized in the above-reviewed studies are unlikely to be appropriate for translation to human portal hypertension. In addition to the well-documented safety concerns of adenoviral vectors in humans, a chronic condition such as cirrhosis and portal hypertension requires a transduction system that allows for longer expression or repeated dosing, neither of which is presently compatible with adenoviral vector use in humans. Significant advances in vector biology, including establishment of alternative expression systems such as lentivirus and adeno-associated virus, as well as improvements in vector safety profile, will be necessary prior to consideration of translation of these gene-delivery approaches to human portal hypertension. However, the types of preclinical studies reviewed in this chapter are important because they provide proof-in-concept for which targets may be useful in treating portal hypertension and provide mechanism data relating to why portal hypertension occurs. In this regard, future studies for consideration include gene delivery of eNOS activation targets upstream of the enzyme such as AKT as recently published[18], approaches to correct caveolin-mediated eNOS dysfunction such as caveolin siRNA, alternative NOS isoforms such as inducible NOS, or targets downstream of eNOS, such as PKG or soluble guanylate cyclase. Cell-based gene delivery therapies are also under active consideration.

### References

1. Bosch J, Abraldes J, Groszmann R. Current management of portal hypertension. J Hepatol. 2003;38(Suppl. 1):S54–68.
2. Clemens M. Nitric oxide in liver injury. Hepatology. 1999;30:1–5.
3. Rockey, DC, Chung JJ. Reduced nitric oxide production by endothelial cells in cirrhotic rat liver: endothelial dysfunction in portal hypertension. Gastroenterology. 1998;114:344–51.
4. Shah V, Cadelina G, Seesa WC, Groszmann RJ. Comparison of eNOS protein levels in SEC from normal and cirrhotic rats. Hepatology. 1997;26:359A.
5. Shah V, Toruner M, Haddad F et al. Impaired endothelial nitric oxide synthase activity associated with enhanced caveolin binding in experimental liver cirrhosis. Gastroenterology. 1999;117:1222–8.
6. Gupta T, Toruner M, Chung M, Groszmann R. Endothelial dysfunction and decreased production of nitric oxide in the intrahepatic microcirculation of cirrhotic rats. Hepatology. 1998;28:926–31.
7. Shah V. Cellular and molecular basis of portal hypertension. Clin Liver Dis Portal Hypertens. 2001;5:629–44.
8. Rockey D, Shah V. Nitric oxide and the liver. Hepatology. 2004;39:250–7.
9. Anderson W. Human gene therapy. Nature. 1998;392:25–30.
10. Van de Casteele M, Omasta A, Janssens S et al. In vivo gene transfer of endothelial nitric oxide synthase decreases portal pressure in anaesthetised carbon tetrachloride cirrhotic rats. Gut. 2002;51:440–5.
11. Yu Q, Shao R, Zian H, George S, Rockey D. Gene transfer of the neuronal NO synthase isoform to cirrhotic rat liver ameliorates portal hypertension. J Clin Invest. 2000;105:741–8.
12. Hendrickson H, Chatterjee S, Cao S et al. Influence of caveolin on a constitutively activated form of recombinant eNOS: insights into eNOS dysfunction in the bile duct ligated rat liver. Am J Gastroenterol. 2003;285:G652–60.
13. Shah V, Chen A, Cao S et al. Gene transfer of recombinant endothelial nitric oxide synthase to liver in vivo and in vitro. Am J Physiol. 2000;279:G1023–30.

14. McCabe T, Fulton D, Roman L, Sessa W. Enhanced electron flux and reduced calmodulin dissociation may explain "calcium-independent" eNOS activation by phosphorylation. J Biol Chem. 2000;275:6123–8.
15. Taimr P, Higuchi H, Kocova E, Rippe R, Friedman S, Gores G. Activated stellate cells express the TRAIL receptor-2/death receptor-5 and undergo TRAIL-mediated apoptosis. Hepatology. 2003;37:87–95.
16. Fulton D, Gratton J-P, Sessa W. Post-translational control of endothelial nitric oxide synthase: why isn't calcium/calmodulin enough? J Pharmacol Exp Ther. 2001;299:818–24.
17. Shah V, Hendrickson H, Cao S, Yao J, Katusic Z. Regulation of hepatic endothelial nitric oxide synthase by caveolin and calmodulin after bile duct ligation in rats. Am J Physiol. 2001;280:G1209–16.
18. Morales-Ruiz M, Cejudo-Martin P, Fernandez-Varo G et al. Transduction of the liver with activated Akt normalizes portal pressure in cirrhotic rats. Gastroenterology. 2003; 125:522–31.

# 16
# Inhibition of nitric-oxide-mediated vasodilation (including K$^+$ channels)

RICHARD MOREAU

## INTRODUCTION

Portal hypertension is associated with a chronic hyperkinetic syndrome[1–3]. This syndrome is characterized by elevated cardiac output, low arterial pressure and low systemic vascular resistance[2,3]. Splanchnic circulation is also hyperdynamic; i.e. blood flow is elevated and vascular resistance is low in arteries that supply splanchnic organs[1,4]. Systemic and splanchnic alterations are interrelated: decreased systemic vascular resistance (systemic vasodilation) is largely due to the decrease in splanchnic arterial resistance (splanchnic vasodilation)[5]. Finally, in portal hypertension, there is *in-vivo* and *ex-vivo* arterial hyporeactivity to different receptor-dependent and -independent vasoconstrictors[6–14]. A hyperkinetic syndrome also occurs in extrahepatic portal hypertension[15], but it is less marked than that observed in cirrhosis.

An arterial overproduction of the vasorelaxant nitric oxide (NO) plays a major role in the pathogenesis of systemic and splanchnic arterial alterations in patients and animals with portal hypertension[16–44].

NO synthases (NOS) are enzymes that produce NO from L-arginine[45]. NOS have been well studied in conditions other than portal hypertension. There are three isoforms of NOS that are regulated by distinct genes. Neuronal NOS (nNOS), also known as NOS-1, is found in neuronal and some non-neuronal tissues. Inducible NOS (iNOS or NOS-2) was first found in macrophages but has been identified in other cell types (e.g. smooth muscle cells (SMC)). Endothelial NOS (eNOS or NOS-3) was first identified as the enzyme producing endothelium-derived relaxing factor. Both nNOS and eNOS are constitutively expressed. iNOS is not a constitutive enzyme and its expression may be induced by stimuli such as lipopolysaccharide (LPS, endotoxin) or proinflammatory cytokines (i.e. tumor necrosis factor alpha (TNF-α), interleukin-1, and interferon-γ).

133

In cirrhotic rats the protein levels of the three NOS isoforms are increased in the aorta[40,46] while only eNOS is up-regulated in the mesenteric vascular bed[35]. In portal vein-stenosed rats, eNOS is the only up-regulated NOS, in the aorta and mesenteric vascular bed[38,39].

NO inhibition can be achieved by molecules that intercept NO signaling in SMC, or by interventions that have NOS *per se* as a target. NO inhibition can also be obtained by acting on mechanisms that induce post-translational eNOS activation. Finally, NO inhibition can be achieved by drugs such as propranolol, norfloxacin or "anti-TNF" therapies whose mechanism of action has not yet been completely elucidated.

The ideal "NO inhibitor" should decrease NO production and/or action in systemic and splanchnic arteries without affecting intrahepatic NO production. Indeed, inhibition of intrahepatic NO leads to an inappropriate increase in intrahepatic vascular resistance (a portal hypertensive effect).

## MOLECULES THAT INTERCEPT NO SIGNALING

### Inhibition of abluminal diffusion of NO

The administration of erythropoietin to portal hypertensive rats causes increased intravascular hemoglobin concentration which is associated with a reduction in NO-induced arterial tone[47]. Hemoglobin is a potent NO scavenger which decreases abluminal NO diffusion (i.e. movement of NO from endothelial cells to SMC). Thus, in portal hypertensive rats, the effects of the erythropoietin-induced increase in hemoglobin concentration is probably due to decreased NO diffusion from the endothelium to SMC.

### Inhibition of NO-induced $K^+$ channel activation in SMC

In normal SMC, NO stimulates soluble guanylyl cyclase to produce the second messenger cyclic 3′,5′-guanosine monophosphate (cGMP)[48]. cGMP then activates a cGMP-dependent serine–threonine protein kinase called PKG. PKG may phosphorylate and activate plasmalemmal high-conductance, calcium ($Ca^{2+}$)-sensitive $K^+$ (BKCa) channels. This causes membrane hyperpolarization which inhibits L-type $Ca^{2+}$ channels and decreases $Ca^{2+}$ entry. The subsequent decrease in cytosolic free $Ca^{2+}$ concentrations ($[Ca^{2+}]_i$) induces SMC relaxation[49]. There is evidence of an enhanced NO/guanylyl cyclase/cGMP/BKCa channel pathway in portal hypertension, at least under *ex-vivo* conditions. In portal vein-stenosed rats, *ex-vivo* experiments have shown that guanylyl cyclase inhibition with methylene blue decreases arterial hyporeactivity to vasoconstrictors[32]. In portal hypertensive rats, with or without cirrhosis, *ex-vivo* experiments have shown that iberiotoxin (a selective BKCa channel blocker)[50] or tetraethylammonium (a nonselective BKCa channel blocker)[32] decreases arterial hyporeactivity to vasoconstrictors. The pathophysiological role of BKCa channels under *in-vivo* conditions needs to be clarified.

It should be emphasized that, in normal arteries, the NO/cGMP/PKG pathway may relax SMC through several other mechanisms leading to decreased $[Ca^{2+}]_i$ (reviewed in refs 49 and 51). First, PKG may decrease

$Ca^{2+}$ entry by directly inhibiting L-type $Ca^{2+}$ channels. Second, PKG may favor $Ca^{2+}$ extrusion outside the cytosol, by stimulating $Ca^{2+}$-ATPases located in the plasma membrane and in the membrane of the sarcoplasmic reticulum. Third, PKG has been shown to inhibit the G protein-coupled receptors (GPCR)/Gq/11/phospholipase C (PLC)-β signaling pathway used by vasoconstrictors to induce SMC contraction. Indeed, PKG may phosphorylate GPCR and thereby uncouple the receptor and G-proteins. PKG may also bind to and phosphorylate regulator of G protein signaling-2 (RGS-2) which increases GTPase activity of Gq/11, terminating vasoconstrictor signaling[52]. PKG may inhibit PLC-b to produce inositol triphosphate (IP3) and diacylglycerol, two important messengers of constrictor signals. Finally, PKG may decrease intracellular $Ca^{2+}$ release by inhibiting the IP3 receptor. On the other hand, PKG may also use "$Ca^{2+}$-independent" mechanisms of relaxation. Indeed, PKG is known to phosphorylate and activate myosin phosphatase, an effect known to cause desensitization of the contractile apparatus to $Ca^{2+}$ (ref. 53). These "$Ca^{2+}$-dependent" and "$Ca^{2+}$-independent" mechanisms of PKG-induced SMC relaxation have not all been investigated in portal hypertensive SMC. A better understanding of the NO/cGMP/PKG pathway may provide clues to novel approaches in the pharmacological manipulation of NO-elicited SMC relaxation.

## INVESTIGATIONS THAT TARGET NOS *PER SE*

In this setting NO inhibition can be achieved by deletion of NOS genes or pharmacological NOS inhibition.

### Genetic studies

A key role for eNOS in the development of hyperdynamic circulation is suggested by the finding that the hyperkinetic syndrome does not occur in portal vein-stenosed mice lacking eNOS (eNOS$^{-/-}$) but not in portal vein-stenosed mice lacking iNOS[54]. However, this hypothesis is not supported by the results of another study showing that hyperkinetic syndrome induced by portal vein stenosis occurred in eNOS$^{-/-}$ mice lacking eNOS or in those lacking both eNOS and iNOS (double-knockout mice)[55].

The reasons for these discrepant results regarding the impact of *eNOS* deletion on the development of hyperdynamic state are unclear. On the other hand, neither of these studies supports a role of iNOS in circulatory alterations associated with portal hypertension.

### Pharmacological inhibition of NOS

Two families of NOS inhibitors have been used in portal hypertensive animals: L-arginine analogs and non-amino acid-based compounds. Among L-arginine analogs, there are Nω-nitro-L-arginine (also known as L-NA), Nω-nitro-L-arginine methyl ester (also known as L-NAME), and Nω-monomethyl-L-arginine (also known as L-NMMA). Studies using L-arginine analogs (which are non-selective NOS inhibitors[56]) show that NO is a main player in the portal hypertension-associated hyperdynamic state and hyporeactivity to vasoconstrictors. However, studies show that, in cirrhotic rats, L-arginine analogs fail to decrease portal hypertension because these compounds inhibit intrahepatic eNOS and thus increase intrahepatic vascular resistance[16].

*In-vivo* studies aimed at inhibiting iNOS have been performed in portal hypertensive rats. Two studies using high doses of the non-amino acid-based compound aminoguanidine (AG) found that AG induced a significant increase in mean arterial pressure[57,58]. Since high doses of AG inhibit not only iNOS but also eNOS[56], the cause of AG-induced vasopressor response is unclear. On the other hand, the administration of L-N6-(1-iminoethyl)lysine (also known as L-NIL), a relatively selective iNOS inhibitor[59], induced no significant changes in arterial pressure[60]. Moreover, long-term administration of dexamethasone, a glucorticoid which inhibits iNOS induction, failed to prevent the development of hyperdynamic state in portal hypertensive rats[61,62]. Along with genetic studies, these findings do not support a major role of iNOS-derived NO in circulatory alterations associated with portal hypertension. However, the effects of W1400, which is the more selective iNOS inhibitor[56], have not yet been studied in portal hypertensive animals. Thus, studies are needed with this compound.

The administration of 7-nitroindazole (a non-amino acid-based compound that selectively inhibits nNOS) decreases the hyperdynamic state in cirrhotic rats[40]. This suggests a role of nNOS-derived NO in portal hypertension. However, this hypothesis should be confirmed because the previous study had been performed in a small number of animals[40].

## BLOCKADE OF $K^+$ CHANNELS INVOLVED IN eNOS ACTIVATION

Under physiological conditions eNOS may be regulated through post-translational mechanisms involving interaction of eNOS with other proteins such as caveolin-1, calmodulin and the chaperone heat-shock protein 90 (Hsp90) (reviewed in refs 63–65). Caveolin-1 inhibits eNOS while calmodulin and Hsp90 stimulate eNOS activity. Endothelial cells express a plasmalemmal small-conductance, $Ca^{2+}$-sensitive $K^+$ (SKCa) channel whose opening is induced by shear stress[66]. SKCa channel opening induces endothelial membrane hyperpolarization which favors the entry of extracellular $Ca^{2+}$ through voltage-independent $Ca^{2+}$ channels. The resulting $Ca^{2+}$ entry increases $[Ca^{2+}]i$. Then, $Ca^{2+}$ binds to calmodulin and the complex $Ca^{2+}$/calmodulin binds to eNOS and activates the enzyme by displacing the inhibitory protein caveolin-1. In cirrhotic rat aortas, endothelial SKCa channels are overexpressed and overactive[50]. Indeed, in cirrhotic aortas, selective SKCa channel blockade induces significant decreases in *ex-vivo* eNOS activity and hyporeactivity to vasoconstrictors[50]. In portal hypertension, increased shear stress participates in eNOS up-regulation. Since shear stress is known to activate endothelial SKCa channels to stimulate eNOS, this mechanism may also participate in portal hypertension-elicited, shear stress-mediated eNOS up-regulation.

In aortas, *in-vivo* Hsp90 protein levels are significantly higher in portal hypertensive rats than in normal rats[46]. In portal vein-stenosed rats the ansamycin antibiotic with antitumor geldanamycin, a specific inhibitor of Hsp90 signaling, decreases the NO-mediated hyporeactivity to vasoconstrictors in the mesenteric vasculature[38]. Together these findings suggest that, in portal hypertension, Hsp90 may play a role in NOS up-regulation. It should be kept in mind that Hsp90 is known to be involved in different processes such as eNOS modulation by shear stress or TNF receptor-1 signaling and many others[65,67]. Both shear stress and TNF-$\alpha$ signaling are enhanced in portal hypertension (see below). Moreover, since geldanamycin is an antitumor agent with marked cytotoxic effects, this substance not only inhibits Hsp90 signaling but may also have several other cellular effects. In other words the exact role of Hsp90 in portal hypertension-associated NOS up-regulation needs to be clarified.

Under normal conditions post-translational regulation of eNOS activity may also occur via protein phosphorylation (reviewed in refs 64 and 65). For example, the serine/threonine kinase Akt phosphorylates eNOS at serine 1177 (Ser$^{1177}$), and Ser$^{1177}$ phosphorylation is known to stimulate eNOS catalytic activity. In the mesenteric arterial bed from portal vein-stenosed rats, early phases of portal hypertension are associated with eNOS phosphorylation at Ser$^{1177}$ (ref. 41). In addition, exposure of mesenteric vascular bed to wortamannin (which blocks phosphatidylinositol-3-OH-kinase-elicited Akt activation) reduces NO-elicited vasodilation[41]. Preliminary results show that cirrhotic rat aortas have increased Akt activity and eNOS phosphorylation at Ser$^{1177}$ (Tazi KA, Moreau R, Lebrec D, unpublished data). In portal hypertensive rats the stimuli responsible for increased Akt activity and subsequent eNOS phosphorylation at Ser$^{1177}$ are unknown. Interestingly, Akt activity may be enhanced by shear stress or by TNF-$\alpha$[43].

Finally, it should be emphasized that eNOS may be phosphorylated at residues other than Ser$^{1177}$ (ref. 65). This needs to be studied in portal hypertension.

## PROPRANOLOL-INDUCED NOS INHIBITION

In cirrhotic and portal vein-stenosed rats a 7-day administration of the non-selective $\beta$-blocker, propranolol, induces a significant decrease in *in-vivo* aortic eNOS mRNA[39], eNOS protein[39,46] and in *ex-vivo* aortic NOS activity[39,46]. In portal vein-stenosed rats treated with propranolol there is normalization of *ex-vivo* aortic reactivity to vasoconstrictors[39]. Propranolol therapy is also associated with a marked decrease in Hsp90 protein expression[46]. The effects of propranolol administration on up-regulated Akt activity and eNOS phosphorylation at Ser$^{1177}$ have not yet been studied in portal hypertension. Interestingly, in cirrhotic rat aortas, propranolol therapy is associated with a 50% decrease in *in-vivo* iNOS protein expression[46].

In normal rats, chronic exercise induces a sustained increase in cardiac ouput causing chronic increases in shear stress forces perceived at the surface of arterial endothelial cells. In response to chronic shear stress there is an increase in the expression and catalytic activity of eNOS. In addition, shear stress may up-regulate Hsp90, Akt activity and eNOS phosphorylation at Ser[1177] (ref. 65). Since portal hypertensive rats have chronic hyperdynamic state, sustained shear stress may explain both eNOS and Hsp90 aortic up-regulation in these animals. Since propranolol reduces the hyperdynamic state this reduction may explain the down-regulation of eNOS and Hsp90 in rats with β-blockers.

To interpret the effects of propranolol therapy one should bear in mind that intestinal translocation of Gram-negative bacteria causing endotoxemia without overt sepsis is common in cirrhosis[35]. This "non-septic endotoxemia" results in increased plasma concentrations of proinflammatory cytokines such as TNF-α[35]. Since endotoxin (i.e. lipopolysaccharide, LPS) and TNF-α are potent iNOS (co-)inducers[56], the presence of iNOS in cirrhotic aortas indicates the existence of bacterial translocation. However, in cirrhotic rats the functional role of iNOS is unclear (see above). Moreover, bacterial products such as LPS may induce mechanisms that stimulate eNOS. First, LPS induces GTP-cyclohydrolase I (GTPCH-I), a key enzyme involved in the production of tetrahydrobiopterin (BH4), which is an essential, rate-limiting cofactor in the synthesis of NO by eNOS[68]. In cirrhotic mesenteric vasculature, bacterial translocation is associated with GTPCH-I up-regulation[68] and increased BH4 levels[35]. Second, TNF-α may activate eNOS by stimulating Akt to phosphorylate eNOS at Ser[1177] (ref. 43). In other words, bacterial translocation may participate in eNOS up-regulation. Since propranolol is known to decrease intestinal bacterial translocation[69], this decrease probably explains the β-blockade-induced reduction in aortic iNOS. Moreover, inhibition of bacterial translocation and subsequent decreases in GTPCH-I/BH4 and/or TNF-α/Akt pathways may participate in propranolol-elicited eNOS down-regulation.

## NORFLOXACIN-INDUCED NOS INHIBITION

Preliminary results show that, in cirrhotic rats, a 5-day therapy with norfloxacin (an antibiotic that causes selective intestinal decontamination and inhibits bacterial translocation[42]) is associated with a marked *in-vivo* decrease in aortic iNOS-inducing cytokines (TNF-α and IFN-γ) and iNOS protein (Tazi KA, Moreau R, Lebrec D, unpublished results). Moreover, norfloxacin therapy induces significant decreases in eNOS protein and activity, eNOS phosphorylation at Ser[1177] and Akt activity. The effects of norfloxacin on Hsp90 are unknown.

Since bacterial translocation may result in both iNOS induction and eNOS up-regulation (see above), the responses obtained with 5-day norfloxacin therapy might be explained by norfloxacin-elicited suppression of bacterial translocation. However, since norfloxacin is also known to decrease the hyperdynamic state in cirrhotic rats[42], this mechanism may contribute to norfloxacin-induced eNOS down-regulation.

In patients with cirrhosis the administration of norfloxacin induces a reduction in plasma levels of TNF-α and NO metabolites, and a decrease in the systemic hyperdynamic syndrome[70]. These effects of norfloxacin may be due to NOS down-regulation.

## "ANTI-TNF THERAPY"-INDUCED NOS INHIBITION

"Anti-TNF therapy" with antibody to TNF[37,71], thalidomide[72] or tyrphostin AG126[73] decreases the systemic hyperdynamic state in portal hypertensive rats. These effects may be due to the inhibition of TNF-α-induced up-regulation of NOS.

The administration of an antibody to TNF results in *in-vivo* down-regulation of eNOS protein and activity in the portal hypertensive rat gastric mucosa[33,43]. These effects are associated with a decrease in eNOS phosphorylation at $Ser^{1177}$ and Akt activity[43].

## FUTURE APPROACHES: INHIBITION OF LPS SIGNALING

LPS, a component of Gram-negative bacteria, is recognized specifically by a receptor located at the surface of immune cells (monocytes/macrophages). This receptor is called toll-like receptor 4 (TLR4)[74]. Engagement of TLR4 leads to tyrosine kinase-dependent activation of mitogen-activated protein kinases (MAPK) such as p38, c-Jun NH2-terminal kinase (JNK) and extracellular-signal regulated kinase. These MAPK have several transcriptional effects via AP-1 (including perhaps increased TNF mRNA transcription). In addition, MAPK increase TNF-α production by stimulating nucleocytoplasmic TNF mRNA transport and increasing TNF mRNA translation, and perhaps stability of the RNA. In addition, TL4 engagement stimulates Iκ-B kinases (IKK, a multiprotein complex containing IKKβ which is indispensable to LPS signaling). IKKβ then activates nuclear factor-κB (NF-κB) which induces the expression of proinflammatory cytokine genes (including *TNF*).

TNF-α produced in response to LPS binds to specific surface receptors (called TNF receptor-1, TNFR-1) in target cells (e.g. SMC, hepatocytes). TNFR-1 engagement stimulates proapoptotic pathways (i.e. MAPK/JNK and procaspase-8), antiapoptotic and proinflammatory pathways (i.e. the IKK/NF-κB pathway) and proinflammatory signals (e.g. MAPK/p38)[67].

It should be noted that thalidomide is an "anti-TNF" therapy because it decreases TNF mRNA stability in immune cells and inhibits IKKβ in target cells[75]. This suggests that the newly developed IKKβ inhibitor may be useful in the treatment of vascular alterations in portal hypertension[75]. However, since the IKK/NF-κB pathway has an important antiapoptotic function, inhibition of this antiapoptotic pathway might induce adverse effects[75].

Tyrphostin AG126 may decrease both TNF-α production and action. Indeed, this tyrphostin has been shown to inhibit tyrosine kinase activation of MAPK (probably p38) which occurs upstream and downstream in TNF-α signaling[76]. Since pharmacological p38 inhibitors are available[77], these molecules may be useful in portal hypertension.

LPS seems to be a main upstream player in the cascade of events leading to NOS up-regulation in portal hypertension. Since antibodies to endotoxin are available[78], these antibodies should be evaluated in the treatment of vascular alterations in portal hypertension.

## CONCLUSIONS

Several strategies can be used to inhibit NO production and/or action in portal hypertension. The use of molecules that inhibit primary mechanisms involved in NOS up-regulation (e.g. intestinal bacterial translocation) is a novel approach in the treatment of vascular alterations due to portal hypertension.

## References

1. Groszmann R. Hyperdynamic circulation of liver disease forty years later: pathophysiology and clinical consequences. Hepatology. 1994;20:1359–63.
2. Moreau R, Lee SS, Soupison T, Roche-Sicot J, Sicot C. Abnormal tissue oxygenation in patients with cirrhosis and liver failure. J Hepatol. 1988;7:98–105.
3. Braillon A, Cales P, Valla D, Gaudy D, Geoffroy P, Lebrec D. Influence of the degree of liver failure on systemic and splanchnic haemodynamics and on response to propranolol in patients with cirrhosis. Gut. 1986;27:1204–9.
4. Lebrec D, Blanchet L. Effects of two models of portal hypertension on splanchnic organ blood flow in the rat. Clin Sci. 1985;68:23–8.
5. Fernandez-Seara J, Prieto J, Quiroga J et al. Systemic and regional hemodynamics in patients with liver cirrhosis and ascites with and without functional renal failure. Gastroenterology. 1989;97:1304–12.
6. Murray BM, Paller MS. Pressor resistance to vasopressin in sodium depletion, potassium depletion, and cirrhosis. Am J Physiol. 1986;251:R525–30.
7. Pinzani M, Marra F, Fusco BM et al. Evidence for $\alpha_1$-adrenoreceptor hyperresponsiveness in hypotensive cirrhotic patients with ascites. Am J Gastroenterol. 1991;86:711–14.
8. Braillon A, Cailmail S, Gaudin C, Lebrec D. Reduced splanchnic vasoconstriction to angiotensin II in conscious rats with biliary cirrhosis. J Hepatol. 1993;17:86–90.
9. Ryan J, Sudhir K, Jennings G, Esler M, Dudley F. Impaired reactivity of the peripheral vascular to pressor agents in alcoholic cirrhosis. Gastroenterology. 1993;105:1167–72.
10. Hartleb M, Moreau R, Cailmail S, Gaudin C, Lebrec D. Vascular hyporesponsiveness to endothelin-1 in rats with cirrhosis. Gastroenterology. 1994;107:1085–93.
11. Hartleb M, Moreau R, Gaudin C, Lebrec D. Lack of vascular hyporesponsiveness to the L-type calcium channel activator, Bay K 8644, in rats with cirrhosis. J Hepatol. 1995; 22:202–7.
12. Liao J, Yu PC, Lin HC, Lee FY, Kuo JS, Yang MCM. Study on the vascular reactivity and $\alpha_1$-adrenoceptors of portal hypertensive rats. Br J Pharmacol. 1994;111:439–44.
13. Huang YT, Wang GF, Yang MCM, Chang SP, Lin HC, Hong CY. Vascular hyporesponsiveness in aorta from portal hypertensive rats: possible sites of involvement. J Pharmacol Exp Ther. 1996;278:535–41.
14. Sogni P, Sabry S, Moreau R, Gadano A, Lebrec D, Din-Xuan AT. Hyporeactivity of mesenteric resistance arteries in portal hypertensive rats. J Hepatol. 1996;24:487–90.
15. Moreau R, Cailmail S, Lebrec D. Haemodynamic effects of vasopressin in portal hypertensive rats receiving clonidine. Liver. 1994;14:45–9.
16. Pizcueta P, Piqué JM, Bosch J, Whittle BJR, Moncada S. Effects of inhibiting nitric oxide biosynthesis on the systemic and splanchnic circulation of rats with portal hypertension. Br J Pharmacol. 1992;105:184–90.
17. Claria J, Jiménez W, Ros J et al. Pathogenesis of arterial hypotension in cirrhotic rats with ascites: role of endogenous nitric oxide. Hepatology. 1992;15:343–9.
18. Sogni P, Moreau R, Ohsuga M et al. Evidence for a normal nitric oxide-mediated vasodilator tone in conscious rats with cirrhosis. Hepatology. 1992;16:980–3.
19. Lee FY, Albillos A, Colombato LA, Groszmann RJ. The role of nitric oxide in the vascular hyporesponsiveness to methoxamine in portal hypertensive rats. Hepatology. 1992; 16:1043–8.
20. Sieber CC, Groszmann RJ. In vitro hyporeactivity to methoxamine in portal hypertensive rats: reversal by nitric oxide blockade. Am J Physiol. 1992;262:G996–1001.

21. Sieber CC, Groszmann RJ. Nitric oxide mediates hyporeactivity to vasopressors in mesenteric vessels of portal hypertensive rats. Gastroenterology. 1992;103:235–9.
22. Pizcueta P, Piqué JM, Fernandez M et al. Modulation of the hyperdynamic circulation of cirrhotic rats by nitric oxide inhibition. Gastroenterology. 1992;103:1909–15.
23. Sieber CC, Lopez-Talavera JC, Groszmann RJ. Role of nitric oxide in the *in vitro* splanchnic vascular hyporeactivity in ascitic cirrhotic rats. Gastroenterology. 1993;104:1750–4.
24. Michielsen PP, Boeckxstaens GE, Sys SU, Herman AG, Pelckmans PA. Role of nitric oxide in hyporeactivity to noradrenaline of isolated aortic rings in portal hypertensive rats. Eur J Pharmacol. 1995;273:167–74.
25. Niederberger M, Ginès P, Tsai P et al. Increased aortic cyclic guanosine monophosphate concentration in experimental cirrhosis in rats: evidence for a role of nitric oxide in the pathogenesis of arterial vasodilation in cirrhosis. Hepatology. 1995;21:1625–31.
26. Cahill PA, Foster C, Redmond EM, Gingalewski C, Wu Y, Sitzmann JV. Enhanced nitric oxide synthase activity in portal hypertensive rabbits. Hepatology. 1995;22:598–606.
27. Kanwar S, Kubes P, Tepperman BL, Lee SS. Nitric oxide synthase activity in portal-hypertensive and cirrhotic rats. J Hepatol. 1996;25:85–9.
28. Martin PY, Xu DI, Niederberger M et al. Upregulation of endothelial constitutive NOS: a major role in the increased NO production in cirrhotic rats. Am J Physiol. 1996;270:F494–9.
29. Pilette C, Moreau R, Sogni P et al. Haemodynamic and hormonal responses to long-term inhibition of nitric oxide synthesis in rats with portal hypertension. Eur J Pharmacol. 1996;312:63–8.
30. Pilette C, Kirstetter P, Sogni P, Cailmail S, Moreau R, Lebrec D. Dose-dependent effects of a nitric oxide biosynthesis inhibitor on hyperdynamic circulation in two models of portal hypertension in conscious rats. J Gastroenterol Hepatol. 1996;11:1–6.
31. Gadano AC, Sogni P, Yang S et al. Endothelial calcium-calmodium dependent nitric oxide synthase in the *in vitro* vascular hyporeactivity of portal hypertensive rats. J Hepatol. 1997;26:678–86.
32. Atucha NM, Ortiz MC, Fortepiani LA, Ruiz FM, Martinez C, Garcia-Estan J. Role of cyclic guanosine monophosphate and $K^+$ channels as mediators of the mesenteric vascular hyporesponsiveness in portal hypertensive rats. Hepatology. 1998;27:900–5.
33. Ohta M, Tarnawski AS, Itani R et al. Tumor necrosis factor a regulates nitric oxide synthase expression in portal hypertensive gastric mucosa of rats. Hepatology. 1998;27:906–13.
34. Pateron D, Oberti F, Lefilliatre P et al. Relationship between vascular reactivity *in vitro* and blood flows in rats with cirrhosis. Clin Sci. 1999;97:313–18.
35. Wiest R, Das S, Gadelina G, Garcia-Tsao G, Milstien S, Groszmann RJ. Bacterial translocation in cirrhotic rats stimulates eNOS-derived NO production and impairs mesentenric vascular contractility. J Clin Invest. 1999;104:1223–33.
36. Wiest R, Shah V, Sessa WC, Groszmann RJ. NO overproduction by eNOS precedes hyperdynamic splanchnic circulation in portal hypertensive rats. Am J Physiol. 1999; 276:G1043–51.
37. Munoz J, Albillos A, Perez-Paramo M, Rossi I, Alvarez-Mon M. Factors mediating the hemodynamic effects of tumor necrosis factor-alpha in portal hypertensive rats. Am J Physiol. 1999;276:G687–93.
38. Shah V, Wiest R, Garcia-Cardena G, Cadelina G, Groszmann RJ, Sessa WC. Hsp90 regulation of endothelial nitric oxide synthase contributes to vascular control in portal hypertension. Am J Physiol. 1999;277:G463–8.
39. Pateron D, Tazi KA, Sogni P et al. Role of aortic nitric oxide synthase 3 (eNOS) in the systemic vasodilation of portal hypertension. Gastroenterology. 2000;119:196–200.
40. Xu L, Carter EP, Ohara M. Neuronal nitric oxide synthase and systemic vasodilation in rats with cirrhosis. Am J Physiol. 2000;279:F1110–15.
41. Iwakiri Y, Tsai MH, McCabe TJ et al. Phosphorylation of eNOS initiates excessive NO production in early phases of portal hypertension. Am J Physiol. 2002;282:H2084–90.
42. Rabiller A, Nunes H, Lebrec D et al. Prevention of Gram-negative translocation reduces the severity of hepatopulmonary syndrome. Am J Respir Crit Care Med. 2002;166:514–17.
43. Kawanaka H, Jones MK, Szabo IL et al. Activation of eNOS in rat portal hypertensive gastric mucosa is mediated by TNF-alpha via the PI 3-kinase-Akt signaling pathway. Hepatology. 2002;35:393–402.
44. Tsai MH, Iwakiri Y, Cadelina G, Sessa WC, Groszmann RJ. Mesenteric vasoconstriction triggers nitric oxide overproduction in the superior mesenteric artery of portal hypertensive rats. Gastroenterology. 2003;125:1452–61.

45. Davis KL, Martin E, Turko IV, Murad F. Novel effects of nitric oxide. Annu Rev Pharmacol Toxicol. 2001;41:203–36.
46. Tazi KA, Barrière E, Moreau R et al. Role of shear stress in aortic eNOS up-regulation in rats with biliary cirrhosis. Gastroenterology. 2002;122:1869–77.
47. Casadevall M, Pique JM, Cirera I et al. Increased blood hemoglobin attenuates splanchnic vasodilation in portal-hypertensive rats by nitric oxide inactivation. Gastroenterology. 1996;110:1156–65.
48. Lincoln TM, Cornwell TL. Intracellular cyclic GMP receptor proteins. FASEB J. 1993;7:328–38.
49. Moreau R, Lebrec D. Endogenous factors involved in the control of arterial tone in cirrhosis. J Hepatol. 1995;22:370–6.
50. Barrière E, Tazi KA, Pessione F, Heller J, Poirel O, Lebrec D, Moreau R. Role of small-conductance $Ca^{2+}$-dependent $K^+$ channels in in vitro NO-mediated aortic hyporeactivity to a-adrenergic vasoconstriction in rats with cirrhosis. J Hepatol. 2001;35:350–7.
51. Moreau R. Heme oxygenase: protective enzyme or portal hypertensive molecule? J Hepatol. 2001;34:936–939.
52. Tang M, Wang G, Lu P et al. Regulator of G-protein signaling-2 mediates vascular smooth muscle relaxation and blood pressure. Nat Med. 2003;9:1506–12.
53. Somlyo AP, Somlyo AV. Signal transduction and regulation in smooth muscle. Nature. 1994;372:231–6.
54. Theodorakis NG, Wang YN, Skill NJ et al. The role of nitric oxide synthase isoforms in extrahepatic portal hypertension: studies in gene-knockout mice. Gastroenterology. 2003;124:1500–8.
55. Iwakiri Y, Cadelina G, Sessa WC, Groszmann RJ. Mice with targeted deletion of eNOS develop hyperdynamic circulation associated with portal hypertension. Am J Physiol. 2002;283:G1074–81.
56. Hobbs AJ, Higgs A, Moncada S. Inhibition of nitric oxide synthase as a potential therapeutic target. Annu Rev Pharmacol Toxicol. 1999;39:191–220.
57. Ortiz MC, Fortepiani LA, Martinez C, Atucha NM, Garcia-Estan J. Renal and pressor effects of aminoguanidine in cirrhotic rats with ascites. J Am Soc Nephrol. 1996;7:2694–9.
58. Criado M, Flores O, Ortiz MC et al. Elevated glomerular and blood mononuclear lympho-cyte nitric oxide production in rats with chronic bile duct ligation: role of inducible nitric oxide synthase activation. Hepatology. 1997;26:268–76.
59. Moore WM, Webber RK, Jerome GM, Tjoeng FS, Misko TP, Currie MG. L-$N^6$-(1-iminoethyl)lysine: a selective inhibitor of inducible nitric oxide synthase. J Med Chem. 1994;37:3886–8.
60. Porst M, Hartner A, Krause H, Hilgers KF, Veelken R. Inducible nitric oxide synthase and glomerular hemodynamics in rats with liver cirrhosis. Am J Physiol Renal Physiol. 2001;281:F293–9.
61. Fernandez M, Garcia-Pagan JC, Casadevall M et al. Evidence against a role for inducible nitric oxide synthase in the hyperdynamic circulation of portal-hypertensive rats. Gastroenterology. 1995;108:1487–95.
62. Albornoz L, Bandi JC, de las Heras M, Mastai R. Dexamethasone, an inhibitor of the expression of inducible nitric oxide synthase, does not modify the hyperdynamic state in cirrhotic rats. Medicina (B Aires). 2000;60:477–81.
63. Shaul PW. Regulation of endothelial nitric oxide synthase: location, location, location. Annu Rev Physiol. 2002;64:749–74.
64. Fleming I, Busse R. Molecular mechanisms involved in the regulation of the endothelial nitric oxide synthase. Am J Physiol. 2003;284:R1–12.
65. Boo YC, Jo H. Flow-dependent regulation of endothelial nitric oxide synthase: role of protein kinases. Am J Physiol. 2003;285:C499–508.
66. Nilius B, Viana F, Droogmans G. Ion channels in vascular endothelium. Annu Rev Physiol. 1997;59:145–70.
67. Chen G, Goeddel DV. TNF-R1 signaling: a beautiful pathway. Science. 2002;296:1634–5.
68. Wiest R, Cadelina G, Milstien S, McCuskey RS, Garcia-Tsao G, Groszmann RJ. Bacterial translocation up-regulates GTP-cyclohydrolase I in mesenteric vasculature of cirrhotic rats. Hepatology. 2003;38:1508–15.
69. Perez-Paramo M, Munoz J, Albillos A et al. Effect of propranolol on the factors promoting bacterial translocation in cirrhotic rats with ascites. Hepatology. 2000;31:43–8.

70. Albillos A, de la Hera A, Gonzalez M et al. Increased lipopolysaccharide binding protein in cirrhotic patients with marked immune and hemodynamic derangement. Hepatology. 2003;37:208–17.
71. Lopez-Talavera JC, Merrill WW, Groszmann RJ. Tumor necrosis factor alpha: a major contributor to the hyperdynamic circulation in prehepatic portal-hypertensive rats. Gastroenterology. 1995;108:761–7.
72. Lopez-Talavera JC, Cadelina G, Olchowski J, Merrill W, Groszmann RJ. Thalidomide inhibits tumor necrosis factor alpha, decreases nitric oxide synthesis, and ameliorates the hyperdynamic circulatory syndrome in portal-hypertensive rats. Hepatology. 1996; 23:1616–21.
73. Lopez-Talavera JC, Levitzki A, Martinez M, Gazit A, Esteban R, Guardia J. Tyrosine kinase inhibition ameliorates the hyperdynamic state and decreases nitric oxide production in cirrhotic rats with portal hypertension and ascites. J Clin Invest. 1997;100:664–70.
74. Medzhitov R. Toll-like receptors and innate immunity. Nat Rev Immunol 2001;135–45.
75. Karin M, Yamamoto Y, Wang QM. The IKK NF-kappa B system: a treasure trove for drug development. Nat Rev Drug Discov. 2004;3:17–26.
76. Levitzki A, Gazit A. Tyrosine kinase inhibition: an approach to drug development. Science. 1995;267:1782–8.
77. Kumar S, Boehm J, Lee JC. p38 MAP kinases: key signalling molecules as therapeutic targets for inflammatory diseases. Nat Rev Drug Discov. 2003;2:717–26.
78. Marshall JC. Such stuff as dreams are made on: mediator-directed therapy in sepsis. Nat Rev Drug Discov. 2003;2:391–405.

# Section V
# Introduction to variceal bleeding

# 17
# Esophageal varices: from appearance to rupture; natural history and prognostic indicators

GENNARO D'AMICO

## BACKGROUND

Bleeding, ascites and encephalopathy are the major clinical manifestations of liver cirrhosis. The appearance of these manifestations marks the *decompensated* stage of the disease. The expected survival rate of patients with compensated disease is nearly 90% after 10 years if they do not develop decompensation, whereas the median survival is about 2 years after decompensation. The progression from compensated to decompensated cirrhosis is parallel to the development and progression of portal hypertension, signaled by the appearance of esophageal varices and/or ascites.

Esophageal varices are among the most serious consequences of portal hypertension. They appear only when the hepatic venous pressure gradient (HVPG)[1] is above 10–12 mmHg, and their increasing size is accompanied by an increasing risk of bleeding. The mortality of variceal bleeding has decreased from about 50% in the late 1970s to around 20% nowadays[2]. After the first bleeding 60% of patients rebleed in the following 1–2 years and about 33% die in the same period. A reappraisal of the clinical course of portal hypertension is here reported according to a review of the current medical literature, and according to individual patient data from two large studies of the natural history of cirrhosis[3,4].

## PREVALENCE OF ESOPHAGEAL VARICES

The prevalence of varices at the diagnosis of cirrhosis is widely variable across the published studies and ranges from 0% in patients with compensated cirrhosis to 80% in those with decompensated cirrhosis in prognostic studies published after 1980. The median prevalence of esophageal varices in these studies is 55%. Although there is a trend toward a relationship

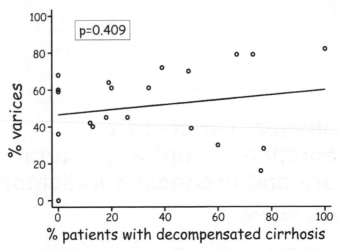

**Figure 1.** Prevalence of varices in cirrhosis, according to the proportion of patients with decompensated cirrhosis. Data from 22 out of 93 prognostic studies published between 1980 and 2003 and reporting complete information

between the prevalence of varices and the prevalence of decompensated disease, this relationship is not statistically significant (Figure 1).

## DEVELOPMENT OF ESOPHAGEAL VARICES

Two recent prospective cohort studies showed that the incidence of esophageal varices in patients with newly diagnosed cirrhosis is nearly 5% per year[5,6]. A similar finding was recently reported also in a large consensus conference after a thorough review of available studies[7]. Therefore, overall, the estimated prevalence of varices at 5 years from the diagnosis may be as high as 75%, assuming that about half of patients may have varices at the diagnosis of cirrhosis. However, the incidence of varices is significantly lower in patients with compensated cirrhosis than in those with decompensated cirrhosis at diagnosis (Figure 2).

Varices do not develop below the threshold hepatic venous pressure gradient (HVPG) value of 10–12 mmHg[1]. Above this threshold the median time to the development of varices and/or bleeding, or other complications of portal hypertension, is about 4 years[8]. Worsening of liver function and continuing exposure to alcohol are factors associated with an increasing risk of developing varices. However, HVPG frequently increases with worsening liver function and continuing alcohol abuse, and may decrease when liver function improves and after alcohol withdrawal[9]. Therefore, an increased HVPG is presently considered the most important risk factor for the development of esophageal varices. This is also confirmed by the reduction of the risk of first bleeding in patients achieving a reduction of HVPG either pharmacologically induced or spontaneously[10].

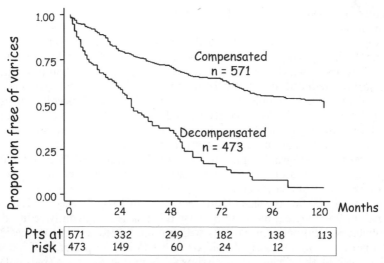

**Figure 2.** Proportion of patients free of varices after diagnosis among 571 patients with compensated and 473 decompensated cirrhosis, without esophageal varices at diagnosis

## PROGRESSION OF ESOPHAGEAL VARICES FROM SMALL TO LARGE

Once developed, varices increase in size from small to large before they eventually rupture and bleed. Prospective studies have reported progression rates ranging from 0.05 to 0.12 per year (median 0.07)[5,6,11]. This variability probably depends on different patient selection criteria across studies, with inclusion of patients with different degrees of progression of the underlying cirrhosis. In this respect it may be worth noting that the one study which included only patients with newly diagnosed cirrhosis reported a variceal progression rate of 0.05 per year[5].

Changes in HVPG may be followed by parallel variations in the size of esophageal varices[9] indicating that HVPG plays a key role both in development and progression of varices, and should be considered a main target in monitoring treatment to prevent variceal bleeding or rebleeding.

The increase in size of esophageal varices is associated with increasing risk of bleeding, of developing ascites and of mortality.

## INCIDENCE OF VARICEAL BLEEDING AND RISK INDICATORS

The incidence of variceal bleeding is approximately 4% per year in nonselected patients who have never bled at the time of diagnosis. The risk is about 2% in patients without varices at diagnosis, and increases to about 5% per year in those with small varices and 15% in those with medium or large varices[12]. Major indicators of the risk of bleeding are Child–Pugh class, variceal size and red weal marks on endoscopy, which have been combined in the NIEC index[13]. Although its accuracy is far from satisfactory, this is the best available system for the prediction of the first variceal bleeding in cirrhosis.

Esophageal varices do not bleed below a threshold HVPG level of 12 mmHg[14]. Importantly, in patients with higher baseline HVPG, the bleeding risk is abolished if HVPG is reduced to levels below 12 mmHg, and is significantly reduced if HVPG is reduced to $\geq 20\%$ from baseline[14,15]. Variceal pressure is significantly related with the risk of bleeding through the wall tension, which is inversely related to variceal wall thickness and is therefore another potential bleeding risk indicator[16]. However, variceal wall tension cannot be measured accurately at present.

Several ultrasonographic parameters have been reported to be related to esophageal varices and the risk of variceal bleeding; however the predictive accuracy is far from satisfactory[17].

In clinical practice the size of varices is the most widely used indicator of the risk of first variceal bleeding because this risk is significantly reduced by prophylactic treatments in patients with medium-sized to large varices[18].

All patients with cirrhosis should be screened for the presence of esophageal varices at the diagnosis of cirrhosis[7]. Non-invasive tests (particularly platelet count and abdominal ultrasound) have not been proven sufficiently accurate to safely avoid endoscopy in patients who are negative for the test[17]. To detect newly developed varices, endoscopy should be repeated every 2–3 years in compensated patients[7]; however, in compensated patients with HVPG $\geq 10$ mmHg, endoscopy should be repeated yearly, as well as in patients with decompensated cirrhosis. In patients with small varices endoscopy should be repeated yearly to detect the progression from small to large size[7].

## ACUTE VARICEAL BLEEDING

Ruptured esophageal varices cause 60–70% of all upper gastrointestinal bleeding episodes in cirrhosis[2]. Data from placebo-controlled clinical trials have shown that variceal bleeding ceases spontaneously in 40–50% of patients. Active treatment achieves control of bleeding within 24 h from admission in nearly 85% of episodes[19]. Active bleeding on endoscopy, bacterial infection and HVPG > 20 mmHg are significant prognostic indicators of failure to control bleeding. Immediate mortality from uncontrolled bleeding is approximately 5%. The incidence of rebleeding is about 20% in the first 6 weeks. Active bleeding at emergency endoscopy, gastric varices, low albumin and/or high blood urea nitrogen and HVPG > 20 mmHg have been reported as significant indicators of early rebleeding risk. Six-week mortality is about 20% with nearly one-half of deaths caused by bleeding or early rebleeding. Albumin, bilirubin, creatininemia, encephalopathy, hepatocellular carcinoma, the number of transfused blood units, bacterial infection and HVPG > 20 mmHg are indicators of the risk of mortality within 6 weeks.

Following a first episode of variceal bleeding there is a 63% rebleeding risk and 33% death risk within 1 year. Rebleeding risk indicators are variceal size, Child–Pugh class, continued alcohol abuse, and hepatocellular carcinoma. Reduction of HVPG to below 12 mmHg totally prevents recurrent

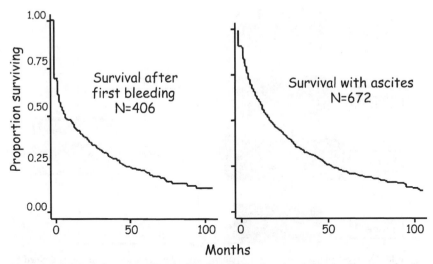

**Figure 3.** Survival after upper digestive bleeding (406 patients) and after development of ascites (672 patients) in patients with cirrhosis. Individual patient data from two large prospective studies (see refs 3 and 4)

bleeding and a reduction of ≥ 20% of the baseline value reduces the risk of recurrent bleeding by nearly 70%[10].

## LONG-TERM OUTCOME OF PORTAL HYPERTENSION AS RELATED TO CLINICAL STAGES

At diagnosis the prevalence of ascites ranges from 20% to 60% according to the referral pattern. The incidence of ascites is about 5% per year, and together with variceal bleeding, represents the most frequent modality of transition from the compensated into the decompensated phase of cirrhosis[3].

A less frequent modality is the development of hepatic encephalopathy with an incidence of approximately 2–3% per year[3]; however, the incidence of encephalopathy in the absence of ascites or previous bleeding is much lower. Therefore, the most important markers of decompensated cirrhosis are bleeding and ascites, while encephalopathy and jaundice mark a very advanced stage of the disease.

After the first variceal bleeding the median survival time is about 1 year, and after the development of ascites it is 2 years[12] (Figure 3). Encephalopathy and jaundice usually appear after bleeding or ascites, and the median survival after the first episode of encephalopathy or after the appearance of jaundice is therefore shorter than for bleeding or ascites, respectively. The most frequent causes of death are bleeding, liver failure with hepatic coma, sepsis, and the hepatorenal syndrome.

By combining individual patient data from two large prospective studies of the natural history of cirrhosis[12], we identified four stages in the progression of the disease (Figure 4).

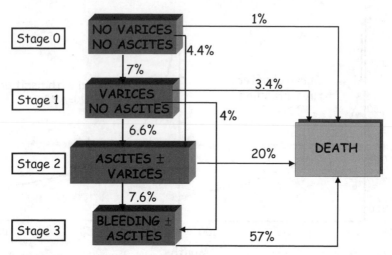

**Figure 4.** One-year outcome in cirrhotic patients according to four clinical stages defined by the presence of esophageal varices, ascites and bleeding. Data from two large prospective studies (see refs 3 and 4)

*Stage 0:* absence of esophageal varices and of ascites. While in this stage, until free of varices and ascites, the mortality rate is as low as 1% per year. However, patients exit from this stage also by developing varices (7% per year) and/or ascites (4.4% per year).

*Stage 1:* varices without ascites and without bleeding. In this stage the mortality rate is 3.4% per year, significantly higher than in stage 0. Patients leave this stage also by developing ascites (6.6% per year) and/or bleeding (4% per year).

*Stage 2:* ascites with or without esophageal varices which have not bled. Mortality in this stage is 20% per year; significantly higher than in the two former stages. Besides death, patients may leave this stage by bleeding at a rate of 7.6% per year.

*Stage 3:* bleeding with or without ascites. In this stage the mortality rate is 57% per year (near half of these deaths occur within 6 weeks from the bleeding episode).

## PROGNOSTIC SCORES

The Child–Pugh score[20] is the most widely used and widely applied in all clinical situations along the course of cirrhosis, and to stratify patients included in clinical trials in portal hypertension. Previously included among the most important criteria for the allocation of livers for transplantation, the Child–Pugh score has been recently substituted with the Model for End stage Liver Disease (MELD)[21], by the United Network for Organ Sharing (the UNOS). The most important reason for doing this was that the MELD is based on objective variables not affected by subjective judgement: etiology of cirrhosis, bilirubin, creatinin and INR (the International Normal Ratio for prothrombin time), whereas the Child–Pugh score includes ascites and encephalopathy. Although the two scores are not significantly different for the predictive accuracy for survival, it should be expected that the interobserver agreement to classify cirrhotic patients in prognostically different subgroups would be higher with MELD.

## References

1. Garcia-Tsao G, Groszmann RJ, Fisher RL, Conn HO, Atterbury CE, Glickman M. Portal pressure, presence of gastroesophageal varices and variceal bleeding. Hepatology. 1985;5: 419–24.
2. D'Amico G, De Franchis R. Upper digestive bleeding in cirrhosis: post-therapeutic outcome and prognostic indicators. Hepatology. 2003;38:599–612.
3. D'Amico G, Morabito A, Pagliaro L, Marubini E. Survival and prognostic indicators in compensated and decompensated cirrhosis. Dig Dis Sci. 1986;31:468–75.
4. Pagliaro L, D'Amico G, Pasta L et al. Portal hypertension in cirrhosis: natural history. In: Bosch J, Groszmann R, editors. Portal Hypertension: Pathophysiology and Treatment. Cambridge, MA: Blackwell Scientific, 1994:72–92.
5. D'Amico G, Pasta L, Madonna S, Tarantino I, Mancuso A, Malizia G. The incidence of esophageal varices in cirrhosis. DDW 2001, Atlanta, 20–23 May 2001.
6. Merli M, Nicolini G, Angeloni S et al. Incidence and natural history of small esophageal varices in cirrhotic patients. J Hepatol. 2003;38:266–72.
7. D'Amico G, Garcia-Tsao G, Calès P et al. Diagnosis of portal hypertension: how and when. In: De Franchis R, editor. Proceedings of the Third Baveno International Consensus Workshop on Definitions, Methodology and Therapeutic Strategies. Oxford: Blackwell Science, 2001;36–63.
8. Groszmann RJ, Garcia-Tsao G, Bosch J et al. Multicenter randomized placebo-controlled trial of non-selective beta-blockers in the prevention of the complications of portal hypertension: final results and identification of a predictive factor. AASLD, Boston, 2003.
9. Vorobioff J, Groszmann RJ, Picabea E et al. Prognostic value of hepatic venous pressure gradient measurements in alcoholic cirrhosis: a 10-year prospective sudy. Gastroenterology. 1996;111:701–9.
10. D'Amico G. The role of vasoactive drugs in the treatment of oesophageal varices. Expert Opin Pharmacother. 2004;5:349–60.
11. Merkel C, Marin R, Angeli P et al. Beta-blockers in the prevention of aggravation of esophageal varices in patients with cirrhosis and small varices: a placebo controlled clinical trial. AASLD, Boston, 2003.
12. D'Amico G, Luca A. Portal hypertension. Natural history. Clinical-hemodynamic correlations. Prediction of the risk of bleeding. Bailliere's Clin Gastroenterol. 1997;11:243–56.
13. North-Italian Endoscopic Club. Prediction of the first variceal hemorrhage in patients with cirrhosis of the liver and esophageal varices. A prospective multicenter study. N Engl J Med. 1988;319:983–9.
14. Groszmann RJ, Bosch J, Grace N et al. Hemodynamic events in a prospective randomized trial of propranolol vs placebo in the prevention of the first variceal hemorrhage. Gastroenterology. 1990;99:1401–7.
15. Feu F. Garcia-Pagan JC, Bosch J et al. Relation between portal pressure response to pharmacotherapy and risk of recurrent variceal haemorrhage in patients with cirrhosis. Lancet. 1995;346:1056–9.
16. Rigau J, Bosch J, Bordas JM et al. Endoscopic measurement of variceal pressure in cirrhosis: correlation with portal pressure and variceal hemorrhage. Gastroenterology. 1989;96: 873–80.
17. D'Amico G, Morabito A. Non invasive markers of esophageal varices. Another round not the last. Hepatology. 2004;39:30–4.
18. D'Amico G, Pagliaro L, Bosch J. Pharmacological treatment of portal hypertension: an evidence based approach. Semin Liver Dis. 1999;19:475–505.
19. D'Amico G, Pietrosi G, Tarantino I, Pagliaro L. Emergency sclerotherapy versus vasoactive drugs for variceal bleeding in cirrhosis: a Cochrane meta-analysis. Gastroenterology. 2003;124:1277–91.

20. Pugh RN, Murray-Lyon IM, Dawson JL, Pietrni MC, Williams R. Transection of the esophagus for bleeding oesophageal varices. Br J Surg. 1973;60:646–9.
21. Kamath PS, Wiesner RH, Malinchoc M et al. A model to predict survival in patients with end-stage liver disease. Hepatology. 2001;33:464–70.

# 18
# Pathophysiology of variceal bleeding

**ÀNGELS ESCORSELL and JAIME BOSCH**

## INTRODUCTION

Variceal formation is an almost unavoidable complication of cirrhosis. Varices are already present in about 40% of compensated, asymptomatic patients at diagnosis, and the incidence increases to up to 90% of patients on long-term follow up[1]. The annual incidence is around 6% per year[2].

This chapter reviews the pathophysiology of variceal formation and rupture in order to provide a rational basis for new therapeutic strategies.

## MECHANISMS OF COLLATERAL DEVELOPMENT

Three mechanisms have been involved in the development of portal–systemic collateral circulation, which includes the gastroesophageal varices[3]. The first is a hemodynamic factor, the increased pressure and blood flow in the portal venous system. The second is an anatomic factor, represented by the existence of embryonic channels communicating the portal and systemic circulation. The third is angiogenesis. A role for angiogenesis was first suggested by the fact that portal–systemic collaterals are not merely dilated vessels, but vessels that have a marked hyperplasia and hypertrophy of their walls, which requires the activation of specific cell factors to develop. Until very recently it was thought that the most important factor in the formation of the portal–systemic collaterals was the dilation of preexistent embryonic channels by the increase in portal venous pressure[4,5]. Very recently, studies performed in portal-hypertensive mice have demonstrated that these animals have a marked and progressive overexpression of vascular endothelial growth factor (VEGF) in splanchnic tissues, and that the administration of a monoclonal antibody against VEGF receptor-2 causes a marked, significant inhibition of the formation of portal–systemic collateral vessels, as indicated by a 40–50% reduction in the extent of portal–systemic shunting of radioactive microspheres injected into the spleen[6]. This finding highlights the importance

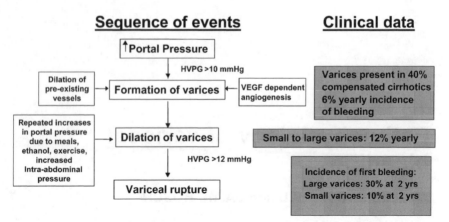

**Figure 1.** Chain of events leading to variceal ruptures

of angiogenesis in portal hypertension and opens new fields for the treatment of this syndrome.

## HEMODYNAMIC FACTORS

As in any vascular system, the pressure gradient along the portal venous system depends on the relationship between the flow within this vascular system and the resistance that impedes that flow. According to Ohm's law:

$$\text{Pressure gradient} = \text{Blood flow} \times \text{Resistance}$$

Therefore, changes in portal pressure can be related to changes in the flow and resistance in the portal system, including the portal vein and the hepatic and portocollateral circulations. When collaterals begin to develop, the portal venous inflow increases because of splanchnic vasodilation. Such an increased portal venous inflow (the sum of the portal and the collateral blood flow) represents an important factor maintaining and worsening the portal pressure elevation[7]. When collateralization is extensive, factors modulating the collateral resistance become important determinants of portal pressure.

### Increased portal pressure

As already stated, increased portal pressure is the initial and most important factor leading to the development of portal–systemic collaterals (Figure 1). Portal hypertension is initiated by an increased resistance to portal blood flow which in cirrhosis is in part due to an insufficient release of nitric oxide in the hepatic circulation and increased release of hepatic vasoconstrictors[8,9].

In patients with cirrhosis and portal hypertension, a threshold increase in the portal pressure gradient (most commonly evaluated in clinical practice by its equivalent, the hepatic venous pressure gradient or HVPG) has been established for the development and rupture of esophageal varices (12 mmHg)[10–13]. The same threshold is probably required to trigger splanchnic vasodilation, with increased portal blood flow and, ultimately, for the hyperkinetic circulatory syndrome of cirrhosis.

The significance of this threshold value has been defined by longitudinal studies showing that patients in whom the portal pressure gradient is reduced below 12 mmHg – by means of pharmacological therapy[14,15], TIPS[16] or spontaneously[17,18] – are almost totally protected from the risk of experiencing variceal bleeding on follow-up. Two of these studies actually reported a prolonged actuarial survival probability in the group of patients decreasing the HVPG to less than 12 mmHg[14,18]. This points out the reversibility of the portal hypertension syndrome; also, even if the HVPG is not reduced below threshold values, patients decreasing HVPG substantially (i.e. more than 20% of baseline) have a pronounced reduction in the risk of variceal bleeding and rebleeding[15,17,19,20].

Above this threshold increase in HVPG, however, there is no clear relationship between the magnitude of the portal pressure elevation and the risk of hemorrhage[13]. However, as shown by recent studies in which the HVPG was measured very early during variceal hemorrhage, the magnitude of HVPG elevation is a strong, independent predictor of failure to control bleeding and of early rebleeding in patients with cirrhosis[21].

On the other hand, it has been suggested that repeated, brisk increases in portal pressure, associated with physiologic circumstances (meals[22], ethanol intake[23], circadian rhythms[24], physical exercise[25] and increased intra-abdominal pressure[26]), and other events (splanchnic angiography[27], hepatic artery to portal vein fistulas and acute alcoholic hepatitis), could play a key role in determining the progressive dilation of the varices.

## Increased blood flow

The amount of blood flow diverted from the portal to systemic circulation through the gastroesophageal collaterals is thought to be another important factor in the formation, dilation and rupture of the varices[13]. This is suggested by the findings of hemodynamic studies evaluating azygos blood flow, an index of blood flow through gastroesophageal collaterals, in portal hypertensive patients. These studies showed a close and exponential relationship between portal pressure and azygos blood flow, as well as a parallelism between the presence and size of the varices and the increase in azygos blood flow[28,29].

## Factors modulating collateral resistance

The vascular resistance of the collateral vessels, although lower than that of the obstructed portal system, is nevertheless higher than normal portal resistance[7,30]. Hence, the development of portal–systemic collaterals does not lead to the normalization of portal pressure, even in the extreme situation in which all portal flow is diverted to the systemic circulation[31].

As expressed by Poiseuille's law, resistance across a vascular system ($R$) can be defined as:

$$R = 8nl/\pi r^4$$

where $n$ is the viscosity of blood, $r$ is the radius of the vessel, and $l$ is the length of the vessel. It follows that changes in vascular resistance mainly depend on variations in the size (radius) of the vessel.

The collateral vessels have vascular smooth muscle cells in their walls, which, by contraction or relaxation, are able to modify vessel diameter according to the presence or absence of different vasoactive stimulus: beta-adrenergic (which mediates vasodilation in portal–systemic collaterals)[32], alpha-adrenergic[33], serotoninergic[33], nitric oxide[34], vasopressin[33], endothelin[33], among others.

The effect of beta-blockers on portal collateral resistance may explain why the administration of propranolol causes greater decreases in portal pressure in animal models and in cirrhotic patients with a small degree of collateralization (i.e. animals with $CCl_4$-induced cirrhosis and cirrhotic patients without gastroesophageal varices, respectively) than in those with extensive collaterals (i.e. portal vein-ligated rats and patients with gastroesophageal varices)[30,35,36].

Nevertheless, a randomized controlled trial of prevention of variceal development in cirrhotic patients without varices has failed to demonstrate the efficacy of timolol, a non-selective beta-blocker, in that setting[37]. This lack of efficacy may be related to the inability of timolol to decrease the HVPG below threshold values in the studied population[37].

## Variceal pressure

Following the development of gastroesophageal varices, variceal pressure plays an important role determining variceal hemorrhage. Previous studies have shown that variceal pressure was greater in patients with large varices compared to those with small varices, and in patients with previous bleeding as compared with those who have never bled[11,38,39]. This suggests that a lower resistance in the collaterals feeding the varices increases variceal pressure and the risk of bleeding.

Variceal pressure has been identified as an independent predictor of the evolution of an acute variceal bleeding episode, of the risk of first variceal hemorrhage, and of the risk of variceal rebleeding during pharmacologic therapy. Ruiz del Árbol et al. showed that variceal pressures greater than 18 mmHg during the acute bleeding episode were frequently associated with failure to control bleeding and early rebleeding[39]. Nevens et al. published the results of a prospective investigation in cirrhotic patients showing that a variceal pressure above 15.2 mmHg is a strong risk factor predicting the first variceal hemorrhage[40].

Finally, in patients receiving pharmacologic therapy, a decrease in variceal pressure from baseline of 20% or more was associated with a very low actuarial probability of variceal bleeding on follow-up (7% at 3 years). Patients considered non-responders by this measurement had a 46% rate of variceal bleeding during the same time-period[20]. Altogether, these findings suggest that transmural variceal pressure plays a major role in the pathogenesis of variceal bleeding.

## Variceal size

Several studies have shown that patients who have previously bled from varices have larger varices that those who have not[11,12,41]. In addition, prospective studies have shown that patients with large varices (defined as those with a diameter $> 5$ mm) have a higher risk of variceal hemorrhage compared to patients with small varices ($< 5$ mm in diameter)[41–43]. As previously mentioned, big varices have also been shown to have higher variceal pressure than small ones[12,44]. However, clinical studies have found that 14–28% of patients with variceal hemorrhage had small varices[11,42], indicating that size *per se* does not allow us to discriminate the risk of bleeding.

Furthermore, it should be taken into account that endoscopy is not the best method for measuring variceal size, due to lack of objectivity and low reproducibility. Miller et al[45]. investigated the value of the cross-sectional area (CSA) of esophageal varices measured by using a 20-MHz endosonographic probe in predicting the risk of variceal bleeding. The authors studied 28 patients with no prior history of variceal bleeding, in whom they calculated the sum of the CSA of all the varices identified at the point where the varices appeared the largest. A cutoff value of CSA of 0.45 cm$^2$ was identified as that having the highest sensitivity (83%) and specificity (75%) for determining future bleeding[45]. This observation is not surprising considering that the size of the varices is a key factor determining variceal wall tension according to Laplace's law (see below).

## Variceal wall thickness

Due to its location in the lamina propria, esophageal varices have a thin wall and lack of tissue support, facilitating their progressive dilation and additional slimming of the vessel wall as flow and pressure inside the varix increase[13]. These findings agree with the clinical observation that presence at endoscopy of red color signs, such as the red wale markings, red spots and reddish discoloration of the variceal wall, is an independent predictor of the risk of bleeding from esophageal or fundal varices[41]. The red color signs are thought to correspond to areas where the variceal wall is extremely thin.

## Variceal wall tension

The above discussion considered several factors involved in the pathophysiology of variceal bleeding, but that by themselves are unable to explain the mechanism of variceal rupture. However, all these factors are mutually interrelated in the concept of variceal wall tension, which is presently accepted as the key factor in variceal rupture[12,13]. Variceal wall tension is the force generated by the variceal wall opposing further distension. According to Frank's modification of Laplace's law, variceal wall tension is directly proportional to the transmural variceal pressure (the difference between intravariceal and esophageal luminal pressure) and the radius of the varix, and inversely proportional to the thickness of the variceal wall (Figure 2). Variceal bleeding is thought to occur when the tension exerted over the thin wall of the varices goes beyond a critical value determined by the elastic limit of the vessel (Figure 3)[13].

This pathophysiologic concept fits perfectly with clinical observations showing that increased variceal pressure, increased variceal size and presence

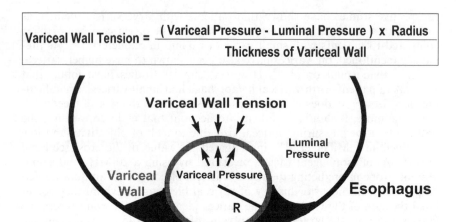

$$\text{Variceal Wall Tension} = \frac{(\text{Variceal Pressure - Luminal Pressure}) \times \text{Radius}}{\text{Thickness of Variceal Wall}}$$

**Figure 2.** Laplace's Law applied to esophageal varices explains how different factors interact in the pathophysiology of variceal bleeding

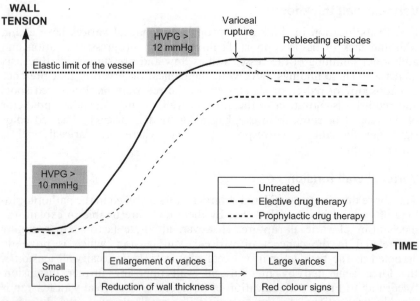

**Figure 3.** Natural history of variceal bleeding as a function of variceal wall tension. The solid line illustrates the evolution of untreated patients. Variceal wall tension increases markedly as a result of an increase in HVPG above threshold for variceal formation, enlargement of the varices, and reduction of variceal wall thickness. Once wall tension increases to values exceeding the elastic limit of the varices, the patient may experience his first bleeding episode. After this the patient remains at a high risk of rebleeding unless wall tension is decreased. This is achieved by reducing HVPG to < 12 mmHg (optimal response) or by > 20% of baseline pretreatment values (good response). Primary prophylaxis protects from the risk of bleeding by preventing or delaying variceal wall tension reaching the rupture point

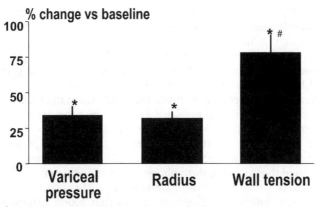

**Figure 4.** Summary of the changes caused by the acute increase of intra-abdominal pressure on variceal pressure, radius and wall tension

of red color signs are, alone or in combination, predictors of the risk of variceal bleeding[12,39–43].

The elastic limit of the varix is influenced by external tissue support, which is almost nil in the varices. Experimental studies using artificial varices have shown that, in vessels without tissue support, wall tension increases disproportionately to rises in transmural pressure[13]. Clinically, this phenomenon explains why esophageal varices bleed and paraesophageal varices and other collaterals, although frequently being greater in size, do not.

Few studies have assessed variceal wall tension in patients with cirrhosis. Rigau et al.[12] estimated variceal wall tension by the combination of the endoscopic measurement of variceal pressure and the semiquantitative estimation of variceal size. Their results showed that bleeders had significantly higher values of "estimated" wall tension than non-bleeders[12]. More recently, wall tension has been calculated from objective measurements of variceal diameter using endosonography, combined with the endoscopic measurement of variceal pressure. Such a combined technique has shown that increasing intra-abdominal pressure, as it occurs in patients with ascites or abdominal muscle strain, significantly increases variceal pressure, variceal volume and variceal wall tension, suggesting that increased intra-abdominal pressure may contribute to the progressive dilation that precedes the rupture of the varices (Figure 4)[26]. Pharmacologic therapy with beta-blockers significantly decreased these parameters, which may correlate with its clinical efficacy[46].

## Increased blood volume

An increased blood volume is a constant finding in portal hypertension. This plays a key role in maintaining the hyperkinetic circulation of portal hypertension[47]. The administration of a low-sodium diet and spironolactone in patients with compensated cirrhosis reverses the increase in blood volume and significantly reduces portal pressure[47,48]. Interestingly, portal hypertensive animals maintained on a low sodium diet since the induction of portal hypertension had a diminished formation of collaterals compared to animals kept on normal sodium intake[47]. Altogether, these results suggest that an increased blood volume may contribute to the formation of collaterals.

Moreover, acute increments of intravascular volume may lead to a further increase in portal and variceal pressure, and thereby promote variceal hemorrhage in patients already with high variceal wall tension (close to the elastic limit of the vessel). This situation is best exemplified by the patient in whom hemostasis from variceal bleeding has recently been achieved. In this case an expansion of the intravascular volume may precipitate variceal rebleeding. Blood volume restitution should be done with great care and very conservatively, since experimental studies have shown that blood volume restitution after a hemorrhage may produce an increase of portal pressure beyond baseline values[49] and that blood replacement worsens the hemorrhage[50]. The hypovolemia caused by bleeding elicits reflex splanchnic vasoconstriction, which reduces portocollateral blood flow and portal pressure, which tends to spontaneously arrest the bleeding. This is reverted, and even aggravated, by blood transfusion.

## ANATOMICAL FACTORS

As previously mentioned, whenever portal pressure rises above normal values, collateral circulation begins to develop in an attempt to decompress the portal system. In humans, different anastomotic venous systems between portal and systemic circulations have been described[3]. The most common and important collaterals are the cephalad vessels, formed through the dilation of the left gastric (coronary) vein and the short gastric veins. The left gastric vein arises from the portal vein and is the main factor responsible for the development of esophageal varices. The short gastric veins, arising from the splenic vein, are responsible for the dilation of fundal and gastroesophageal varices, in association with the polar gastric vein when present.

The palisade zone of the esophagus acts as the critical area for variceal rupture[4] due to its physiologic role as spontaneous communication between the portal and systemic circulations, through the azygos venous system. In chronic portal hypertension this zone becomes congestive due to an increased pressure and blood flow[5]. The perforating or transitional zone is characterized by having tortuous and dilated vessels running in the submucosa and connected with the paraesophageal venous system by perforating veins. In portal hypertension these vessels dilate, become incompetent and, due to the continuous variations in pressure with the respiratory cycle, allow retrograde and turbulent blood flow from the paraesophageal to the submucosal veins. This has been proposed as another important mechanism for the development of esophageal varices (Figure 5)[51].

It has been further hypothesized that decreases in lower esophageal sphincter (LES) pressure may play a role in the development of varices[51]. In that regard some studies suggest a beneficial effects of drugs such as metoclopram-

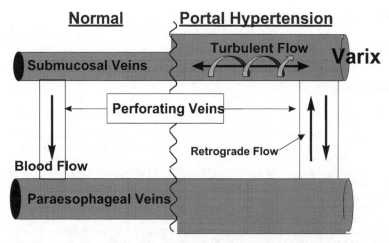

**Figure 5.** The perforating veins connect the paraesophageal and submucosal venous plexuses. These veins are dilated in portal hypertension and become incompetent, facilitating retrograde flow from the paraesophageal veins into the esophageal varices and creating turbulences. These factors, together with the increased portal pressure and collateral blood flow, contribute to the dilation of the varices.

ide, domperidone and pentagastrin, that increase LES pressure and reduce blood flow through the esophageal varices, azygos blood flow and variceal pressure[52,53].

## PERSISTENCE OF VARICEAL HEMORRHAGE

Once varices bleed, the factors determining the severity and continuation of the hemorrhage may differ from those that have initiated the bleeding[13]. Although multiple factors could be involved, the severity of bleeding is thought to be directly proportional to variceal pressure and to the area of the varix rent and inversely proportional to blood viscosity[13]. Blood viscosity is inversely related to the hematocrit. Thus, expansion with crystalloid fluids or anemia may decrease viscosity and increase bleeding after variceal rupture. In addition, experimental studies have shown that changes in blood hemoglobin result in nitric oxide-mediated changes in vascular tone, due to the fact that hemoglobin is an important physiologic inactivator of nitric oxide[54]. Thus, a reduced hemoglobin concentration contributes to aggravate splanchnic vasodilation.

The area of variceal rent can be physiologically modified by an efficient primary hemostasis. This may explain why advanced cirrhotics, with more severe coagulopathy, usually have more severe bleeding episodes. Interestingly, the coagulopathy of cirrhosis is markedly improved by rFVIIa[55,56], which in a recent double-blind placebo-controlled randomized controlled trial has been shown to improve the outcome of bleeding in Child–Pugh B and C cirrhotic patients[57].

## Acknowledgements

This work was supported in part by grants from the Instituto de Salud Carlos III (C03/02) and the Fondo de Investigación Sanitaria (PI 02/0739).

## References

1. D'Amico G, Pagliaro L, Bosch J. Pharmacological treatment of portal hypertension: an evidence-based approach. Semin Liver Dis. 1999;19:475–505.
2. Pagliaro L, D'Amico G, Pasta L et al. Portal hypertension in cirrhosis: natural history. In: Bosch J, Groszmann RJ, editors. Portal Hypertension: Pathophysiology and Treatment. Oxford: Blackwell Science, 1992:72–92.
3. Vianna A. Anatomy of the portal venous system in portal hypertension. In: McIntyre N, Benhamou JP, Bircher J, Rizzetto M, Rodés J, editors. Oxford Textbook of Clinical Hepatology. Oxford: Oxford University Press, 1991:393–9.
4. Noda T. Angioarchitectural study of esophageal varices (with special reference to variceal rupture). Virchows Arch A. 1984;404:381–92.
5. Spence RAJ. The venous anatomy of the lower esophagus in normal subjects and in patients with varices: an image analysis study. Br J Surg. 1984;71:739–44.
6. Fernández M, Vizzutti F, García-Pagán JC et al. Anti-VEGF receptor-2 monoclonal antibody prevents portal–systemic collateral vessel formation in portal hypertensive mice. Gastroenterology. 2004;126:886–94.
7. Vorobioff J, Bredfeldt JE, Groszmann RJ. Increased blood flow through the portal system in cirrhotic rats. Gastroenterology. 1984;87:1120–6.
8. Gupta TK, Toruner M, Chung MK, Groszmann RJ. Endothelial dysfunction and decreased production of nitric oxide in the intrahepatic microcirculation of cirrhotic rats. Hepatology. 1988;28:926–31.
9. Rockey DC, Chung JJ. Reduced nitric oxide production by endothelial cells in cirrhotic rat liver: endothelial dysfunction in portal hypertension. Gastroenterology. 1998;114:344–51.
10. Viallet A, Marleau D, Huet PM et al. Hemodynamic evaluation of patients with intrahepatic portal hypertension. Relationship between bleeding varices and the portohepatic gradient. Gastroenterology. 1975;69:1297–300.
11. García-Tsao G, Groszmann RJ, Fisher Rl et al. Portal pressure, presence of gastroesophageal varices and variceal bleeding. Hepatology. 1985;5:419–24.
12. Rigau J, Bosch J, Bordas JM et al. Endoscopic measurement of variceal pressure in cirrhosis: correlation with portal pressure and variceal hemorrhage. Gastroenterology. 1989;96: 873–80.
13. Polio J, Groszmann RJ. Hemodynamic factors involved in the development and rupture of esophageal varices: a pathophysiologic approach to treatment. Semin Liver Dis. 1986; 6:318–31.
14. Groszmann RJ, Bosch J, Grace N et al. Hemodynamic events in a prospective randomized trial of propranolol vs placebo in the prevention of the first variceal hemorrhage. Gastroenterology. 1990;99:1401–7.
15. Feu F, García-Pagán JC, Bosch J et al. Relation between portal pressure response to pharmacotherapy and risk of recurrent variceal hemorrhage in patients with cirrhosis. Lancet. 1995;346:1056–9.
16. Casado M, Bosch J, García-Pagán JC et al. Clinical events following TIPS: correlation with hemodynamic findings. Gastroenterology. 1998;114:1296–303.
17. Villanueva C, Balanzó J, Novella MT et al. Nadolol plus isosorbide-5-mononitrate compared to sclerotherapy for the prevention of variceal rebleeding. N Engl J Med. 1996;334:1624–34.
18. Villanueva C, Minana J, Ortiz J et al. Endoscopic ligation compared with combined treatment with nadolol and isosorbide mononitrate to prevent recurrent variceal bleeding. N Engl J Med. 2001;345:647–55.
19. Vorobioff J, Groszmann RJ, Picabea E et al. Prognostic value of hepatic venous pressure gradient measurements in alcoholic cirrhosis: a 10-year prospective study. Gastroenterology. 1996;111:701–9.

20. Escorsell A, Bordas JM, Castañeda B et al. Predictive value of the variceal pressure response to continued pharmacogical therapy in patients with cirrhosis and portal hypertension. Hepatology. 2000;31:1061–7.
21. Moitinho E, Escorsell A, Bandi JC et al. Prognostic value of early measurements of portal pressure in acute variceal hemorrhage. Gastroenterology. 1999;117:626–31.
22. McCormick PA, Dick R, Graffeo M et al. The effect of non-protein liquid meals on the hepatic venous pressure gradient in patients with cirrhosis. J Hepatol. 1990;11:221–5.
23. Luca A, García-Pagán JC, Bosch J et al. Effects of ethanol consumption on hepatic hemodynamics in patients with alcoholic cirrhosis. Gastroenterology. 1997;112:1291–6.
24. García-Pagán JC, Feu F, Castells A et al. Circadian variations of portal pressure and variceal hemorrhage in patients with cirrhosis. Hepatology. 1994;19:595–601.
25. García-Pagán JC, Santos C, Barberá JA et al. Physical exercise increases portal pressure in patients with cirrhosis and portal hypertension. Gastroenterology. 1996;111:1300–6.
26. Escorsell A, Ginès A, Llach J et al. Increasing intra-abdominal pressure increases pressure, volume and wall tension in esophageal varices. Hepatology. 2002;36:936–40.
27. Bredfeldt JE, Bosch J, Groszmann RJ. Splanchnic angiography increases portal pressure in portal-hypertensive patients. Hepatology. 1982;2:684 (abstract).
28. Bosch J, Groszmann RJ. Measurement of azygos venous blood flow by a continuous thermodilution technique: an index of blood flow through gastroesophageal collaterals in cirrhosis. Hepatology. 1984;4:424–9.
29. Bosch J, Mastai R, Kravetz D et al. Measurement of azygos venous blood flow in the evaluation of portal hypertension in patients with cirrhosis: clinical and hemodynamic correlations in 100 patients. J Hepatol. 1985;1:125–39.
30. Kroeger RJ, Groszmann RJ. Increased portal venous resistance hinders portal pressure reduction during the administration of beta-adrenergic blocking agents in a portal hypertensive model. Hepatology. 1985;5:97–101.
31. Sikuler E, Kravetz D, Groszmann RJ. Evolution of portal hypertension and mechanisms involved in its maintenance in a rat model. Am J Physiol. 1985;248:G618–25.
32. Mosca P, Lee FY, Kaumann AJ, Groszmann RJ. Pharmacology of portal–systemic collaterals in portal hypertensive rats: role of endothelium. Am J Physiol. 1992;263:G544–50.
33. Moreno L, Martínez-Cuesta MA, Piqué JM et al. Anatomical differences in responsiveness to vasoconstrictors in the mesenteric vein from normal and portal-hypertensive rats. Naunyn-Schmiedeberg's Arch Pharmacol. 1996;354:474–80.
34. Lee FY, Albillos A, Colombato LA, Groszmann RJ. The role of nitric oxide in the vascular hyporesponsiveness to methoxamine in portal hypertensive rats. Hepatology. 1992;16: 1043–8.
35. Pizcueta MP, de Lacy AM, Kravetz D et al. Propranolol decreases portal pressure without changing portocollateral resistance in cirrhotic rats. Hepatology. 1989;10:953–7.
36. Escorsell A, Ferayorni L, Bosch J et al. The portal pressure response to beta-blockade is greater in cirrhotic patients without varices than in those with varices. Gastroenterology. 1997;112:2012–16.
37. Groszmann RJ, García-Tsao G, Makuch R et al. Multicenter randomized placebo-controlled trial of non-selective beta-blockers in prevention of the complications of portal hypertension: final results and identification of a predictive factor. Hepatology. 2003;38 (Suppl. 1):206A.
38. Feu F, Bordas JM, Luca A et al. Reduction of variceal pressure by propranolol: comparison of the effects on portal pressure and azygos blood flow in patients with cirrhosis. Hepatology. 1993;18:1082–9.
39. Ruiz del Árbol L, Martín de Argila C, Vázquez M et al. Endoscopic measurement of variceal pressure during hemorrhage from esophageal varices. Hepatology. 1992;16:147 (abstract).
40. Nevens F, Fevery J. Variceal pressure predicts a first variceal hemorrhage: a prospective cohort study. Hepatology. 1996;24:209 (abstract).
41. North Italian Endoscopic Club for the Study and Treatment of Esophageal Varices. Prediction of the first variceal hemorrhage in patients with cirrhosis of the liver and esophageal varices. N Engl J Med. 1988;13:983–9.
42. Lebrec D, De Fleuny P, Rueff B et al. Portal hypertension, size of the varices and risk of gastrointestinal bleeding in alcoholic cirrhosis. Gastroenterology. 1980;79:1139–44.
43. Zoli M, Merkel C, Magalotti D et al. Evaluation of a new endoscopic index to predict first bleeding from the upper gastrointestinal tract in patients with cirrhosis. Hepatology. 1996;24:1047–52.

44. Nevens F, Sprengers D, Feu F et al. Measurement of variceal pressure with an endoscopic pressure sensitive gauge: validation and effect of propranolol therapy in chronic conditions. J Hepatol. 1996;24:66–73.
45. Miller L, Banson FL, Bazir K et al. Risk of esophageal variceal bleeding based on endoscopic ultrasound evaluation of the sum of esophageal variceal cross-sectional surface area. Am J Gastroenterol. 2003;98:454–9.
46. Escorsell A, Bordas JM, Feu F et al. Endoscopic assessment of variceal volume and wall tension in cirrhotic patients: effects of pharmacological therapy. Gastroenterology. 1997;113:1640–6.
47. Genecin P, Polio J, Groszmann RJ. Na restriction blunts expansion of plasma volume and ameliorates hyperdynamic circulation in portal hypertension. Am J Physiol. 1990;259: G498–503.
48. García-Pagán JC, Salmerón JM, Feu F et al. Effects of low sodium diet and spironolactone on portal pressure in patients with compensated cirrhosis. Hepatology. 1994;19:1095–9.
49. Kravetz D, Bosch J, Arderiu M et al. Hemodynamic effects of blood volume restitution following a hemorrhage in rats with portal hypertension due to cirrhosis of the liver: influence of the extent of portal–systemic shunting. Hepatology. 1989;9:808–14.
50. Castañeda B, Morales J, Lionetti R et al. Effects of blood volume restitution following a portal hypertensive-related bleeding in anesthetized cirrhotic rats. Hepatology. 2001;33:821–5.
51. McCormack TT, Rose JD, Smith PM, Johnson AG. Perforating veins and blood flow in esophageal varices. Lancet. 1983;2:1442–4.
52. Mastai R, Grande L, Bosch J et al. Effects of metoclopramide and domperidone on azygos venous blood flow in patients with cirrhosis and portal hypertension. Hepatology. 1986;6:1244–7.
53. Saraya A, Sarin SK. Effects of intravenous nitroglycerin and metoclopramide on intravariceal pressure: a double-blind, randomized study. Am J Gastroenterol. 1993;88:1850–3.
54. Casadevall M, Piqué JM, Cirera I et al. Increased blood hemoglobin attenuates splanchnic vasodilation in portal-hypertensive rats by nitric oxide inactivation. Gastroenterology. 1996;110:1156–65.
55. Bernstein DE, Jeffers L, Erhardtsen E et al. Recombinant factor VIIa corrects prothrombin time in cirrhotic patients: a preliminary study. Gastroenterology. 1997;113:1930–7.
56. Ejlersen E, Melsen T, Ingerslev J et al. Recombinant activated factor VII (rFVIIa) acutely normalizes prothrombin time in patients with cirrhosis during bleeding from oesophageal varices. Scand J Gastroenterol. 2001;36:1081–5.
57. Thabut D, de Franchis R, Bendtsen F et al. Efficacy of activated recombinant factor VII (rFVIIa; Novoseven) in cirrhotic patients with upper gastrointestinal bleeding: a randomised placebo-controlled double-blind multicenter trial. J Hepatol. 2003;38(Suppl. 2):13A.

# 19
# Approaches to the management of pediatric portal hypertension: results of an informal survey

BENJAMIN L. SHNEIDER

## INTRODUCTION

Portal hypertension and its related complications are major clinical issues in pediatric hepatology. The leading cause of significant liver disease in children is biliary atresia. The biliary injury in this disorder is associated with prominent portal hypertension at disease stages where synthetic liver function is typically intact. Thus the relative contribution of complications of portal hypertension to morbidity and mortality in liver disease is greater in children than in adults. In children with biliary atresia, prominent portal hypertension is often present at the time of corrective hepatoportoenterostomy (Kasai procedure) and it progresses over relatively short periods of time[1]. The rate of progression of the portal hypertension is related to outcome after hepatoportoenterostomy, with more accelerated progression in children with failed procedures or with recurrent cholangitis[2]. Complications that are a direct result of this portal hypertension are common. Variceal hemorrhage occurs in a large percentage of children, often within the first 5 years of life[2-7]. Ascites, hepatopulmonary syndrome, rectal varices/colopathy, stomal hemorrhage, and pulmonary hypertension have also been described in children with biliary atresia[8-13].

Evidence-based approaches to the management of portal hypertension in children do not exist[14]. This is in stark contrast to the extensive array of randomized trials and meta-analyses that have been performed in adults[15]. Pediatric hepatologists must instead rely on their clinical experience and a growing anecdotal pediatric literature in the context of the previously mentioned adult experience. In order to ascertain current management approaches in pediatric portal hypertension, a survey was recently sent to 35 pediatric gastroenterologists at 35 different centers who have practices that concentrate on the care of children with liver disease. Anonymous responses were obtained from 30 of these individuals. The survey was not intended to ascertain the "correct" approach, but instead to investigate the range of practices that exist in the setting of a lack of pediatric-specific evidence-based approaches.

The survey, which investigated several aspects of portal hypertension, was conducted in the context of the following case:

> The following questions pertain to an 8-year-old child who is status post-portoenterostomy for biliary atresia. He is clinically well with the exception of portal hypertension. In particular he has normal growth and development and no history of complications of his liver disease. Pertinent laboratory findings include: platelet count 65 000, albumin 3.3 g/dl, total bilirubin 1.6 mg/dl, prothrombin time 13.2 s.

Several questions were then asked related to surveillance, primary prophylaxis, acute management, and secondary prophylaxis.

## SURVEILLANCE

### Esophageal varices

> Do you perform surveillance procedures to look for esophageal varices? (yes 63%, no 37%). If yes, what procedure do you use? (endoscopy 79%, esophagram 5%, ultrasound 26%). If yes, what is the frequency of your surveillance? (6 months 15%, 12 months 78%, 24 months 7%).

Surveillance for varices in children is typically performed by endoscopy (79%). Surveillance endoscopy in children typically requires significant sedation and/or general anesthesia. As an invasive procedure it is justified only if there is a significant benefit to be derived from the identification of varices. Presumably the 37% of centers that do not perform surveillance have chosen this method because of a lack of perceived benefit, while the remainder have concluded that there are potential benefits. One benefit might be prognostic, especially in children who live in remote locations where documentation of presumably worrisome varices might impact on management approaches and counseling. In adults the finding of large varices portends a poor immediate prognosis[16]. Special care must be taken in direct application of this finding to children, as the types of diseases that predispose to the development of cirrhosis in adults are quite different from those in children. In most circumstances cirrhosis in adults is the result of hepatocellular diseases such as hepatitis C or alcohol-related disease. In these disorders complications of portal hypertension are late manifestations and occur at a time when hepatic reserve may be low. In contrast, pediatric cholestatic disorders such as biliary atresia appear to have much more significant portal hypertension early in the course of the disease. Variceal hemorrhage alone does not necessarily predict higher mortality in children with biliary atresia[6].

### Hepatopulmonary syndrome

> Do you perform screening for hepatopulmonary syndrome? (yes 58%, no 42%). If yes, what method do you use for screening? (oxygen satura-

tion 87%, contrast echocardiography 27%, macroaggregated albumin scanning 13%).

The prevalence of hepatopulmonary syndrome in children with cirrhosis is not well characterized, although two large studies have revealed markedly different results[9,17]. Universal screening might, at a minimum, clarify the prevalence of this problem. Transcutaneous oxygen saturation measurement in the upright position (87%) is a simple and reliable screening method for physiologically significant desaturation, while contrast echocardiography (27%) is exceptionally sensitive in identifying intrapulmonic shunting. Macroaggegated albumin scanning (13%) is an involved nuclear imaging study that can quantify the degree of shunting and may clarify the role of shunting in children with underlying pulmonary disease (e.g. cystic fibrosis). Despite the potential simplicity of screening, 42% of centers do not do so, presumably because of the lack of consensus of the management of affected children. The natural history of the child with mild shunting has not been well described; however, identification of significant hepatopulmonary syndrome may ultimately impact on management decisions, especially as they pertain to portosystemic shunting and liver transplantation.

## PRIMARY PROPHYLAXIS

Do you institute prophylactic treatment prior to variceal bleeding? (yes 84%, no 16%). If yes, please list your approach (β-blocker 88%, sclerotherapy 6%, band ligation 38%).

Surveillance endoscopy is typically predicated upon the concept of primary prophylaxis of variceal hemorrhage. Interestingly 16% of respondents performed surveillance procedures presumably for purposes of determining prognosis, as there was no plan for primary prophylaxis. The use of non-specific β-blockers for primary prophylaxis of varices, which is well accepted in adults, leads to a statistically significant reduction in the risk of variceal hemorrhage; however, one must treat 10 patients for life in order to prevent one episode of bleeding[18,19]. A beneficial effect on mortality is more difficult to demonstrate. Unfortunately, the hemodynamic parameters for effective β-blockade in children are unknown. Eighty-eight percent of the respondents depend upon anecdotal studies that suggest dosing ranges and indicate presumed safety[20-23]. The use of prophylactic band ligation in adults is controversial. The reduced rates of complications associated with band ligation therapy relative to sclerotherapy have increased the enthusiasm for banding as an endoscopic approach to primary prophylaxis. In adults it appears that risk of hemorrhage after ligation is reduced relative to β-blocker therapy, although this does not translate into a change in mortality[24]; therefore it appears that the use of prophylactic band ligation in children (38%) is in response to results of published studies in adults. This is a relatively invasive approach in children, where the benefit is not known.

## ACUTE THERAPY

In the event of hemodynamically significant acute gastrointestinal bleeding do you perform endoscopy? (yes 100%, no 0%). If yes, immediately

(20%) or after medical treatment (80%). What is included in your approach to hemodynamically significant acute gastrointestinal bleeding (check all that are used)? Nasogastric tube (80%), intravenous antibiotics (13%), vasopressin (10%), somatostatin (10%), octreotide (93% typically 1–2 μg/kg per hour), occlusion tube (13%), endoscopic (7%).

In one of the only universally agreed-upon management issues, endoscopy was recommended for all patients. The importance of identification of the source of hemorrhage is well understood[25]. Few centers (20%) prefer to perform emergent endoscopy, but instead most medically stabilize patients prior to diagnostic/therapeutic endoscopy. The lack of uniform use of nasogastric tubes (20% not recommending) in the early management of variceal hemorrhage is surprising. There is clear benefit to monitoring the rate of bleeding. More importantly, removal of gastric blood may reduce portal pressures and therefore reduce on-going bleeding and/or the risk of recurrent hemorrhage[26]. Octreotide appears to be the vasoactive agent of choice (93%), despite a lack of clear data in adults demonstrating efficacy in the setting of acute variceal hemorrhage[27]. Antibiotic usage (13%) was not typically part of the management of acute variceal hemorrhage, although there is growing evidence that this is being reconsidered by many centers[28].

## SECONDARY PROPHYLAXIS

The following questions pertain to the same 8-year-old child who is status post-portoenterostomy for biliary atresia. He has had a hemodynamically significant esophageal varix bleed, which required a single red blood cell transfusion. He is clinically stable after initial medical management. Your recommendation for secondary prophylaxis of variceal hemorrhage for this particular patient would include which of the following: β-blockade (54%), sclerotherapy (15%), band ligation (88%), TIPS (0%), surgical shunt (4%), transplantation (0%).

A combination of β-blocker therapy and endoscopic band ligation appears to be the general consensus (54%) to the approach for prevention of recurrent hemorrhage. The use of band ligation over sclerotherapy is supported by the only randomized pediatric portal hypertension related trial that has been published to date[29]. Although this study examined children with extra-hepatic portal vein obstruction, the findings are likely to be applicable to biliary atresia. The use of combined therapy is in line with current approaches for adults, although it is not clear if β-blockade alone (one center) is a potentially less invasive option for initial secondary prophylaxis in children. It is worth noting that no center views variceal hemorrhage as an indication for immediate transplantation. This is consistent with a recent report that indicates a favorable long-term prognosis after first variceal hemorrhage in children with functioning portoenterostomies[6].

## SECONDARY PROPHYLAXIS: RECURRENT HEMORRHAGE

In the circumstance of recurrent esophageal varix hemorrhage 8 months after successful prior therapy (above) what is your recommendation for this specific patient (other clinical parameters unchanged); β-blockade (15%), sclerotherapy (4%), band ligation (38%), TIPS (38%), surgical shunt (15%), transplantation (38%).

The prevention of recurrent hemorrhage is clearly the most controversial. A significant number of respondents chose to continue and/or reapply the previous treatment strategy, despite this early rebleeding episode. TIPS is a common choice (38%) in spite of concerns about long-term patency in both children and adults. Recurrent hemorrhage is an apparent indication for some (38%) to proceed with liver transplantation in the setting of relatively intact liver function and evidence of adequate bile flow. Interestingly, only 13% of centers recommended the use of surgical portosystemic shunting, despite its potential long-term palliation of the portal hypertension in this child[30–32]. It is unclear whether this represents excessive concern for the risk of the development of encephalopathy, or whether it indicates a lack of recent surgical expertise with this procedure in young children.

In summary, the lack of consensus in the approach to the management of portal hypertension in children is understandable given the absence of evidence-based studies. This survey and review of the pediatric literature clearly highlight the great need for prospective collaborative investigations of optimal treatment of pediatric portal hypertension.

## Acknowledgements

The insights, guidance and assistance of Dr William Balistreri in the compilation and interpretation of the survey is greatly appreciated. The author also thanks the survey respondents for their cooperation and input with this questionnaire. This work was presented in part at the 51st Annual Meeting of the American Association for the Study of Liver Disease, 10 November 2001, Dallas, TX.

## References

1. Kasai M, Okamoto A, Ohi R, Yabe K, Matsumura Y. Changes of portal vein pressure and intrahepatic blood vessels after surgery for biliary atresia. J Pediatr Surg. 1981;16:152–9.
2. Miyata M, Satani M, Ueda T, Okamoto E. Long-term results of hepatic portoenterostomy for biliary atresia: special reference to postoperative portal hypertension. Surgery. 1974;76:234–7.
3. Lilly JR, Stellin G. Variceal hemorrhage in biliary atresia. J Pediatr Surg. 1984;19:476–9.
4. Ohi R, Mochizuki I, Komatsu K, Kasai M. Portal hypertension after successful hepatic portoenterostomy in biliary atresia. J Pediatr Surg. 1986;21:271–4.
5. Stringer M, Howard E, Mowat A. Endoscopic sclerotherapy in the management of esophageal varices in 61 children with biliary atresia. J Pediatr Surg. 1989;24:438–92.
6. Miga D, Sokol R, MacKenzie T, Narkewicz M, Smith D, Karrer F. Survival after first esophageal variceal hemorrhage in patients with biliary atresia. J Pediatr. 2001;139:291–6.
7. van Heurn LW, Saing H, Tam PK. Portoenterostomy for biliary atresia: long-term survival and prognosis after esophageal variceal bleeding. J Pediatr Surg. 2004;39:6–9.
8. Beath S, Pearmain G, Kelly D, McMaster P, Mayer A, Buckels J. Liver transplantation in babies and children with extrahepatic biliary atresia. J Pediatr Surg. 1993;28:1044–7.
9. Yonemura T, Yoshibayashi M, Uemoto S, Inomata Y, Tanaka K, Furusho K. Intrapulmonary shunting in biliary atresia before and after living-related liver transplantation. Br J Surg. 1999;86:1139–43.
10. Heaton ND, Davenport M, Howard ER. Incidence of haemorrhoids and anorectal varices in children with portal hypertension. Br J Surg. 1993;80:616–18.

11. Smith S, Wiener ES, Starzl TE, Rowe MI. Stoma-related variceal bleeding: an under-recognized complication of biliary atresia. J Pediatr Surg. 1988;23:243–5.
12. Schuijtvlot ET, Bax NM, Houwen RH, Hruda J. Unexpected lethal pulmonary hypertension in a 5-year-old girl successfully treated for biliary atresia. J Pediatr Surg. 1995;30:589–90.
13. Soh H, Hasegawa T, Sasaki T et al. Pulmonary hypertension associated with postoperative biliary atresia: report of two cases. J Pediatr Surg. 1999;34:1779–81.
14. Shneider B. Portal hypertension. In: Suchy F, Sokol R, Balistreri W, editors. Liver Disease in Children. Philadelphia: Lippincott Williams & Wilkins; 2001:129–51.
15. D'Amico G, Pagliaro L, Bosch J. The treatment of portal hypertension: a meta-analytic review. Hepatology. 1995;22:332–54.
16. Lay C, Tsai Y, Teg C et al. Endoscopic variceal prophylaxis of first variceal bleeding in cirrhotic patients with high-risk esophageal varices. Hepatology. 1997;25:1346–50.
17. Barbe T, Losay J, Grimon G et al. Pulmonary arteriovenous shunting in children with liver disease. J Pediatr. 1995;126:571–9.
18. D'Amico G, Pagliaro L, Bosch J. Pharmacological treatment of portal hypertension: an evidence-based approach. Semin Liver Dis. 1999;19:475–505.
19. Abraczinskas DR, Ookubo R, Grace ND et al. Propranolol for the prevention of first esophageal variceal hemorrhage: a lifetime commitment? Hepatology. 2001;34:1096–102.
20. Ozsoylu S, Kocak N, Yuce A. Propranalol therapy for portal hypertension in children. J Pediatr. 1985;106:317–20.
21. Shashidhar H, Langhans N, Grand RJ. Propranalol in prevention of portal hypertensive hemorrhage in children: a pilot study. J Pediatr Gastroenterol Nutr. 1999;29:12–17.
22. de Kolster C, Rapa de Higuera M, Carvajal A, Castro J, Callegari C, Kolster J. Propranolol in children and adolescents with portal hypertension: its dosage and the clinical, cardiovascular and biochemical effects. G.E.N. 1992;46:199–207.
23. Ozsoylu S, Kocak N, Demir H, Yuce A, Gurakan F, Ozen H. Propranalol for primary and secondary prophylaxis of variceal bleeding in children with cirrhosis. Turk J Pediatr. 2000;42:31–3.
24. Imperiale T, Chalasani N. A meta-analysis of endoscopic variceal ligation for primary prophylaxis of esophageal variceal bleeding. Hepatology. 2001;33:802–7.
25. Sokal E, Van Hoorebeeck N, Van Obbergh L, Otte JB, Buts JP. Upper gastro-intestinal tract bleeding in cirrhotic children candidates for liver transplantation. Eur J Pediatr. 1992;151:326–8.
26. Chen L, Groszmann RJ. Blood in the gastric lumen increases splanchnic blood flow and portal pressure in portal-hypertensive rats. Gastroenterology. 1996;111:1103–10.
27. Corley D, Cello J, Adkisson K, Ko W, Kerlikowske K. Octreotide for acute esophageal variceal bleeding: a meta-analysis. Gastroenterology. 2001;120:946–54.
28. Bernard B, Grange J, Khac E, Amiot X, Opolon P, Poynard T. Antibiotic prophylaxis for the prevention of bacterial infections in cirrhotic patients with gastrointestinal bleeding: a meta-analysis. Hepatology. 1999;29:1655–61.
29. Zargar SA, Javid G, Khan BA et al. Endoscopic ligation compared with sclerotherapy for bleeding esophageal varices in children with extrahepatic portal venous obstruction. Hepatology. 2002;36:666–72.
30. Botha J, Grant W, Chinnakotla S et al. Is there still a role for shunt surgery in children during the era of liver transplantation. Hepatology. 2001;34:201A.
31. Evans S, Stovroff M, Heiss K, Ricketts R. Selective distal splenorenal shunts for intractable variceal bleeding in pediatric portal hypertension. J Pediatr Surg. 1995;30:1115–18.
32. Fonkalsrud EW. Surgical management of portal hypertension in childhood. Arch Surg. 1980;115:1042–5.

# Section VI
# Therapeutic tools

# 20
# Therapeutic tools in portal hypertension: drugs

**AGUSTÍN ALBILLOS**

## INTRODUCTION

Portal hypertension often complicates the course of chronic liver disease and is a principal cause of mortality. Improvements in treating this complication made towards the end of the past century have been the consequence of several major achievements in our understanding of the pathophysiology of portal hypertension:

1. Increased intrahepatic vascular resistance (IHVR) to portal blood flow is the factor that initiates portal hypertension, but increased splanchnic blood flow due to splanchnic vasodilation contributes to maintain and aggravate this portal hypertension. Based on this finding, splanchnic vasoconstrictors are currently used to treat portal hypertension. As do beta-blockers, these reduce portal pressure, decreasing splanchnic blood flow.

2. In the cirrhotic liver, increased IHVR is the result of fixed elements (i.e. extracellular matrix, regenerative nodules, and vascular thrombosis) and elements that can be modulated (i.e. endothelial and stellate cells)[1]. Although the resistance provided by each of these modulatable and fixed elements is difficult to quantify precisely, vasodilators can reduce portal resistance up to 15% in the perfused cirrhotic rat liver[2]. This drop represents about 30% of the difference in resistance between the cirrhotic and normal liver. The dynamic component of the IHVR is a consequence of an enhanced vascular tone, secondary to an imbalance between vasoconstrictor and vasodilatory stimuli. Recent evidence indicates that a deficient intrahepatic release of nitric oxide (NO) plays a key role in the hepatic endothelial dysfunction of cirrhosis[3,4]. In the normal liver the sinusoidal endothelial cells basally produce NO and increase its production in response to flow[5,6]. In contrast, the cirrhotic liver fails to produce NO in response to incremental flow[7]. Endothelial(e)-NO synthase (NOS) and protein levels are unaltered, but endothelial-derived NO

175

is impaired[6]. Since eNOS is extensively modified at the post-translational level, deficient NO release could be the consequence of an abnormality in one of these biochemical modifications occurring after injury to sinusoidal endothelial cells. For example, caveolin-1 controls eNOS activity, and increased binding of caveolin to eNOS in cirrhosis is associated with reduced eNOS activity[7]. In addition, protein kinase B (Akt) phosphorylates eNOS and enhances its ability to generate NO. Down-regulation of Akt activity is responsible, in part, for the diminished NO production observed in cirrhotic livers, and constitutes another potential target for restoring hepatic endothelial function[8]. The hepatic vascular tone of the cirrhotic liver is also influenced by an increased production and exaggerated response to vasoconstrictors, such as endothelin-1[9], angiotensin II[10], norepinephrine[11-14], thromboxane and leukotrienes[15,16]. Knowing that an increased intrahepatic vascular tone contributes toward increasing portal pressure has provided a rational basis for the use of vasodilators to treat portal hypertension.

3. The third important concept is the correlation between the value or change in portal pressure, as measured by the hepatic venous pressure gradient (HVPG), and clinical events (i.e. variceal formation and bleeding). Pharmacological or spontaneous reduction in portal pressure to below 12 mmHg, or more than 20% from baseline, leads to a null or low ($\sim 10\%$) risk of variceal bleeding, respectively[17-22]. Pharmacological treatment seeks to achieve this reduction in portal pressure since it is known that this will lessen the risk of variceal bleeding and other complications of cirrhosis[23]. Non-response to vasoactive therapy is the most important independent risk factor for variceal bleeding[23].

This chapter will briefly overview the spectrum of drugs available for the long-term treatment of portal hypertension.

## DRUGS THAT REDUCE SPLANCHNIC BLOOD FLOW: SPLANCHNIC VASOCONSTRICTORS

Non-selective beta-adrenergic blockers (propranolol, nadolol) are still the mainstay long-term medical treatment for portal hypertension. However, only 30–40% of the patients under long-term beta-blocker therapy reduce their portal pressure $> 20\%$ from baseline or to levels $< 12$ mmHg (responders)[22,24,25]. The HVPG response during continuous beta-blocker therapy is unpredictable. Individual sensitivity to beta-blockers varies, and is determined by factors such as age and genetic beta-adrenoceptor polymorphism and, in the cirrhotic patient, by the extent of liver damage and of portal–systemic collaterals and varices[26,27]. Related to this, previous variceal bleeding is an independent risk factor for the non-response of portal pressure to beta-blockade[28]. There are several issues we can consider to minimize non-response to beta-blockers. The first relates to the optimal dose of beta-blockers in the portal hypertensive patient. The beneficial effect of beta-blockers on portal hypertension stems both from the portal pressure reduction achieved by lowering portal venous inflow through cardiac output

176

reduction (by blockade of beta-1 cardiac receptors) and through splanchnic arteriolar vasoconstriction (by blockade of beta-2 vascular receptors), and from portal–collateral (variceal) blood flow reduction through portal venous inflow reduction and constriction of the collateral vessels (by beta-2 blockade)[26]. Currently the dose of beta-blockers is titrated against the degree of beta-1-adrenoceptor blockade, by stepwise increases in dose until the heart rate decreases by 25% or below 55 bpm, or the appearance of arterial hypotension or clinical intolerance. However, the fall in portal pressure depends not only on the degree of beta-1 blockade, but also on beta-2 blockade; indeed, early studies in which patients received incremental doses of propranolol irrespective of the heart rate response showed that the higher the dose, the higher the number of responders[29]. The dose of propranolol has recently been identified as an independent predictor of the portal pressure response to this drug[23]. This suggests that the number of responders can be increased by titrating beta-blockers against clinical tolerance up to the maximum tolerated dose. The choice of the type of beta-blocker is another aspect to consider. The hemodynamics and clinical efficacy of the two non-cardioselective beta-blockers used in portal hypertensive patients seem to be similar, although we have more experience with the use of propranolol. Theoretically, nadolol has the advantages of single-day dosing, and causing less asthenia because of reduced lipid solubility and entry into the central nervous system[30]. Timolol, a beta-blocker with low liposolubility and greater beta-2 adrenoceptor blocking effect, has been associated with a high incidence of adverse effects requiring drug reduction or withdrawal in a recent placebo-controlled trial on pre-primary prophylaxis of variceal bleeding[31]. Finally, beta-blockers have been combined with other synergistically acting drugs (nitrates, prazosin, spironolactone) as a way of enhancing their effectiveness in lowering portal pressure and increasing the number of responders.

## DRUGS THAT DECREASE INTRAHEPATIC VASCULAR RESISTANCE: VASODILATORS

The armamentarium for the therapy of portal hypertension has expanded in the direction of vasodilators. Although the spectrum of available agents is ever broader, only nitrovasodilators, which were the first used to treat portal hypertension in 1982[32], have so far been tested in randomized trials with clinical end-points (i.e. variceal bleeding). The ideal vasodilator should reduce portal pressure by selectively relaxing the increased vascular resistance of the cirrhotic liver, while enhancing or maintaining hepatic blood flow. Hepatic vascular relaxation can be attempted by restoring the deficient hepatic NO delivery, or blocking the increased activity of vasoconstrictors. However, most of the available agents are not selective of the hepatic microcirculation, and worsen systemic and splanchnic vasodilation[33].

### Specific and non-specific liver NO donors

Nitrovasodilators, specifically organic nitrates such as isosorbide mononitrate (ISMN), were used to lower portal pressure long before the discovery of NO. Organic nitrates are prodrugs from which NO is liberated enzymatically[34]. Hemodynamic studies in human and experimental cirrhosis suggest that nitrates reduce portal pressure by: decreasing the IHVR; inducing a baroreflex-mediated splanchnic arterial vasoconstriction (secondary to a decrease in arterial pressure) with a consequent reduction in portal blood flow; reducing vascular resistance in the collateral circulation; or most likely a variable combination of these mechanisms[35,36]. ISMN is inadequate as single therapy, since it reduces arterial pressure even at the minimum dose capable of decreasing portal pressure[37]; indeed, when compared with propranolol or placebo, ISMN fails to show a benefit for the primary prevention of variceal bleeding and may even increase mortality in patients older than 50 years[38,39]. The prevailing systemic rather than intrahepatic vasodilation achieved by organic nitrates stems from three factors: impaired metabolizing of nitroglycerin to NO by the cirrhotic liver, bypass of liver microcirculation through portal–systemic collaterals of orally administered ISMN, and the up-regulation of endothelial NO pathways in the splanchnic and systemic circulation[4,33,40]. The real benefit of ISMN is observed when this agent is combined with beta-blockers. Combination therapy enhances the fall in portal pressure by beta-blockers alone, increasing the number of responders by about one-third[24,25]. To achieve this effect, ISMN counteracts the increase in portohepatic outflow resistance (secondary to unopposed beta-adrenergic activity) and in portocollateral resistance (secondary to passive collapse and active beta-2 blockade mediated constriction of the collaterals) caused by beta-blockers, which hinder their portal pressure-lowering action[26]. The benefit of combined therapy in terms of portal pressure reduction is restricted to subjects not responding to beta-blockers alone; portal pressure does not fall further after the addition of ISMN in beta-blocker responders[25]. Further, beta-blockers limit the untoward effects of ISMN on renal function and arterial pressure, since beta-blockade increases peripheral vascular resistance and blocks renin secretion[25]. However, side-effects requiring withdrawal of therapy are almost twice as likely in patients on combined therapy as in those receiving beta-blockers alone[41,42].

These data indicate that the lack of hepatic selectivity of organic nitrates puts them in a position far from being the ideal drugs for the treatment of portal hypertension. Research has focused on the development of agents that selectively deliver NO to the liver and restore conditions of low NO release in the microcirculation of the cirrhotic liver. A highly selective hepatic NO donor could be used as a single drug at doses high enough to effectively reduce portal pressure, without the need for combination with other drugs. For the time being, these strategies have only been developed in the experimental setting:

1. *Liver-specific donors.* NCX-1000 is a stable compound obtained by adding a NO-releasing moiety to ursodeoxycholic acid (UDCA)[43]. Two recently published studies have tested the hemodynamic effects of the long-term administration of NCX-1000 in rats with established cirrhosis and portal hypertension. One study uses the $CCl_4$ cirrhotic rat model (considered as the model that best mimics the disease in humans), and the other uses the bile duct-ligated (BDL) model[44,45]. In both studies, NCX-1000 attenu-

ated the hyperresponse to alpha-adrenergic stimulation of the perfused cirrhotic rat liver. In BDL rats, NCX-1000 markedly reduced baseline portal pressure[43], while in $CCl_4$ cirrhotic rats the compound failed to modify portal pressure, and only blunted the portal pressure increase induced by blood volume expansion[44]. The published results are promising, but preliminary; they show that it is possible to selectively deliver NO to the liver and modify hepatic, but not systemic, hemodynamics. If the results of the study on $CCl_4$ cirrhotic rats are confirmed, as a NO donor, it is thought that NCX-1000 may prevent further increases in portal pressure secondary to increases in portal blood flow, and may be of use as a adjuvant to portal pressure-lowering agents.

2. *Gene transfer of NO-synthase.* Hepatic gene transfer of the endothelial and neuronal isoforms of NOS enhanced NOS expression and NO synthesis, and reduced portal pressure in two different models of cirrhosis and portal hypertension[46-48]. Gene therapy is, nevertheless, complex and risky, and for the time being this approach can only be considered experimental.

3. *Activation of Akt-dependent eNOS phosphorylation.* Adenoviral delivery of constitutively activated Akt has been found to restore hepatic eNOS phosphorylation and NO synthesis, lowering portal pressure[8]. Akt-dependent endothelial NOS phosphorylation in cirrhosis can also be pharmacologically increased with simvastatin. In the short term simvastatin increases the hepatosplanchnic output of NO and decreases hepatic resistance in patients with cirrhosis[49].

NO is not the only therapeutic target that will modulate the increased hepatic vascular tone that arises from an imbalance between a lack of vasodilators (i.e. NO) and surplus of vasoconstrictors in cirrhosis.

## Alpha-1-adrenergic blockers

The rationale for the use of alpha-1-adrenergic blockers in portal hypertension lies in the enhanced systemic and splanchnic sympathetic nervous activity that occurs in cirrhosis, as well as in the hypersensitivity of the hepatic vasculature to norepinephrine[14]. Long-term prazosin administration markedly lowers portal pressure by reducing hepatic vascular resistance; the extent of the fall in portal pressure comparing favorably with that achieved by propranolol[12,13]. However, prazosin also lowers arterial pressure and peripheral vascular resistance, promoting sodium retention, plasma volume expansion and, in some patients, ascites formation. These findings preclude the use of this drug as a single agent. Interestingly, the combination of beta-blockers (propranolol) with prazosin has a synergistic effect on lowering portal pressure, whereas it attenuates the effects of prazosin on systemic hemodynamics[25]; indeed, proportions of patients responding to prazosin plus propranolol (85%) have been greater than to propranolol and ISMN. However, tolerance to the combination of propranolol and prazosin was worse than to propranolol and ISMN, and a greater number of patients required discontinuation of the drugs because of side-effects. Based on these findings the most recent approach has been to test carvedilol, a non-selective beta-blocker with intrinsic anti alpha-1-adrenergic activity[50-53]; as such its effects mimic those of the propranolol/prazosin combination. When carvedilol was compared to propranolol in a randomized trial it gave rise to a greater reduction in portal pressure and a larger number of responders, but also induced greater arterial hypotension and derived systemic effects[53]. Thus, carvedilol would need to be tested in randomized controlled trials with clinical endpoints before widespread use.

## Renin–angiotensin system blockers

Angiotensin-II (AT-II) is a powerful vasoconstrictor formed by activation of the renin–angiotensin system, commonly observed in patients with advanced cirrhosis and found to be related to portal pressure[54]. AT-II can contribute to the genesis of portal hypertension in several ways: it increases hepatic resistance in isolated perfused cirrhotic livers[9,55], which is probably the result of contraction of vascular smooth muscle cells and hepatic stellate cells, and it promotes the formation of transforming growth factor beta and liver fibrogenesis, which may worsen portal hypertension[10,56]. Further possible mechanisms contributing to the portal hypertensive effect of AT-II are: increasing the adrenergic vasoconstrictor effects on the portal system, and sodium and fluid retention, induced by the stimulation of aldosterone secretion[57]. These mechanisms are all consistent with the idea of blocking the activity of AT-II as a way of decreasing portal pressure. However, activation of the renin–angiotensin system is a homeostatic response that maintains arterial pressure when faced with ongoing vasodilator synthesis. An initial non-randomized trial reported a dramatic effect of the long-term administration of losartan, an AT-II receptor blocker, in patients with portal hypertension[58]. These results were not, however, confirmed in four randomized trials comparing losartan and ibersartan (another AT-II receptor blocker) with propranolol or placebo[59-62]. Losartan and ibersartan caused a null or only slight decrease in portal pressure in three of these trials, but caused marked arterial hypotension and renal function impairment in patients with advanced disease and high plasma renin activity[59,60]. In a fourth, recently published trial, including a large number of alcoholic patients, the lowering effect on portal pressure by losartan was similar to that shown by propranolol[63]. In view of all these data, AT-II receptor blockers are not recommended for the treatment of portal hypertension.

## Endothelin receptor blockers

Apart from NO, endothelin-1 is the most potent regulator of hepatic vascular tone. Endothelin-1 receptors are particularly numerous on stellate cells, where they affect vascular tone[64]. In cirrhosis the increased local production of endothelin and enhanced endothelin-1 receptor expression in stellate cells contribute toward increasing IHVR[9,64,65]. Selective blockade of $ET_A$ receptors, which mediate the contraction and proliferation of hepatic stellate cells, would be a good approach to treating portal hypertension. Attempts to block endothelin-1 receptors have been made in several experimental settings and designs, including different models of cirrhosis, acute and chronic blockade, mixed $ET_A$–$ET_B$ receptors or selective $ET_A$ blockers[66-70]. To date these studies have yielded conflicting results precluding any firm conclusions.

## Acknowledgements

This work was supported in part by grants BFI2003–03858 from the Plan Nacional de Investigación y Desarrollo, and from the Instituto de Salud Carlos III (C03/02).

## References

1. McCuskey RS. Morphological mechanisms for regulating blood flow through hepatic sinusoids. Liver. 2000;20:3–7.
2. Bhathal PS, Grossman HJ. Reduction of the increased portal vascular resistance of the isolated perfused cirrhotic rat liver by vasodilators. J Hepatol. 1985;1:325–37.
3. Gupta TK, Toruner M, Chung MK, Groszmann RJ. Endothelial dysfunction and decreased production of nitric oxide in the intrahepatic microcirculation: effects on portal hemodynamics and on liver and renal function. Hepatology. 1998;28:926–31.
4. Wiest R, Groszmann RJ. The paradox of nitric oxide in cirrhosis and portal hypertension: too much, not enough. Hepatology. 2002;35:478–91.
5. Shah V, Haddad F, Garcia-Cardena G et al. Liver sinusoidal endothelial cells are responsible for nitric oxide modulation of resistance in the hepatic sinusoids. J Clin Invest. 1997;100:2923–30.
6. Rockey DC, Chung JJ. Reduced nitric oxide production by endothelial cells in cirrhotic rat liver: endothelial dysfunction in portal hypertension. Gastroenterology. 1998;114:344–51.
7. Shah V, Toruner M, Haddad F et al. Impaired endothelial nitric oxide synthase activity associated with enhanced caveolin binding in experimental cirrhosis in the rat. Gastroenterology. 1999;117:1222–8.
8. Morales-Ruiz M, Cejudo-Martin P, Fernandez-Varo G et al. Transduction of the liver with activated Akt normalizes portal pressure in cirrhotic rats. Gastroenterology. 2003;125:522–31.
9. Rockey DC, Weisiger RA. Endothelin induced contractility of stellate cells from normal and cirrhotic rat liver: implications for regulation of portal pressure and resistance. Hepatology. 1996;24:233–40.
10. Bataller R, Gines P, Nicolas JM et al. Angiotensin II induces contraction and proliferation of human hepatic stellate cells. Gastroenterology. 2000;118:1149–56.
11. Albillos A, Bañares R, Barrios C et al. Oral administration of clonidine in patients with alcoholic cirrhosis: hemodynamic and liver function effects. Gastroenterology. 1992;102:248–54.
12. Albillos A, Lledo JL, Banares R et al. Hemodynamic effects of α-adrenergic blockade with prazosin in cirrhotic patients with portal hypertension. Hepatology. 1994;20:611–17.
13. Albillos A, Lledo JL, Rossi I et al. Continuous prazosin administration in cirrhotic patients: effects on portal hemodynamics and on liver and renal function. Gastroenterology. 1995;109:1257–65.
14. Marteau P, Ballet F, Chazouilleres O et al. Effect of vasodilators on hepatic microcirculation in cirrhosis: a study in the isolated perfused rat liver. Hepatology. 1989;9:820–3.
15. Titos E, Claria J, Bataller R et al. Hepatocyte-derived cysteinyl leukotrienes modulate vascular tone in experimental cirrhosis. Gastroenterology. 2000;119:794–805.
16. Graupera M, Garcia-Pagan JC, Titos E et al. 5-Lipoxygenase inhibition reduces intrahepatic vascular resistance of cirrhotic rat livers: a possible role of cysteinyl-leukotrienes. Gastroenterology. 2002;122:387–93.
17. Groszmann RJ, Bosch J, Grace ND et al. Hemodynamic events in a prospective randomized trial of propranolol versus placebo in the prevention of a first variceal hemorrhage. Gastroenterology. 1990;99:1401–7.
18. Feu F, Garcia-Pagan JC, Bosch J et al. Relation between portal pressure response to pharmacotherapy and risk of recurrent variceal haemorrhage in patients with cirrhosis. Lancet. 1995;346:1056–9.
19. Merkel C, Bolognesi M, Sacerdoti D et al. The hemodynamic response to medical treatment of portal hypertension as a predictor of clinical effectiveness in the primary prophylaxis of variceal bleeding in cirrhosis. Hepatology. 2000;32:930–4.

20. Villanueva C, Balanzo J, Novella MT et al. Nadolol plus isosorbide mononitrate compared with sclerotherapy for the prevention of variceal rebleeding. N Engl J Med. 1996;334:1624–9.
21. Villanueva C, Minana J, Ortiz J et al. Endoscopic ligation compared with combined treatment with nadolol and isosorbide mononitrate to prevent recurrent variceal bleeding. N Engl J Med. 2001;345:647–55.
22. Bosch J, Arroyo V, Betriu A et al. Hepatic hemodynamics and the renin–angiotensin–aldosterone system in cirrhosis. Gastroenterology. 1980;78:92–9.
23. Abraldes JG, Tarantino I, Turnes J, Garcia-Pagan JC, Rodes J, Bosch J. Hemodynamic response to pharmacological treatment of portal hypertension and long-term prognosis of cirrhosis. Hepatology. 2003;37:902–8.
24. Garcia-Pagan JC, Feu F, Bosch J, Rodés J. Propranolol compared with propranolol plus isosorbide-5-mononitrate for portal hypertension in cirrhosis. A randomized controlled study. Ann Intern Med. 1991;114:869–73.
25. Albillos A, Garcia-Pagan JC, Iborra J et al. Propranolol plus prazosin compared with propranolol plus isosorbide-5-mononitrate in the treatment of portal hypertension. Gastroenterology. 1998;115:116–23.
26. Kroeger RJ, Groszmann RJ. Increased portal venous resistance hinders portal pressure reduction during the administration of beta-adrenergic blocking agents in a portal hypertensive model. Hepatology. 1985;5:97–101.
27. Escorsell A, Ferayorni L, Bosch J et al. The portal pressure response to beta-blockade is greater in cirrhotic patients without varices than in those with varices. Gastroenterology. 1997;112:2012–16.
28. Albillos A, Pérez M, Cacho G, Calleja JL, Escartín P. Accuracy of portal and forearm blood flow measurements in the assessment of portal pressure response to propranolol. J Hepatol. 1997;27:496–504.
29. Garcia-Tsao G, Grace ND, Groszmann RJ et al. Short-term effects of propranolol on portal venous pressure. Hepatology. 1986;6:101–6.
30. Gengo FM, Huntoon L, McHugh WB. Lipid-soluble and water-soluble beta-blockers. Comparison of the central nervous system depressant effect. Arch Intern Med. 1987;147: 39–43.
31. Groszmann RJ, Garcia-Tsao G, Bosch J et al. Multicenter randomized placebo-controlled trial of non-selective beta-blockers in the prevention of the complications of portal hypertension: final results and identification of a predictive factor. Hepatology. 2003;38:206A.
32. Groszmann RJ, Kravetz D, Bosch J et al. Nitroglycerin improves the hemodynamic response to vasopressin in portal hypertension. Hepatology. 1982;2:757–62.
33. Groszmann R. Beta-adrenergic blockers and nitrovasodilators for the treatment of portal hypertension: the good, the bad, the ugly. Gastroenterology. 1997;113:1794–7.
34. Harrison D, Bates J. The nitrovasodilators: new ideas about old drugs. Circulation. 1993;87:1461–7.
35. Garcia-Tsao G, Groszmann RJ. Portal hemodynamics during nitroglycerin administration in cirrhotic patients. Hepatology. 1987;7:805–9.
36. Navasa M, Chesta J, Bosch J, Rodes J. Reduction of portal pressure by isosorbide-5-mononitrate in patients with cirrhosis. Effects on splanchnic and systemic hemodynamics and liver function. Gastroenterology. 1989;96:1110–18.
37. Bellis L, Berzigotti A, Abraldes JG et al. Low doses of isosorbide mononitrate attenuate the postprandial increase in portal pressure in patients with cirrhosis. Hepatology. 2003;37:378–84.
38. Angelico M, Carli L, Piat C, Gentile S, Capocaccia L. Effects of isosorbide-5-mononitrate compared with propranolol on first bleeding and long-term survival in cirrhosis. Gastroenterology. 1997;113:1632–9.
39. Garcia-Pagan JC, Villanueva C, Vila MC et al. Isosorbide mononitrate in the prevention of first variceal bleed in patients who cannot receive beta-blockers. Gastroenterology. 2001;121:908–14.
40. Dudenhoefer AA, Loureiro-Silva MR, Cadelina GW, Gupta T, Groszmann RJ. Bioactivation of nitroglycerin and vasomotor response to nitric oxide are impaired in cirrhotic rat livers. Hepatology. 2002;36:381–5.
41. Gournay J, Masliah C, Martin T, Perrin D, Galmiche JP. Isosorbide mononitrate and propranolol compared with propranolol alone for the prevention of variceal rebleeding. Hepatology. 2000;31:1239–45.

42. Garcia-Pagan JC, Morillas R, Banares R et al. Spanish Variceal Bleeding Study Group. Propranolol plus placebo versus propranolol plus isosorbide-5-mononitrate in the prevention of a first variceal bleed: a double-blind RCT. Hepatology. 2003;37:1260–6.
43. Fiorucci S, Antonelli E, Morelli O et al. NCX-1000, a NO-releasing derivative of ursodeoxycholic acid, selectively delivers NO to the liver and protects against development of portal hypertension. Proc Natl Acad Sci USA. 2001;98:8897–902.
44. Fiorucci S, Antonelli E, Brancaleone V et al. NCX-1000, a nitric oxide-releasing derivative of ursodeoxycholic acid, ameliorates portal hypertension and lowers norepinephrine-induced intrahepatic resistance in the isolated and perfused rat liver. J Hepatol. 2003;39:932–9.
45. Loureiro-Silva MR, Cadelina GW, Iwakiri Y, Groszmann RJ. A liver-specific nitric oxide donor improves the intra-hepatic vascular response to both portal blood flow increase and methoxamine in cirrhotic rats. J Hepatol. 2003;39:940–6.
46. Yu Q, Shao R, Qian HS, George SE, Rockey DC. Gene transfer of the neuronal NO synthase isoform to cirrhotic rat liver ameliorates portal hypertension. J Clin Invest. 2000;105:741–8.
47. Van de Casteele M, Omasta A, Janssens S et al. In vivo gene transfer of endothelial nitric oxide synthase decreases portal pressure in anaesthetised carbon tetrachloride cirrhotic rats. Gut. 2002;51:440–5.
48. Van de CM, Van Pelt JF, Nevens F, Fevery J, Reichen J. Low NO bioavailability in CCl4 cirrhotic rat livers might result from low NO synthesis combined with decreased superoxide dismutase activity allowing superoxide-mediated NO breakdown: a comparison of two portal hypertensive rat models with healthy controls. Comp Hepatol. 2003;2:2.
49. Zafra C, Abraldes J, Turnes J et al. Simvastatin enhances hepatic nitric oxide production and decreases the hepatic vascular tone in patients with cirrhosis. Gastroenterology. 2004;126:749–55.
50. Stanley AJ, Therapondos G, Helmy A, Hayes PC. Acute and chronic haemodynamic and renal effects of carvedilol in patients with cirrhosis. J Hepatol. 1999;30:479–84.
51. Banares R, Moitinho E, Piqueras B et al. Carvedilol, a new nonselective beta-blocker with intrinsic anti-alpha-1 adrenergic activity, has a greater portal hypotensive effect than propranolol in patients with cirrhosis. Hepatology. 1999;30:79–83.
52. Tripathi D, Therapondos G, Lui HF, Stanley AJ, Hayes PC. Haemodynamic effects of acute and chronic administration of low-dose carvedilol, a vasodilating beta-blocker, in patients with cirrhosis and portal hypertension. Aliment Pharmacol Ther. 2002;16:373–80.
53. Banares R, Moitinho E, Piqueras B et al. Randomized comparison of long-term carvedilol and propranolol administration in the treatment of portal hypertension in cirrhosis. Hepatology. 2002;36:1367–73.
54. Bosch J, Arroyo V, Betriu A et al. Hepatic hemodynamics and the renin–angiotensin–aldosterone system in cirrhosis. Gastroenterology. 1980;78:92–9.
55. Ballet F, Chretien Y, Rey C et al. Differential response of normal and cirrhotic liver to vasoactive agents. A study in the isolated perfused rat liver. J Pharmacol Exp Ther. 1988;244:233–5.
56. Blobe GC, Schiemann WP, Lodish HF. Role of transforming growth factor $\beta$ in human disease. N Engl J Med. 2000;342:1350–8.
57. Goodfriend TL, Elliott ME, Catt KJ. Angiotensin receptors and their antagonists. N Engl J Med. 1996;25:1649–54.
58. Schneider AW, Friedrich J, Klein CP. Effect of losartan, an angiotensin II receptor antagonist, on portal pressure in cirrhosis. Hepatology. 1999;29:334–9.
59. Gonzalez-Abraldes J, Albillos A, Banares R et al. Randomized comparison of long-term losartan versus propranolol in lowering portal pressure in cirrhosis. Gastroenterology. 2001;121:382–8.
60. Schepke M, Werner E, Biecker E et al. Hemodynamic effects of the angiotensin II receptor antagonist irbesartan in patients with cirrhosis and portal hypertension. Gastroenterology. 2001;121:389–95.
61. Venon WD, Baronio M, Leone N et al. Effects of long-term irbesartan in reducing portal pressure in cirrhotic patients: comparison with propranolol in a randomised controlled study. J Hepatol. 2003;38:455–60.
62. Debernardi-Venon W, Barletti C, Alessandria C et al. Efficacy of irbesartan, a receptor selective antagonist of angiotensin II, in reducing portal hypertension. Dig Dis Sci. 2002;47:401–4.

63. De BK, Bandyopadhyay K, Das TK et al. Portal pressure response to losartan compared with propranolol in patients with cirrhosis. Am J Gastroenterol. 2003;98:1371–6.
64. Rockey DC, Fouassier L, Chung JJ et al. Cellular localization of endothelin-1 and increased production in liver injury in the rat: potential for autocrine and paracrine effects on stellate cells. Hepatology. 1998;27:472–80.
65. Leivas A, Jimenez W, Bruix J et al. Gene expression of endothelin-1 and ET(A) and ET(B) receptors in human cirrhosis: relationship with hepatic hemodynamics. J Vasc Res. 1998;35:186–93.
66. Reichen J, Gerbes AL, Steiner MJ, Sagesser H, Clozel M. The effect of endothelin and its antagonist bosentan on hemodynamics and microvascular exchange in cirrhotic rat liver. J Hepatol. 1998;28:1020–30.
67. Sogni P, Moreau R, Gomola A et al. Beneficial hemodynamic effects of bosentan, a mixed ET(A) and ET(B) receptor antagonist, in portal hypertensive rats. Hepatology. 1998;28:655–9.
68. Poo JL, Jimenez W, Munoz R et al. Chronic blockade of endothelin receptors in cirrhotic rats: hepatic and hemodynamic effects. Gastroenterology. 1999;116:161–7.
69. Cho JJ, Hocher B, Herbst H et al. An oral endothelin-A receptor antagonist blocks collagen synthesis and deposition in advanced rat liver fibrosis. Gastroenterology. 2000;118:1169–78.
70. Kojima H, Sakurai S, Kuriyama S et al. Endothelin-1 plays a major role in portal hypertension of biliary cirrhotic rats through endothelin receptor subtype B together with subtype A in vivo. J Hepatol. 2001;34:805–11.

184

# 21
# Endoscopy in the management of portal hypertension

**GREGORY J. MONKEWICH and NORMAN E. MARCON**

## INTRODUCTION

Endoscopy plays a central role in the management of portal hypertension contributing to: early detection of esophageal and gastric varices (EGV); stratification of patients in terms of their risk of bleeding; primary or secondary prophylactic therapy; monitoring the effect of prophylactic therapies on bleeding risk; and treatment of acute variceal bleeding, portal hypertensive gastropathy (PHG), and ectopic varices. The goal of this chapter is to provide an evidence-based approach to the endoscopic management of portal hypertension.

## ENDOSCOPY IN PRIMARY PROPHYLAXIS

### Screening

The detection of esophageal varices (EV) in patients with cirrhosis has been used to direct therapy for the primary prevention of variceal bleeding. Up to 90% of patients with cirrhosis develop EGV during their lives and up to 40% develop variceal bleeding[1]. Variceal bleeding is a major cause of death in patients with cirrhosis[2] and the mortality rate with the first episode of bleeding is high (20–50%)[3,4]. Several randomized controlled trials (RCTs) have confirmed that medical and endoscopic therapies may reduce the risk of variceal bleeding and possibly death[5]. Therefore, a strategy of endoscopic screening followed by primary prophylactic therapy has the potential to reduce morbidity, increase survival and lessen attendant health care costs.

Whether all patients with cirrhosis should undergo endoscopic screening (universal screening) is controversial. The American College of Gastroenterology (ACG) and the American Association for the Study of Liver Disease (AASLD) recommend a screening endoscopy in patients with cirrhosis every 2 years followed by medical prophylactic therapy in patients with large varices[6,7]. However, the efficacy of endoscopic screening in an unselected population of patients with cirrhosis is unproved. In contrast, a benefit is established for high-risk patients selected according to clinical criteria. A recent cost-effectiveness analysis has shed more light: empiric β-blocker therapy for the primary prophylaxis of variceal bleeding was a cost-effective strategy while the use of screening endoscopy to guide therapy added a significant cost with only a marginal increase in effectiveness[8]. Prospective comparisons of empiric versus screening-directed prophylaxis are needed.

## Selective screening endoscopy

What means are available to select high risk patients for endoscopic screening? The clinical factors that correlate with a higher bleeding risk are Child–Pugh classes B and C (in particular, the parameters ascites and encephalopathy), advanced age, and alcohol-induced cirrhosis[9]. One should also consider the patient's life expectancy, comorbid illnesses (e.g. hepatocellular carcinoma), and motivation. The ratio of the platelet count to the maximum spleen diameter measured ultrasonographically may predict the presence or absence of EV. This ratio was independently associated with the presence of EV in a multivariate analysis of cirrhotic patients including those with compensated cirrhosis[10]. A platelet count ($n/mm^3$) to spleen diameter (mm) ratio $> 909$ confers a negative predictive value of 100% for the diagnosis of EV while a ratio $\leq 909$ confers a positive predictive value of 74%.

Screening initiatives require affordable screening methods. Screening cirrhotic patients according to the platelet count/spleen diameter ratio was far more cost effective than uniform endoscopic screening[11]. Unsedated transnasal endoscopy, an attractive alternative to conventional endoscopy because of its lower cost, was compared to conventional endoscopy in 15 patients with cirrhosis[12]. Both methods detected 10 EV and 2 GV, but the transnasal approach missed one case of PHG.

Although the efficacy of screening is apparent in high risk patients, physicians' implementation of screening is far from complete. Only 46% of patients referred to a liver transplant center had undergone either endoscopy or radiological studies to detect varices[13].

## Risk stratification of esophageal and gastric varices

Once varices are identified on screening, the endoscopist must stratify the patients according to their risk of experiencing first bleeding in order to direct therapy targeted at reducing this risk. Stratification is based on endoscopic appearance, clinical and laboratory parameters.

*Esophageal varices*

Overall, unselected patients with known EGV have a low risk of variceal bleeding in the first year (3.5%) and the benefit of medical therapy is likely not better than placebo[14]. Propranolol did not prevent the development of large varices in patients with small or absent varices[15]. Therefore, a careful selection of patients who are most likely to benefit from β-blocker therapy is important in order to effectively manage their illness. Patients with large

**Table 1.** Bleeding risk based on the observed endoscopic findings

| Endoscopic finding | Bleeding risk (%) |
|---|---|
| Proximal extension | |
|    Proximal 1/3 of esophagus | 62.6 |
|    Distal 1/3 of esophagus alone | 26.3 |
| Size ("form") | |
|    F1 (small and non-tortuous) | 15.0 |
|    F2 (tortuous, < 50% of the radius of the esophagus) | 31.8 |
|    F3 (very large and tortuous) | 67.6 |
| Color | |
|    Blue | 79.4 |
|    White | 45.7 |
| Red color sign | |
|    Both RWM and CRS present | 75.7 |
|    Both RWM and CRS absent | 17.4 |
| Hematocystic spots | |
|    present | 100 |
|    absent | 48.8 |

RWM = Red wheal markings; CRS = Cherry-red spots
Adapted and reprinted with permission from Beppu et al.[124]

varices should be considered for prophylactic therapy, either medical or endoscopic.

Several classifications of EV are published and are used for risk stratification. Most employ endoscopic criteria with or without clinical and laboratory criteria. Unfortunately, most are subjective and limited by significant inter-observer variability.

The Japanese Research Society for Portal Hypertension (JRSPH) employs in its classification the variceal size, the variceal extension as measured proximally from the gastroesophageal junction, and the presence or absence of "red signs"[16,17]. The size or "Form" parameter is defined as: F0, no varices; F1, small and non-tortuous; F2, tortuous but less than 50% of the radius of the esophagus; and F3, very large and tortuous. The "red signs" are: red wheal markings (longitudinal dilated venules resembling whip marks), cherry red spots, and hematocystic spots. Red signs represent a small area of a varix with a thin weak wall, likely due to maximum distension of the vessel. These are suspected to be the actual sites of rupture of the varices. Hematocystic spots are thought to have the highest risk of rupture (see Table 1) and represent saccular out-pouches of the varix similar to aneurysmal dilations[18]. Variceal growth over time carries an increased risk of bleeding.

The Northern Italian Endoscopic Club (NIEC) developed a prognostic index to predict the risk of bleeding and thereby identify candidates for prophylactic therapy[19]. The index is based on data from a prospective study that followed 321 patients with cirrhosis and EV without prior bleeding. By multivariate analysis, the risk of bleeding was significantly related to the Child–Pugh class, the variceal size, and the presence of red wheal markings. A prognostic index based on these variables was devised to identify a subset of patients with a one-year incidence of bleeding > 65%.

Objective determinants of bleeding risk are needed to lessen our reliance upon subjective evaluations which are prone to substantial inter-observer variability. The reference standard for the measurement of intravariceal pressure is direct intravariceal needle puncture. Unfortunately, this technique risks initiating bleeding; consequently, it is used only for investigational purposes. The hepatic venous wedge pressure gradient (HVWPG) is an indirect measure of intravariceal pressure. Several studies demonstrated that a HVWPG threshold exists such that a measurement greater than 12 mmHg predicts bleeding from varices, while a measurement less than 12 mmHg is associated with a minimal or absent risk. During β-blocker therapy, the risk of bleeding may become absent or markedly diminished if the HVWPG is reduced below 12 mmHg or more than 25% below the pre-treatment HVWPG measurement. The HVWPG measurement is not widely available and not cost-effective for a majority of patients with large EV[20].

Endoscopic methods are being studied to measure esophageal variceal pressures indirectly. Rigau et al.[21] used a hemispheric latex membrane gauge that could be applied over a varix and perfused with a constant flow of nitrogen. Gertsch et al.[22] used a non-expandable transparent balloon fixed to the end of a regular endoscope. Miller et al.[23] used EUS to measure the cross-sectional surface area (CSA) of all of the EV in the distal esophagus in patients with no prior history of bleeding ($n = 28$). Using a cutoff of 0.45 cm$^2$, the sensitivity and specificity for future variceal bleeding was 83% and 75%, respectively. Miller et al.[24] also use EUS to measure the compression of a varix by a latex balloon applied against it, while simultaneously measuring the balloon pressures. Other interesting techniques under development include: endoscopic Doppler imaging to guide the manometry of EV[25]; and computer analysis of the red component of digital images to objectively quantify red signs[26].

Until these techniques are validated and more widely available, most clinicians must rely on the subjective endoscopic parameters in addition to the clinical and laboratory criteria.

*Gastric varices*

Several classifications are published[27,28]. The most popular classification is that by Sarin et al.[29,30] GV that are associated with EV are sub-classified into Type 1 (GOV1) and Type 2 (GOV2). GOV1 appears as a continuation of EV and extends 2–5 cm below the gastroesophageal junction. GOV2 extends into the fundus of the stomach. Isolated GV (IGV) occur in the absence of EV and are further sub-classified: Type 1 IGV (IGV1) (Figure 3A) are located in the fundus and fall short of the cardia by a few centimeters. Type 2 IGV (IGV2) include ectopic varices that can appear anywhere in the stomach.

Is there a need to stratify GV in terms of their risk for bleeding? In view of the high mortality rate associated with bleeding, it may be argued that large GV, especially those with red signs, should be eradicated endoscopically. This is controversial and there are no compelling studies available to support this approach.

## Endoscopic therapy

β-Blockers are the mainstay of medical therapy, although nitrates may also be used. Endoscopic therapy is an alternative for patients in whom medical therapy is contraindicated because of heart block, asthma, diabetes, or severe heart failure.

Endoscopic therapy is also indicated when medical therapy fails. Intolerance of β-blockers requiring discontinuation of therapy occurs in approximately 30% of treated patients. Poor compliance represents another obstacle. Furthermore, medical therapy is unable to achieve a reduction in HVWPG to < 12 mmHg or more than 25% from baseline in up to 50% of patients. A potential strategy in these settings is to offer endoscopic therapy to achieve the desired reduction in portal pressure. However, this strategy demands reliable noninvasive methods for the measurement of variceal and/or portal pressures.

The optimal treatment strategy has been sought in a number of comparative trials of various combinations of medical therapy and the endoscopic modalities. Important published studies are summarized below:

### EVS

EVS is not recommended for the primary prophylaxis of EGV on its own[31] or in combination with β-blockers[32].

### EVL versus no treatment

New treatment modalities should be tested against the current standard. EVL was compared to no treatment in several small studies[33-38] despite the availability of β-blocker therapy as the standard for primary prophylaxis. A meta-analysis of 5 RCTs including comparing banding with no treatment confirmed that banding reduced first variceal bleeding (RR 0.36; 95% CI [0.26–0.5]), bleeding related mortality (RR 0.20; 95% CI [0.11–0.39]), and overall mortality (RR 0.55; 95% CI [0.43–0.71])[39].

### EVL versus medical therapy

Sarin et al.[40] randomized 89 high-risk patients (variceal diameter > 5 mm) to either EVL ($n = 45$) or propranolol ($n = 44$) for the primary prevention of variceal bleeding. After 18 months, the actuarial probability of bleeding was significantly less with EVL than propranolol (15% vs. 43%). In 3 of the 4 patients from the EVL group who bled, first bleeding occurred before their varices had been obliterated. Nine patients (20%) in the EVL group had recurrent varices 3.7 months after the initial treatment. There was no significant difference in mortality and there were no serious complications of EVL. Propranolol therapy was stopped in 2 patients because of side effects. It was concluded by the authors that in patients with high-risk EV, EVL is safe and more effective than propranolol for the primary prevention of variceal bleeding. This study was criticized for its small sample size and the fact that low doses of propranolol were used.

The meta-analysis by Imperiale et al.[41] examined 4 RCTs ($n = 283$) of EVL versus β-blockers. The only observed benefit for EVL was a reduction of first variceal bleeding (RR 0.48; 95% CI [0.24–0.96]). Bleeding related mortality and overall mortality were similar for EVL and propranolol.

A randomized study grouped 172 patients with cirrhosis and grade II/III EV that had never bled to receive either EVL ($n = 44$), propranolol ($n = 66$) or ISMN ($n = 62$)[42]. On an intention-to-treat analysis, variceal bleeding occurred after 2 years in 7%, 14%, and 23% of those patients randomized to EVL, propranolol, and ISMN, respectively. The 2-year actuarial risks of first variceal bleeding were 6.2% for EVL, 19.4% for propranolol, and 27.7% for ISMN. There were no statistically significant differences in the mortality rates between the groups. More patients reported side effects with drug therapy (propranolol, 45%; ISMN, 42%) compared to EVL (2%), resulting in withdrawal from treatment in 30% of propranolol-treated and 21% of ISMN-treated patients. In an as-treated analysis, there was a statistically significant difference in actuarial risk for bleeding at 2 years between EVL and ISMN, but not between EVL and propranolol. EVL was equivalent to propranolol and superior to ISMN in preventing first variceal bleed.

*Cost effectiveness of prophylactic therapy*

It is uncertain which of β-blockers and EVL is more cost-effective for primary prophylaxis. An empiric β-blocker strategy cost an incremental USD 12408 (US dollars) per additional variceal bleed prevented[43]. Compared with this strategy, the strategies using screening endoscopy followed by either β-blocker or EVL cost over USD 175000 more per additional bleed prevented. Strategies with selective screening endoscopy in high-risk patients followed by either β-blocker or EVL were more expensive and less effective than the empiric β-blocker strategy. Universal prophylaxis with β-blockers (without endoscopic screening) was associated with the lowest cost (USD 34100) and the highest (6.65) quality-adjusted life-years (QALYs)[44]. Endoscopic screening followed by β-blocker prophylaxis was associated with a cost of USD 37300 and 5.72 QALYs.

## ENDOSCOPIC GUIDANCE OF PRIMARY AND SECONDARY PROPHYLAXIS

### Surveillance

In general, patients with no or small varices represent 66–75% of cirrhotics screened by endoscopy and should undergo surveillance endoscopy every 2 years as the risk of developing bleeding in this population is low. Some recommend endoscopy every 1–2 years based on severity of liver disease.

For surveillance during endoscopic eradication therapy, the optimal time interval between endoscopic sessions is generally weekly during the first 3–4 weeks, followed by every 2 weeks until eradication is achieved. Recurrent bleeding is usually related to the development of new esophageal variceal columns. Currently, there are no studies to suggest that long-term follow-up after endoscopic eradication is superior to short-term treatment aimed at eradication, especially if patients are maintained on β-blockers[45].

## EUS for the guidance of endoscopic therapy

EUS probes have been used as an objective measure of EV recurrence[46,47], and may be used to monitor variceal eradication following EVS[48,49]. The identification of perforating veins by color Doppler EUS (CD-EUS) may allow more effective targeting of these sites and therefore reduced variceal recurrence[50,51]. CD-EUS may detect persistent blood flow following endoscopic cyanoacrylate injection of GV[52]. Scheduled repeated EUS-guided cyanoacrylate injection therapy can reduce the risk of recurrent bleeding relative to patients receiving "on-demand" injections[53].

## ENDOSCOPY IN ACUTE VARICEAL BLEEDING

Acute bleeding from EGV in the setting of portal hypertension continues to carry a substantial mortality rate despite the remarkable advances in medical and endoscopic therapies and intensive care. The literature of several decades past reports mortality rates with each bleeding episode between 30 and 60%[54]. A recent large study compared two cohorts a decade apart and suggested improved survival among the later cohort[55]. A recent retrospective multicenter study observed the in-hospital, 6 week, and overall mortality rates to be 14.2%, 17.5% and 33.5%, respectively[56].

Prospective controlled trials are needed to best assess the survival rate associated with variceal bleeding. The duration of time between the onset of bleeding and the starting point for analysis may be an important confounder when determining survival and recurrent bleeding rates and should be considered when comparing outcomes across trials. This effect may be greatest in centers where patients are referred from other hospitals at variable times from the onset of their bleeding[57]. In addition, patients' characteristics should be closely matched, especially with regard to hepatic functional reserve. The prognosis is better in patients without significant liver impairment such as those with non-cirrhotic portal vein thrombosis[58] or idiopathic portal hypertension[59]. In cirrhotic patients, the prognosis is worse with concomitant alcoholic hepatitis, hepatocellular carcinoma, portal vein thrombosis or ascites.

When is the critical time to intervene? The high early mortality rate is the rationale for primary prophylaxis. In an acute bleed, the risk of recurrent bleeding or death rapidly diminishes over the first few days, and early survival may be the best marker for later survival. Improving survival in the early period (the first 2 weeks after the onset of bleeding) is vital to improving long-term survival[60].

## Preparation for endoscopic therapy

The successful management of acute variceal GI bleeding relies on early resuscitation which is best initiated in the emergency department. Endoscopy is best performed either in a high-level therapeutic endoscopy unit with experienced nurses or in the ICU. Management is multidisciplinary involving endoscopists, intensivists, anesthesiologists, surgeons and interventional radiologists.

Patients with massive bleeding, severe lactic acidosis, severe agitation, or altered mental status should be considered for early endotracheal intubation to protect from aspiration. Central venous access is preferable, though access via multiple large-bore peripheral venous catheters is acceptable.

Blood should be grouped and cross-matched immediately. Volume replacement should begin as soon as possible, since hypovolemic shock is an independent predictor of renal failure, which, together with shock, is associated with a higher risk of mortality[61]. This is best achieved by replacing blood loss directly with packed red blood cells rather than crystalloid. Excessive crystalloid may result in overexpansion of the extracellular fluid (ECF) volume and a rebound increase in the portal pressure accompanied by continued bleeding or recurrent bleeding[62].

Correction of a coexisting coagulopathy with plasma and vitamin K is imperative. Recombinant activated factor VII (rFVIIa) normalizes the prothrombin time in patients with cirrhosis and has been assessed as an adjunct to endoscopic and medical therapy[63]. In patients with Child's class B and C cirrhosis, rFVIIa achieves hemostasis in bleeding EV unresponsive to standard treatment[64]. Further research is needed to confirm these results. Severe thrombocytopenia (platelets < 5000) is uncommon and may require platelet transfusions. Antibiotics must be administered to those patients with cirrhosis in order to reduce the risk of bacterial infection and mortality[65]. A flouroquinolone administered orally for 7 days is simple and cost-effective.

Endoscopy should be performed as soon as possible after admission for diagnosis and therapy. Evacuation of blood clots and food is necessary for the accurate identification of the bleeding site(s). A therapeutic endoscope with a 6 mm suction channel (e.g. Olympus GIF-XTQ160) is ideal. An overtube may facilitate rapid re-entry for lavage and ligation.

Prevention of hepatic encephalopathy following acute bleeding may be achieved with administration of lactulose. This may be delivered endoscopically into the duodenum.

## Esophageal varices

Once varices are present, the risk of bleeding is approximately 10% per year. At 2 years, the risk of first variceal bleeding is 24% for all size varices and 33% if one considers only medium- or large-sized varices. In 20% of cirrhotic patients with acute bleeding, the source is from causes other than varices, such as Mallory-Weiss tears, peptic ulcer disease, PHG and cancer.

After an index bleed, the risk of recurrent bleeding is 30–40% within the next 6 weeks[66]. The risk of recurrent bleeding within 1 year is 70%. The risk is maximal within the first 5 days and declines slowly over the next 6 weeks. Thereafter, the risk is nearly equal to the risk prior to the bleed. The risk of recurrent bleeding decreases in patients with spontaneous or treatment-induced reduction of portal pressure gradient or variceal pressure.

The mortality rate per bleeding episode is 30–50%. Among survivors, 30% will die within the following year. Early recurrent bleeding is associated with a higher risk of mortality.

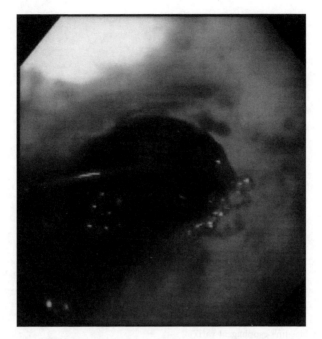

**Figure 1.** An actively bleeding esophageal varix in the distal esophagus

*Endoscopic variceal sclerotherapy (EVS)*

EVS has been supplanted by EVL for the management of acute variceal bleeding.

*Endoscopic variceal ligation (EVL)*

Van Stiegmann et al. in 1986 first described EVL as an alternative to EVS with fewer nonbleeding complications. Multiband ligators became available in 1996 and have greatly simplified the success of EVL.

Bands are applied starting at or just below the GE junction and continuing proximally in the distal 7–10 cm of the esophagus. The number of bands placed during the initial session can be up to 20. Ligated varices become thrombosed with subsequent fibrosis with healing. A ligated varix usually sloughs off in 3–7 days leaving a superficial ulcer that will heal in another 14–21 days.

Ideally, the actively bleeding varix is identified (Figure 1) and a band is placed over it to achieve hemostasis. However, precise localization is not always necessary and placement of bands near the GE junction reduces flow and facilitates further banding. In the absence of active spurting, one should search for a nipple or fibrin plug and ligate it first (Figure 2).

*Efficacy of endoscopic therapy*

Acute variceal hemorrhage can be stopped with either EVL or EVS in 90% of patients. Recurrent bleeding occurs in 20–50% of those treated with EVS and this rate is reduced by 40–50% if EVL is used.

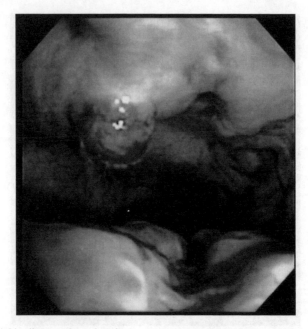

**Figure 2A.** A bleeding esophageal varix

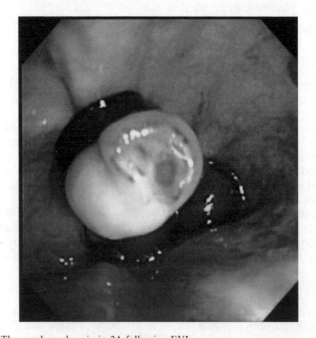

**Figure 2B.** The esophageal varix in 2A following EVL

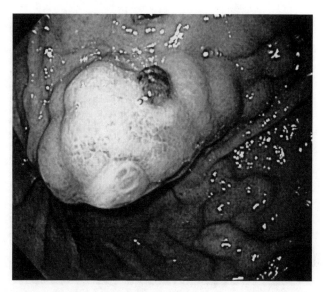

**Figure 3A.** A large gastric varix with an ulceration and platelet plug

*Salvage therapy*

When either EVL or EVS fail to control actively bleeding EV, injection therapy with cyanoacrylate is an effective alternative that can be life-saving. Cyanoacrylate is also useful if recurrent bleeding is from a site of previous ligation that is not easy to re-ligate.

The success of endoscopic therapy depends on the expertise of the endoscopist. When endoscopy fails to control the bleeding, options for salvage therapy include transfer to an advanced therapeutic endoscopy unit, TIPS, or surgical portacaval shunt. Balloon tamponade (Sengstaken-Blakemore, Linton-Nachlas, and Minnesota tubes) can be used as a temporizing measure prior to embarking on any of these alternatives. In centers with advanced therapeutic endoscopy, it is rare that bleeding cannot be controlled endoscopically; consequently, balloon tamponade, TIPS and surgery are rarely needed.

## Gastric varices

GV usually are located in the fundus and account for up to 30% of acute variceal bleeds (Figure 3A). Kim et al.[67] followed 117 patients with fundal varices that had never bled and observed that 34 developed bleeding over 5 years. The cumulative risks for bleeding at 1, 3, and 5 years were 16%, 36%, and 44%, respectively. The endoscopic predictors for bleeding include red signs and variceal size while a clinical predictor is hepatic function as measured by the Child–Pugh class.

Cardiac varices develop as an extension of EV and are amenable to EVS and/or EVL.

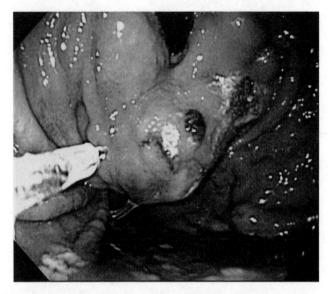

**Figure 3B.** The gastric varix in 3A treated with cyanoacrylate injection therapy

## Cyanoacrylate injection therapy

Cyanoacrylate (Histoacryl®, Glubran®: *n*-butyl-2-cyanoacrylate; Bucrylate®: isobutyl-2-cyanoacrylate) polymerizes and hardens within seconds of its exposure to blood. In 1986, endoscopic injection of cyanoacrylate into GV and EV was introduced (Figure 3B)[68-70]. Injection results in the formation of a cast that sloughs off in weeks or months resulting in late ulceration that ultimately heals. Rapid solidification of cyanoacrylate may be prevented by diluting it with the oily contrast medium, Lipiodol® (Laboratoire Guerbet, Aulnay-sous-Bois Cdx., France). In Europe, Glubran® (GEM, Viareggio, Italy) is available, polymerizes a little more slowly and therefore does not require dilution with Lipiodol®. Over-dilution of cyanoacrylate prolongs the polymerization time and the risk of embolization. We use Histoacryl® and Lipiodol® in a 1:1 mixture. The risk of embolization is also reduced if no more than 1 ml of the mixture is injected at a time. Thus, one must avoid flushing the catheter with a volume greater than its dead space when the needle is in the varix.

An injection catheter with a needle length of at least 5 mm is necessary to puncture a varix deeply during injection. The catheter is first flushed with Lipiodol®. Then the glue mixture is loaded in the catheter and advanced close to the tip of the needle (Figure 3B). With the endoscope retroflexed, the catheter and needle are injected into the varix and the glue mixture is injected. The catheter is then flushed with distilled water as the needle is removed from the varix. To protect the endoscope, its suction source may be disconnected during each injection. In addition, one may lubricate the endoscope channel and external covering with silicone oil. Treated varices should be probed with the catheter's tip to check their consistency. Firmness

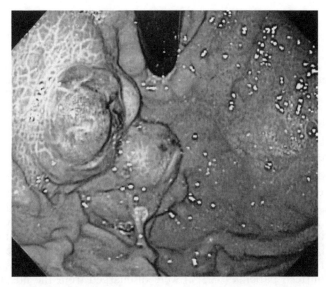

**Figure 3C.** Isolated gastric varices in Figure 3A, 3 weeks after injection therapy with cyanoacrylate

indicates variceal obliteration. A soft and supple consistency indicates the need for more injections. One to eight injections is usually sufficient depending on the size of the varices.

Endoscopic cyanoacrylate injection is approved in most countries. The complications include gastric ulceration, secondary bleeding at the injection site, needle fixation within the glued varix, systemic embolization, retrosternal discomfort, fever, and dysphagia. Embolization may result in stroke[71,72], pulmonary embolism[73–76], multiple systemic emboli[77,78], or splenic infarction[79]. Septicemia[80], splenic or portal vein thrombosis[81], and visceral fistulae[82] have also been reported. Fever and pain are due to the inflammatory response and usually resolve within a few hours.

Follow-up examination is necessary to determine if further therapy is needed. Figure 3C illustrate gastric varices 3 weeks after therapy.

Several studies confirm that cyanoacrylate is effective for initial hemostasis of bleeding GV. Soehendra et al.[83] reported on 202 patients with EGV in whom cyanoacrylate was used. The overall hospital mortality decreased from 31.5% to 17.5%.

Sarin et al.[84] randomized 37 patients with portal hypertension and isolated GVs (17 with histories of active bleeding) to EVS with either alcohol ($n =$ 17) or cyanoacrylate ($n = 20$). Cyanoacrylate was more effective in achieving variceal obliteration (100% vs. 44%) in a significantly shorter period of time (2.0 vs. 4.7 wk). Cyanoacrylate achieved primary hemostasis more often than alcohol (89% vs. 62%). Six patients died from uncontrolled GV bleeding, four from the alcohol group. After a mean follow-up period of 15 months there was no recurrence of GV in either group.

*Thrombin*

The largest study available is retrospective and examined 52 patients with bleeding GV who were treated by intravariceal injection with bovine thrombin[85]. They underwent follow-up endoscopy at 72 hours and then at two-week intervals. The initial hemostasis rate was 94% and the bleeding-related mortality rate at 72 hours after the index bleed was 6%. Gastric variceal ablation was achieved after a median of 2 treatment sessions. At six weeks, 18% rebled and the mortality rate was 8%. No adverse drug effects were observed, but anaphylaxis to bovine thrombin is a known danger.

*Fibrin glue*

Beriplast® (Aventis Behring) is a solution of fibrinogen and thrombin. Patients with gastric variceal bleeding ($n = 15$) were entered into an open trial of gastric intravariceal injection treatment with Beriplast® and followed for up to 1 month after endoscopic treatment[86]. There was failure to control bleeding in one patient (6.7%). Four patients (26.7%) had recurrent bleeding after the index bleed. Each was re-injected with Beriplast®, and the bleeding was controlled in three. The 30-day mortality following therapy was 6.7% (1/15). Fourteen patients (93.3%) were discharged from the hospital after the first episode of gastric variceal bleeding. None of the patients had injection-induced complications.

*Detachable snares*

Lee et al.[87] treated GV ( > 2 cm diameter) with detachable snares and treated adjacent small varices with EVL. Ten of 12 patients with active bleeding and 28 of 29 patients with red color signs were successfully treated. The overall hemostatic rate for endoscopic ligation was 82.9% (34/41). Variceal eradication was nearly complete in 91.7% (33/36) of patients who underwent repeated ligation treatments. Thirty of these patients, after a mean follow-up of 16.4 months, did not have recurrent bleeding. No serious complications were observed.

*EVS*

Paravariceal and intravariceal injection of absolute alcohol is not effective for isolated fundal varices and is actually dangerous[88].

*Balloon-occluded endoscopic injection sclerotherapy (BO-EIS)*

Balloon-occluded retrograde transvenous obliteration (B-RTO) was described by Kanagawa et al.[89] for the treatment of GV with a known gastrorenal shunt (85% of patients with GV) which may be determined using MR angiography. Shiba et al.[90] developed balloon-occluded endoscopic injection sclerotherapy (BO-EIS) that may be used even in patients without a gastrorenal shunt.

## ENDOSCOPY IN SECONDARY PROPHYLAXIS

The options for the prevention of recurrent bleeding are: medical therapy and endoscopic therapy or a combination of the two; TIPS; and surgical portacaval shunt.

*EVL versus EVS*

EVL has essentially replaced EVS as the endoscopic method of choice to control variceal bleeding. Laine et al. confirmed the superiority of EVL over EVS for the outcomes of recurrent bleeding, complications, time to variceal obliteration, and mortality[91].

*EVL versus EVL plus medical therapy*

Combining β-blockade and nitrate therapy is superior to EVL alone[92]. Combining EVL and β-blockade is superior to EVL alone in terms of reduction of recurrent bleeding, lower variceal recurrence, and a trend toward improved survival[93].

*Combination therapy (EVL plus EVS)*

Contradictory results are published on the benefit of adding low-dose EVS to EVL in terms of standard outcomes measures such as variceal eradication and variceal recurrence rates. The available studies are heterogeneous in their methodologies which may be classified according to the timing of delivery of treatments. For example, the two modalities may be delivered either simultaneously during the same session or consecutively on separate sessions. Furthermore, the available studies are likely to be highly operator dependent. The best approach remains to be determined.

*Detachable snares*

A small study by Hepworth et al. ($n = 11$) used modified detachable nylon snares for ligation of esophageal varices[94]. A ridged endcap and snares with modified angulations were developed. The snares were effective and no complications were observed.

Shim et al. randomized 103 patients with recent or active esophageal variceal bleeding to EVL or ligation by a new mini-detachable snare[95]. No differences were observed in the initial hemostasis rates ($\sim 85\%$), the recurrent bleeding rates ($\sim 5\%$), the number of sessions needed to eradicate varices ($\sim 4.5$), and the rates of variceal recurrence ($11\%$). Furthermore, no serious complications were observed.

*APC for the prevention of recurrent esophageal varices*

APC was examined as a potential modality to prevent the recurrence of esophageal varices. APC of the distal esophageal mucosa was shown to be safe and effective for reducing the rate of variceal recurrence following obliteration by EVL[96]. The sample size from this preliminary study is too small to demonstrate a difference in recurrent bleeding and mortality compared to no therapy.

## ENDOSCOPY IN PORTAL HYPERTENSIVE GASTROPATHY

PHG is characterized by ectasia of the gastric mucosal capillaries and submucosal veins without inflammation. Traditional endoscopic descriptive terms have included "pink speckling", "mosaic pattern", "scarlatina rash", "superficial reddening", "snake-skin rash", "cherry-red mucosal spots", and "diffuse hemorrhagic gastritis". Fifty to eighty percent of patients with cirrhosis and portal hypertension develop PHG. The incidence correlates with the duration of portal hypertension, presence and size of esophagogastric varices, and a previous history of EVS.

The role of endoscopy in the management of PHG is primarily diagnostic. It is seen mainly in the body, fundus, and cardia and rarely in the antrum. Similar changes can be seen in the small bowel and colon. Histologically one sees dilated capillaries and venules in the mucosa and submucosa without erosion, inflammation, or fibrinous thrombi.

PHG is generally divided into mild and severe forms, determined subjectively at endoscopy. Severe PHG is manifested by cherry-red spots of gastric mucosa which frequently bleed. D'Amico et al. revealed that 13% of patients with mild and 75% of patients with severe PHG experienced gastric bleeding. There is a lower prevalence of endoscopic findings of PHG in patients with non-cirrhotic portal hypertension such as hepatosplenic schistosomiasis[97]. This difference could not be explained by the underlying histologic changes, which appear similar in both groups.

The optimal management of bleeding PHG is unclear. APC may not be effective in patients with PHG in contrast to those with gastric antral vascular ectasia (GAVE). Medical therapy for bleeding PHG involves the use of agents that reduce portal pressure. The choice of agent is controversial but includes β-blockers, octreotide, omeprazole, vasopressin and oral prednisolone. TIPS has not proved useful. Liver transplantation is the definitive solution.

## ENDOSCOPY IN ECTOPIC VARICES

### Duodenal varices (DV) and small intestinal varices

The incidence in patients with portal hypertension is estimated to be 0.4%[98]. The etiology is either cirrhosis or extrahepatic portal hypertension for which the reported cases have included: schistosomiasis, AVM, pancreatic cancer, non-Hodgkin's lymphoma, previous gastrointestinal surgery, splenic and portal vein thrombosis. The duodenal cap is the most frequent site followed by the second part of the duodenum; however they may be located more distally.

DV either present with severe bleeding or are discovered at endoscopy. Bleeding is associated with a mortality rate of up to 40% because of the difficulty of endoscopic localization and management. The incidence of bleeding is 1–5% in patients with cirrhosis[99] and 30–40% in patients with extrahepatic portal hypertension[100]. The bleeding risk may be higher at anastomotic sites[101].

Tazawa et al.[102] first reported EVL for bleeding DV in 1995. Other case reports and series are available[103–105]. Injection therapy with cyanoacrylate is safe and effective for the treatment of bleeding DV. Several case reports are published on its use[106–109]. Injection therapy with other agents (ethanolamine, sodium tetradecyl sulfate[110], and thrombin[111]) have shown mixed success.

Other therapeutic approaches include surgery and interventional radiology. The surgical approach is generally an enterotomy with oversewing[112]. Interventional radiologic techniques include B-RTO, percutaneous transhepatic obliteration (PTO)[113], transileocolic vein obliteration (TIO)[114], and TIPS. Haskal et al.[115] reported on 9 patients with small intestinal varices who received TIPS. The five with active bleeding achieved initial hemostasis and only one had recurrent bleeding which was managed by coil embolization.

Double-balloon enteroscopy enables endoscopic access to the entire small intestine[116]. The Fujinon EN-450P5/20 enteroscope has a 2.2 mm working channel and injection needles are available for injection of cyanoacrylate compounds. EVL is currently not available for this endoscope. Endoscopic tattooing is possible to aid the surgeon in locating the lesion.

## Colorectal varices

Most cases are associated with portal hypertension[117]. Rarely cases are congenital or idiopathic. Colorectal varices may be found anywhere in the colon, especially in the anorectum and cecum[118]. They may be found at ileocolonic anastomoses in the absence of portal hypertension. They are usually isolated; however, there are reports of extensive cases involving either large segments or the entire colon.

Colonic varices may be the cause of recurrent, massive and sometimes fatal lower gastrointestinal hemorrhage. The incidence of colonic varices as a cause of lower GI bleeding is 1–8%.[119,120]

EVL is useful for anorectal varices[121]. Chen et al.[122] used cyanoacrylate to control active bleeding from colorectal varices but was unable to achieve long-term hemostasis. APC was used successfully to stop bleeding and eradicate ectopic varices at the ileocolonic anastomosis[123].

Alternatives to endoscopic treatment include portosystemic shunt (TIPS) and surgery. Cecectomy, right hemicolectomy, and sigmoid resection are reported. Colorectal varices are difficult to identify at surgery, therefore preoperative localization is important.

## CONCLUSION

Advances in endoscopy have increased the role of endoscopy in the management of portal hypertension. The most valuable recent advances have been: improved stratification of varices according to variceal bleeding risk; endoscopic variceal ligation; and intravariceal injection therapy with cyanoacrylate. Transnasal endoscopy has increased the ease of screening, but its role remains to be determined. Objective endoscopic measurements of variceal bleeding risk need to be developed further so that they are reliable and universally available. With respect to acute variceal bleeding, future research is best directed at decreasing the mortality in the critical early period following the acute bleed. Until the underlying causes of portal hypertension are curable, endoscopy is likely to play an increasing role in the treatment of portal hypertension.

## References

1. Jensen DM. Endoscopic screening for varices in cirrhosis: findings, implications, and outcomes. [Review] [55 refs]. Gastroenterology. 2002;122:1620–30.
2. D'Amico G, Morabito A, Pagliaro L, Marubini E. Survival and prognostic indicators in compensated and decompensated cirrhosis. Dig Dis Sci. 1986;31:468–75.
3. El Serag HB, Everhart JE. Improved survival after variceal hemorrhage over an 11-year period in the Department of Veterans Affairs. Am J Gastroenterol. 2000;95:3566–73.
4. Graham DY, Smith JL. The course of patients after variceal hemorrhage. Gastroenterology. 1981;80:800–9.
5. Poynard T, Cales P, Pasta L et al. β-Adrenergic-antagonist drugs in the prevention of gastrointestinal bleeding in patients with cirrhosis and esophageal varices. An analysis of data and prognostic factors in 589 patients from four randomized clinical trials. Franco-Italian Multicenter Study Group. N Engl J Med. 1991;324:1532–8.
6. Grace ND. Diagnosis and treatment of gastrointestinal bleeding secondary to portal hypertension. American College of Gastroenterology Practice Parameters Committee. Am J Gastroenterol. 1997;92:1081–91.
7. Grace ND, Groszmann RJ, Garcia-Tsao G et al. Portal hypertension and variceal bleeding: an AASLD single topic symposium. Hepatology. 1998;28:868–80.
8. Spiegel BM, Targownik L, Dulai GS, Karsan HA, Gralnek IM. Endoscopic screening for esophageal varices in cirrhosis: Is it ever cost effective? Hepatology. 2003;37:366–77.
9. Jensen DM. Endoscopic screening for varices in cirrhosis: findings, implications, and outcomes. [Review] [55 refs]. Gastroenterology. 2002;122:1620–30.
10. Giannini E, Botta F, Borro P et al. Platelet count/spleen diameter ratio: proposal and validation of a non-invasive parameter to predict the presence of oesophageal varices in patients with liver cirrhosis. Gut. 2003;52:1200–5.
11. Giannini E, Botta F, Borro P et al. Platelet count/spleen diameter ratio: proposal and validation of a non-invasive parameter to predict the presence of oesophageal varices in patients with liver cirrhosis. Gut. 2003;52:1200–5.
12. Saeian K, Staff D, Knox J et al. Unsedated transnasal endoscopy: a new technique for accurately detecting and grading esophageal varices in cirrhotic patients. Am J Gastroenterol. 2002;97:2246–9.
13. Arguedas MR, McGuire BM, Fallon MB, Abrams GA. The use of screening and preventive therapies for gastroesophageal varices in patients referred for evaluation of orthotopic liver transplantation. Am J Gastroenterol. 2001;96:833–7.
14. Plevris JN, Elliot R, Mills PR et al. Effect of propranolol on prevention of first variceal bleed and survival in patients with chronic liver disease. Aliment Pharmacol Ther. 1994;8:63–70.
15. Cales P, Oberti F, Payen JL et al. Lack of effect of propranolol in the prevention of large oesophageal varices in patients with cirrhosis: a randomized trial. French-Speaking Club for the Study of Portal Hypertension. Eur J Gastroenterol Hepatol. 1999;11:741–5.
16. Beppu K, Inokuchi K, Koyanagi N et al. Prediction of variceal hemorrhage by esophageal endoscopy. Gastrointest Endosc. 1981;27:213–18.
17. Idezuki Y. General rules for recording endoscopic findings of esophagogastric varices (1991). Japanese Society for Portal Hypertension. World J Surg. 1995;19:420–2.
18. Schiano TD, Adrain AL, Vega KJ, Liu JB, Black M, Miller LS. High-resolution endoluminal sonography assessment of the hematocystic spots of esophageal varices. Gastrointest Endosc. 1999;49:424–7.
19. Prediction of the first variceal hemorrhage in patients with cirrhosis of the liver and esophageal varices. A prospective multicenter study. The North Italian Endoscopic Club for the Study and Treatment of Esophageal Varices.[see comment]. N Engl J Med. 1988; 319:983–9.
20. Thuluvath PJ, Krishnan A. Primary prophylaxis of variceal bleeding. [Review] [59 refs]. Gastrointest Endosc. 2003;58:558–67.

21. Rigau J, Bosch J, Bordas JM et al. Endoscopic measurement of variceal pressure in cirrhosis: correlation with portal pressure and variceal hemorrhage. Gastroenterology. 1989; 96:873–80.
22. Gertsch P, Fischer G, Kleber G, Wheatley AM, Geigenberger G, Sauerbruch T. Manometry of esophageal varices: comparison of an endoscopic balloon technique with needle puncture. Gastroenterology. 1993;105:1159–66.
23. Miller L, Banson FL, Bazir K et al. Risk of esophageal variceal bleeding based on endoscopic ultrasound evaluation of the sum of esophageal variceal cross-sectional surface area. Am J Gastroenterol. 2003;98:454–9.
24. Miller ES, Kim JK, Gandehok J et al. A new device for measuring esophageal variceal pressure. Gastrointest Endosc. 2002;56:284–91.
25. Pontes JM, Leitao MC, Portela F, Nunes A, Freitas D. Endosonographic Doppler-guided manometry of esophageal varices: experimental validation and clinical feasibility. Endoscopy. 2002;34:966–72.
26. Ichikawa S, Okamura S, Tujigami K et al. Quantitative analysis of red color sign in the endoscopic evaluation of esophageal varices. Endoscopy. 2001;33:747–53.
27. Hosking SW, Johnson AG. Gastric varices: a proposed classification leading to management. Br J Surg. 1988;75:195–6.
28. Hashizume M, Kitano S, Yamaga H, Koyanagi N, Sugimachi K. Endoscopic classification of gastric varices. Gastrointest Endosc. 1990;36:276–80.
29. Sarin SK, Kumar A. Gastric varices: profile, classification, and management. [Review] [72 refs]. Am J Gastroenterol. 1989;84:1244–9.
30. Sarin SK, Jain AK, Lamba GS, Gupta R, Chowdhary A. Isolated gastric varices: prevalence, clinical relevance and natural history. Dig Surg. 2003;20:42–7.
31. Thuluvath PJ, Krishnan A. Primary prophylaxis of variceal bleeding. [Review] [59 refs]. Gastrointest Endosc. 2003;58:558–67.
32. Avgerinos A, Armonis A, Manolakopoulos S et al. Endoscopic sclerotherapy plus propranolol versus propranolol alone in the primary prevention of bleeding in high risk cirrhotic patients with esophageal varices: a prospective multicenter randomized trial. Gastrointest Endosc. 2000;51:652–8.
33. Lo GH, Lai KH, Cheng JS, Lin CK, Hsu PI, Chiang HT. Prophylactic banding ligation of high-risk esophageal varices in patients with cirrhosis: a prospective, randomized trial. J Hepatol. 1999;31:451–6.
34. Sarin SK, Guptan RK, Jain AK, Sundaram KR. A randomized controlled trial of endoscopic variceal band ligation for primary prophylaxis of variceal bleeding [see comment]. Eur J Gastroenterol Hepatol. 1996;8:337–42.
35. Sarin SK, Lamba GS, Kumar M, Misra A, Murthy NS. Comparison of endoscopic ligation and propranolol for the primary prevention of variceal bleedin [see comment]. N Engl J Med. 1999;340:988–93.
36. Lay CS, Tsai YT, Teg CY et al. Endoscopic variceal ligation in prophylaxis of first variceal bleeding in cirrhotic patients with high-risk esophageal varices [see comment]. Hepatology. 1997;25:1346–50.
37. Svoboda P, Kantorova I, Ochmann J, Kozumplik L, Marsova J. A prospective randomized controlled trial of sclerotherapy vs ligation in the prophylactic treatment of high-risk esophageal varices. Surg Endosc. 1999;13:580–4.
38. Burroughs AK, Patch D. Primary prevention of bleeding from esophageal varices [comment]. N Engl J Med. 1999;340:1033–5.
39. Imperiale TF, Chalasani N. A meta-analysis of endoscopic variceal ligation for primary prophylaxis of esophageal variceal bleeding [see comment]. Hepatology. 2001;33:802–7.
40. Sarin SK, Lamba GS, Kumar M, Misra A, Murthy NS. Comparison of endoscopic ligation and propranolol for the primary prevention of variceal bleeding [see comment]. N Engl J Med. 1999;340:988–93.
41. Imperiale TF, Chalasani N. A meta-analysis of endoscopic variceal ligation for primary prophylaxis of esophageal variceal bleeding [see comment]. Hepatology. 2001;33:802–7.
42. Lui HF, Stanley AJ, Forrest EH et al. Primary prophylaxis of variceal hemorrhage: a randomized controlled trial comparing band ligation, propranolol, and isosorbide mononitrate [see comment]. Gastroenterology. 2002;123:735–44.
43. Spiegel BM, Targownik L, Dulai GS, Karsan HA, Gralnek IM. Endoscopic screening for esophageal varices in cirrhosis: Is it ever cost effective? Hepatology. 2003;37:366–77.

44. Saab S, DeRosa V, Nieto J, Durazo F, Han S, Roth B. Costs and clinical outcomes of primary prophylaxis of variceal bleeding in patients with hepatic cirrhosis: a decision analytic model. Am J Gastroenterol. 2003;98:763–70.
45. Thuluvath PJ, Krishnan A. Primary prophylaxis of variceal bleeding. [Review] [59 refs]. Gastrointest Endosc. 2003;58:558–67.
46. Leung VK, Sung JJ, Ahuja AT et al. Large paraesophageal varices on endosonography predict recurrence of esophageal varices and rebleeding. Gastroenterology. 1997; 112:1811–16.
47. Konishi Y, Nakamura T, Kida H, Seno H, Okazaki K, Chiba T. Catheter US probe EUS evaluation of gastric cardia and perigastric vascular structures to predict esophageal variceal recurrence. Gastrointest Endosc. 2002;55:197–203.
48. Ziegler K, Gregor M, Zeitz M, Zimmer T, Habermann F, Riecken EO. Evaluation of endosonography in sclerotherapy of esophageal varices [see comment]. Endoscopy. 1991;23:247–50.
49. Pontes JM, Leitao MC, Portela FA, Rosa AM, Ministro P, Freitas DS. Endoscopic ultrasonography in the treatment of oesophageal varices by endoscopic sclerotherapy and band ligation: do we need it? Eur J Gastroenterol Hepatol. 1995;7:41–6.
50. Nagamine N, Ueno N, Tomiyama T et al. A pilot study on modified endoscopic variceal ligation using endoscopic ultrasonography with color Doppler function [see comment]. Am J Gastroenterol. 1998;93:150–5.
51. Nagamine N, Ido K, Ueno N et al. The usefulness of ultrasonic microprobe imaging for endoscopic variceal ligation. Am J Gastroenterol. 1996;91:523–9.
52. Iwase H, Suga S, Morise K, Kuroiwa A, Yamaguchi T, Horiuchi Y. Color Doppler endoscopic ultrasonography for the evaluation of gastric varices and endoscopic obliteration with cyanoacrylate glue. Gastrointest Endosc. 1995;41:150–4.
53. Lee YT, Chan FK, Ng EK et al. EUS-guided injection of cyanoacrylate for bleeding gastric varices [see comment]. Gastrointest Endosc. 2000;52:168–74.
54. Burroughs AK. The natural history of varices. [Review] [12 refs]. J Hepatol. 1993;17:Suppl-3.
55. El Serag HB, Everhart JE. Improved survival after variceal hemorrhage over an 11-year period in the Department of Veterans Affairs. Am J Gastroenterol. 2000;95:3566–73.
56. Chalasani N, Kahi C, Francois F et al. Improved patient survival after acute variceal bleeding: a multicenter, cohort study. Am J Gastroenterol. 2003;98:653–9.
57. Burroughs AK, Mezzanotte G, Phillips A, McCormick PA, McIntyre N. Cirrhotics with variceal hemorrhage: the importance of the time interval between admission and the start of analysis for survival and rebleeding rates. Hepatology. 1989;9:801–7.
58. Valla DC, Condat B. Portal vein thrombosis in adults: pathophysiology, pathogenesis and management. [Review] [45 refs]. J Hepatol. 2000;32:865–71.
59. Ludwig J, Hashimoto E, Obata H, Baldus WP. Idiopathic portal hypertension. Hepatology. 1993;17:1157–62.
60. Graham DY, Smith JL. The course of patients after variceal hemorrhage. Gastroenterology. 1981;80:800–9.
61. Cardenas A, Gines P, Uriz J et al. Renal failure after upper gastrointestinal bleeding in cirrhosis: incidence, clinical course, predictive factors, and short-term prognosis. Hepatology. 2001;34:671–6.
62. Castaneda B, Morales J, Lionetti R et al. Effects of blood volume restitution following a portal hypertensive-related bleeding in anesthetized cirrhotic rats. Hepatology. 2001; 33:821–5.
63. Ejlersen E, Melsen T, Ingerslev J, Andreasen RB, Vilstrup H. Recombinant activated factor VII (rFVIIa) acutely normalizes prothrombin time in patients with cirrhosis during bleeding from oesophageal varices. Scand J Gastroenterol. 2001;36:1081–5.
64. Romero-Castro R, Jimenez-Saenz M, Pellicer-Bautista F et al. Recombinant-activated factor VII as hemostatic therapy in eight cases of severe hemorrhage from esophageal varices. Clin Gastroenterol Hepatol. 2004;2:78–84.
65. Bernard B, Grange JD, Khac EN, Amiot X, Opolon P, Poynard T. Antibiotic prophylaxis for the prevention of bacterial infections in cirrhotic patients with gastrointestinal bleeding: a meta-analysis. Hepatology. 1999;29:1655–61.
66. D'Amico G, Luca A. Natural history. Clinical-haemodynamic correlations. Prediction of the risk of bleeding. [Review] [71 refs]. Baillieres Clin Gastroenterol. 1997;11:243–56.

67. Kim T, Shijo H, Kokawa H et al. Risk factors for hemorrhage from gastric fundal varices. Hepatology. 1997;25:307–12.
68. Ramond MJ, Valla D, Gotlib JP, Rueff B, Benhamou JP. [Endoscopic obturation of esophagogastric varices with bucrylate. I. Clinical study of 49 patients]. [French]. Gastroenterol Clin Biol. 1986;10:575–9.
69. See A, Florent C, Lamy P, Levy VG, Bouvry M. [Cerebrovascular accidents after endoscopic obturation of esophageal varices with isobutyl-2-cyanoacrylate in 2 patients]. [French]. Gastroenterol Clin Biol. 1986;10:604–7.
70. Soehendra N, Nam VC, Grimm H, Kempeneers I. Endoscopic obliteration of large esophagogastric varices with bucrylate. Endoscopy. 1986;18:25–6.
71. See A, Florent C, Lamy P, Levy VG, Bouvry M. [Cerebrovascular accidents after endoscopic obturation of esophageal varices with isobutyl-2-cyanoacrylate in 2 patients]. [French]. Gastroenterol Clin Biol. 1986;10:604–7.
72. Gallet B, Zemour G, Saudemont JP, Renard P, Hillion ML, Hiltgen M. Echocardiographic demonstration of intracardiac glue after endoscopic obturation of gastroesophageal varices. J Am Soc Echocardiogr. 1995;8:t-61.
73. Hwang SS, Kim HH, Park SH et al. N-butyl-2-cyanoacrylate pulmonary embolism after endoscopic injection sclerotherapy for gastric variceal bleeding. J Comp Assist Tomogr. 2001;25:16–22.
74. Tsokos M, Bartel A, Schoel R, Rabenhorst G, Schwerk WB. [Fatal pulmonary embolism after endoscopic embolization of downhill esophageal varix]. [German]. Deutsche Med Wochenschr. 1998;123:691–5.
75. Palejwala AA, Smart HL, Hughes M. Multiple pulmonary glue emboli following gastric variceal obliteration. Endoscopy. 2000;32:S1-S2.
76. Kull E, Hernandez M, Richer JP, Borderie C, Silvain C, Beauchant M. [Severe pulmonary embolism after obturation of gastric varices with a butyl-cyanoacrylate and lipiodol combination]. [French]. Gastroenterol Clin Biol. 1999;23:1095–6.
77. Tan YM, Goh KL, Kamarulzaman A et al. Multiple systemic embolisms with septicemia after gastric variceal obliteration with cyanoacrylate [see comment]. Gastrointest Endosc. 2002;55:276–8.
78. Roesch W, Rexroth G. Pulmonary, cerebral and coronary emboli during bucrylate injection of bleeding fundic varices. Endoscopy. 1998;30:S89-S90.
79. Cheng PN, Sheu BS, Chen CY, Chang TT, Lin XZ. Splenic infarction after histoacryl injection for bleeding gastric varices. Gastrointest Endosc. 1998;48:426–7.
80. Turler A, Wolff M, Dorlars D, Hirner A. Embolic and septic complications after sclerotherapy of fundic varices with cyanoacrylate. Gastrointest Endosc. 2001;53:228–30.
81. Shim CS, Cho YD, Kim JO et al. A case of portal and splenic vein thrombosis after Histoacryl injection therapy in gastric varices. Endoscopy. 1996;28:461.
82. Battaglia G, Morbin T, Patarnello E, Merkel C, Corona MC, Ancona E. Visceral fistula as a complication of endoscopic treatment of esophageal and gastric varices using isobutyl-2-cyanoacrylate: report of two cases. Gastrointest Endosc. 2000;52:267–70.
83. Soehendra N, Grimm H, Nam VC, Berger B. N-butyl-2-cyanoacrylate: a supplement to endoscopic sclerotherapy. Endoscopy. 1987;19:221–4.
84. Sarin SK, Jain AK, Jain M, Gupta R. A randomized controlled trial of cyanoacrylate versus alcohol injection in patients with isolated fundic varices. Am J Gastroenterol. 2002;97:1010–15.
85. Przemioslo RT, McNair A, Williams R. Thrombin is effective in arresting bleeding from gastric variceal hemorrhage. Dig Dis Sci. 1999;44:778–81.
86. Datta D, Vlavianos P, Alisa A, Westaby D. Use of fibrin glue (beriplast) in the management of bleeding gastric varices. Endoscopy. 2003;35:675–8.
87. Lee MS, Cho JY, Cheon YK et al. Use of detachable snares and elastic bands for endoscopic control of bleeding from large gastric varices [see comment]. Gastrointest Endosc. 2002;56:83–8.
88. Sarin SK. Long-term follow-up of gastric variceal sclerotherapy: an eleven-year experience. Gastrointest Endosc. 1997;46:8–14.
89. Kanagawa H, Mima S, Kouyama H, Gotoh K, Uchida T, Okuda K. Treatment of gastric fundal varices by balloon-occluded retrograde transvenous obliteration. J Gastroenterol Hepatol. 1996;11:51–8.

90. Shiba M, Higuchi K, Nakamura K et al. A case of huge gastric varices successfully treated with endoscopic injection sclerotherapy with occlusion of both supplying and draining veins with balloons. Gastrointest Endosc. 2000;52:104–7.
91. Laine L, Cook D. Endoscopic ligation compared with sclerotherapy for treatment of esophageal variceal bleeding. A meta-analysis [see comment]. Ann Intern Med. 1995;123:280–7.
92. Villanueva C, Minana J, Ortiz J et al. Endoscopic ligation compared with combined treatment with nadolol and isosorbide mononitrate to prevent recurrent variceal bleeding [see comment] [summary for patients in Gastrointest Endosc. 2002 May; 55:761–4; PMID: 12085777]. N Engl J Med. 2001;345:647–55.
93. Lo GH, Lai KH, Cheng JS et al. Endoscopic variceal ligation plus nadolol and sucralfate compared with ligation alone for the prevention of variceal rebleeding: a prospective, randomized trial [see comment]. Hepatology. 2000;32:461–5.
94. Hepworth CC, Burnham WR, Swain CP. Development and application of endoloops for the treatment of bleeding esophageal varices. Gastrointest Endosc. 1999;50:677–84.
95. Shim CS, Cho JY, Park YJ et al. Mini-detachable snare ligation for the treatment of esophageal varices. Gastrointest Endosc. 1999;50:673–6.
96. Cipolletta L, Bianco MA, Rotondano G, Marmo R, Meucci C, Piscopo R. Argon plasma coagulation prevents variceal recurrence after band ligation of esophageal varices: preliminary results of a prospective randomized trial [see comment]. Gastrointest Endosc. 2002;56:467–71.
97. Chaves DM, Sakai P, Mucenic M, Iriya K, Iriya Y, Ishioka S. Comparative study of portal hypertensive gastropathy in schistosomiasis and hepatic cirrhosis. Endoscopy. 2002;34:199–202.
98. Hashizume M, Tanoue K, Ohta M et al. Vascular anatomy of duodenal varices: angiographic and histopathological assessments. Am J Gastroenterol. 1993;88:1942–5.
99. Heaton ND, Khawaja H, Howard ER. Bleeding duodenal varices. Br J Surg. 1991;78:1450–1.
100. Lebrec D, Benhamou JP. Ectopic varices in portal hypertension. Clin Gastroenterol. 1985;14:105–21.
101. Heaton ND, Khawaja H, Howard ER. Bleeding duodenal varices. Br J Surg. 1991;78:1450–1.
102. Tazawa J, Sakai Y, Koizumi K et al. Endoscopic ligation for ruptured duodenal varices. Am J Gastroenterol. 1995;90:677–8.
103. Fayad N, Nammour F, Elfant A. Endoscopic variceal ligation for bleeding duodenal varices. J Clin Gastroenterol. 2004;38:467.
104. Shiraishi M, Hiroyasu S, Higa T, Oshiro S, Muto Y. Successful management of ruptured duodenal varices by means of endoscopic variceal ligation: report of a case. Gastrointest Endosc. 1999;49:255–7.
105. Bosch A, Marsano L, Varilek GW. Successful obliteration of duodenal varices after endoscopic ligation. Dig Dis Sci. 2003;48:1809–12.
106. Bhasin DK, Sharma BC, Sriram PV, Makharia G, Singh K. Endoscopic management of bleeding ectopic varices with histoacryl. HPB Surg. 1999;11:171–3.
107. Ota K, Shirai Z, Masuzaki T et al. Endoscopic injection sclerotherapy with n-butyl-2-cyanoacrylate for ruptured duodenal varices. J Gastroenterol. 1998;33:550–5.
108. Yoshida Y, Imai Y, Nishikawa M et al. Successful endoscopic injection sclerotherapy with N-butyl-2-cyanoacrylate following the recurrence of bleeding soon after endoscopic ligation for ruptured duodenal varices. Am J Gastroenterol. 1997;92:1227–9.
109. D'Imperio N, Piemontese A, Baroncini D et al. Evaluation of undiluted N-butyl-2-cyanoacrylate in the endoscopic treatment of upper gastrointestinal tract varices. Endoscopy. 1996;28:239–43.
110. Wu CS, Chen CM, Chang KY. Endoscopic injection sclerotherapy of bleeding duodenal varices. J Gastroenterol Hepatol. 1995;10:481–3.
111. Rai R, Panzer SW, Miskovsky E, Thuluvath PJ. Thrombin injection for bleeding duodenal varices. Am J Gastroenterol. 1994;89:1871–3.
112. Cottam DR, Clark R, Hayn E, Shaftan G. Duodenal varices: a novel treatment and literature review. Am Surg. 2002;68:407–9.
113. Menu Y, Gayet B, Nahum H. Bleeding duodenal varices: diagnosis and treatment by percutaneous portography and transcatheter embolization. Gastrointest Radiol. 1987; 12:111–13.

114. Ota K, Okazaki M, Higashihara H et al. Combination of transileocolic vein obliteration and balloon-occluded retrograde transvenous obliteration is effective for ruptured duodenal varices. J Gastroenterol. 1999;34:694–9.
115. Haskal ZJ, Scott M, Rubin RA, Cope C. Intestinal varices: treatment with the transjugular intrahepatic portosystemic shunt. Radiology. 1994;191:183–7.
116. Yamamoto H, Sekine Y, Sato Y et al. Total enteroscopy with a nonsurgical steerable double-balloon method. Gastrointest Endosc. 2001;53:216–20.
117. Goenka MK, Kochhar R, Nagi B, Mehta SK. Rectosigmoid varices and other mucosal changes in patients with portal hypertension. Am J Gastroenterol. 1991;86:1185–9.
118. Hamlyn AN, Morris JS, Lunzer MR, Puritz H, Dick R. Portal hypertension with varices in unusual sites. Lancet. 1974;2:1531–4.
119. Hosking SW, Smart HL, Johnson AG, Triger DR. Anorectal varices, haemorrhoids, and portal hypertension. Lancet. 1989;1:349–52.
120. Ganguly S, Sarin SK, Bhatia V, Lahoti D. The prevalence and spectrum of colonic lesions in patients with cirrhotic and noncirrhotic portal hypertension. Hepatology. 1995; 21:1226–31.
121. Levine J, Tahiri A, Banerjee B. Endoscopic ligation of bleeding rectal varices. Gastrointest Endosc. 1993;39:188–90.
122. Chen WC, Hou MC, Lin HC, Chang FY, Lee SD. An endoscopic injection with $N$-butyl-2-cyanoacrylate used for colonic variceal bleeding: a case report and review of the literature. Am J Gastroenterol. 2000;95:540–2.
123. Schafer TW, Binmoeller KF. Argon plasma coagulation for the treatment of colonic varices. Endoscopy. 2002;34:661–3.
124. Beppu K, Inokuchi K, Koyanagi N et al. Prediction of variceal hemorrhage by esophageal endoscopy. Gastrointest Endosc. 1981;27:213–18.

# 22
# Transjugular intrahepatic portosystemic shunt (TIPS): current indications

ZIAD HASSOUN and GILLES POMIER-LAYRARGUES

## INTRODUCTION

The transjugular intrahepatic portosystemic shunt (TIPS) is a new non-surgical therapeutic modality used to treat complications of portal hypertension[1,2]. It allows the creation of a communication between one hepatic vein and an intrahepatic branch of the portal vein by using a transjugular approach. The first TIPS implantation was reported in 1989 by Ritcher et al.[3]; it is a hemodynamic equivalent of the small-diameter side-to-side surgical portacaval shunt. This procedure has been widely used all around the world for more than 15 years. After an initial wave of enthusiasm its exact place in the treatment of portal hypertension is now better defined as clinical controlled trials are available for the main potential indications. The major drawbacks of TIPS are stent dysfunction and hepatic encephalopathy, but progress has been made to decrease their clinical impact.

## CONTRAINDICATIONS

TIPS placement is contraindicated in several circumstances: cardiac failure, polycystic liver, bile duct dilation, severe liver failure, or chronic recurrent encephalopathy. Portal vein thrombosis represents a relative contraindication because in some cases it is still possible to recanalize the thrombosed portal vein and to decrease portal hypertension after stent placement[4].

## ACUTE COMPLICATIONS

The TIPS procedure is usually well tolerated, with a mortality rate less than 1–2%. Perioperative complications are most often minor and transient[5]: neck hematoma, cardiac arrhythmia, stent migration, hemolysis. Bilhemia may occur due to a communication between a biliary radicle and the portal

**Table 1.** Potential indications for TIPS

---

1. Gastrointestinal bleeding: esophageal varices, gastric varices, ectopic varices
2. Refractory ascites (pleural effusion)
3. Budd–Chiari syndrome
4. Hepatorenal syndrome
5. Miscellaneous: hepatopulmonary syndrome? Preoperative TIPS?

---

vein, and can be cured by the use of a covered stent[6]. Life-threatening complications including hemoperitoneum, hemobilia, liver ischemia, cardiac failure and septicemia are rare. Portal vein thrombosis can be observed early after the procedure and is most often related to inadequate placement of the stent.

## LONG-TERM COMPLICATIONS

TIPS is a portacaval shunt; therefore, not surprisingly, the rates of progressive liver failure and chronic recurrent encephalopathy that can be observed after the procedure are quite similar to those reported after surgical portacaval shunt[7]. However, decreasing the diameter of the shunt with a reducing stent or balloon occlusion of the shunt is efficient to treat post-TIPS disabling encephalopathy, but the ensuing recurrence of portal hypertension may lead to clinical complications.

TIPS stenosis is frequently observed and is related to pseudointimal hyperplasia that develops inside the stent. The 1-year stenosis rate is 50–70%[8]. Monitoring of the stent function with Doppler ultrasound should be done routinely[9], and repeated vascular interventions are needed. The use of new polytetrafluoroethylene-covered stents appears very promising to prevent this complication, and this technical advance will be discussed later.

## INDICATIONS

Potential indications for the TIPS procedure are listed in Table 1. The analysis of the literature allows us to determine if TIPS is indicated or not in a given complication of portal hypertension[1,2,10]; however, in some circumstances the role of TIPS is still undetermined given the absence of convincing trials available so far.

### Gastrointestinal bleeding

*Esophageal varices*

Prevention of rebleeding from esophageal varices is the most extensively studied indication for TIPS. It is now well established that either endoscopic or pharmacologic therapies can decrease the risk of rebleeding and improve survival. The TIPS procedure has been compared with endoscopic sclerotherapy, endoscopic variceal ligation and pharmacologic treatment in controlled clinical trials[11–22]. TIPS markedly decreased the risk of bleeding as compared to the other study groups; however, the mortality rate was not affected and the incidence of encephalopathy was increased after the TIPS procedure. These findings were established from results of individual studies as well as from a meta-analysis[23]. As a result TIPS cannot be recommended as a first-line treatment in this situation but it can be used in patients who fail endoscopic and/or pharmacologic treatments (nearly 20% of patients with bleeding varices).

TIPS used as a salvage therapy can be placed successfully in more than 90% of patients, and can control bleeding in a vast majority of them[24]. The target pressure to avoid rebleeding has been established at 12 mmHg, which is the threshold value associated with variceal rupture[8]. There is no controlled trial comparing TIPS and shunt surgery used as a salvage therapy; however, it is well known that surgical portacaval shunt is usually contraindicated in Child C cirrhotic patients, and might be hazardous in Child B patients. Surgery could have a place in Child A patients because the operative risk is lower and the long-term rate of patency of the shunt is very high. However, the use of PTFE-covered stents for the TIPS procedure may lead to abandonment of surgery even in patients with good liver function.

### Gastric varices

It has been proposed to classify gastric varices according to their localization and to the presence of fundal varices which remain a major problem if bleeding occurs[25]. Available treatment for bleeding gastric varices includes endoscopic sclerotherapy with different sclerosing agents, pharmacological treatment, TIPS and shunt surgery. The literature does not allow us to determine which is the best approach, and what could be the optimal treatment algorithm. Given this absence of data it is generally agreed that endoscopic sclerotherapy using either intravariceal thrombin or cyanoacrylate is the best first-line treatment, followed by TIPS when bleeding cannot be controlled, or if early rebleeding occurs[26]. TIPS allows good control of bleeding in the majority of cases; however, rebleeding may occur even if the post-TIPS gradient is lower than 12 mmHg, a threshold value associated with the bleeding risk for esophageal varices[27]. This is probably related to the larger size of fundal varices, as variceal diameter is a major determinant of variceal tension and, therefore, of the risk of variceal rupture.

### Ectopic varices

Varices may develop anywhere along the gastrointestinal tract, in the peritoneum or near the umbilicus. Bleeding may occur from these ectopic varices (duodenal, jejunal, ileal, colic, rectal, stomal varices) which cannot be treated endoscopically. There are no data showing that pharmacological treatment is helpful. Some uncontrolled series suggest that TIPS is a good approach to prevent rebleeding in this situation[28].

### Gastric antral vascular ectasia (GAVE)

GAVE is observed occasionally in cirrhotic patients; recurrent chronic bleeding may occur and may represent a significant problem. It was thought originally that GAVE was related to portal hypertension; however, this concept has been challenged because two recent studies have demonstrated that the TIPS procedure had no beneficial effect on acute or chronic bleeding related to GAVE[29,30].

## Refractory ascites

Ascites may become resistant to diuretic therapy in nearly 10% of patients. A standardized definition has been provided by a panel of experts during a consensus conference[31] allowing better evaluation of the therapeutic modalities available for this condition, including repeated large-volume paracentesis with albumin replacement (the reference treatment), the TIPS procedure and liver transplantation. As previously stated, TIPS is a hemodynamic equivalent of side-to-side surgical portacaval shunt; not surprisingly ascites improves in a vast majority of patients several days or weeks after TIPS[32]. Relief of portal hypertension and shunting of splanchnic blood flow results in a correction of systemic hypovolemia with a concomitant decrease in plasma aldosterone, renin activity and catecholamine levels, leading to an improvement of glomerular filtration rate[33]; however, shunting may also induce liver failure and hepatic encephalopathy. Several uncontrolled series suggested that TIPS was useful to control refractory ascites; thereafter four controlled trials comparing TIPS and paracentesis in the management of refractory ascites were published[34–37]; all of these concluded that TIPS was more efficient in controlling ascites than large-volume paracentesis, but that survival was not different for both groups and that hepatic encephalopathy was higher in TIPS patients. However, given the small size of the patient population, one cannot exclude that TIPS may be beneficial in a subgroup of patients with moderately impaired liver function and a good renal function[38]. These studies also confirm the poor prognosis of cirrhotic patients with refractory ascites which makes them potential candidates for liver transplantation; accordingly, TIPS probably has a role as a bridge to surgery.

## Refractory hepatic hydrothorax

Ascitic fluid may leak from the abdominal cavity into the pleural space through diaphragmatic defects. Small amounts of fluid can lead to respiratory distress and some of these patients require repeated thoracentesis despite diuretic therapy. Several uncontrolled series suggest that the use of TIPS is helpful in these patients[39]; however, the onset of refractory hydrothorax carries the same poor prognosis as refractory ascites, and liver transplantation remains the best option in suitable candidates[40].

## Budd–Chiari syndrome

Budd–Chiari syndrome results from partial or complete obstruction of the hepatic venous outflow system, and in a majority of cases a thrombophilic disorder can be demonstrated. Clinical presentation may be hyperacute with fulminant hepatic failure, or subacute with massive ascites and sometimes bleeding from esophageal varices. TIPS can be used in the treatment of Budd–Chiari syndrome when other treatments fail. When fulminant hepatic failure occurs, liver transplantation is the best option. In subacute cases, when ascites is not controlled by medical therapy, TIPS represents a good option, as demonstrated by several recent series[41,42]. TIPS placement remains a technical challenge in this situation given the obstruction of major hepatic veins; portal vein catheterization must be performed most often by using a transcaval approach. Anticoagulation must be prescribed in all patients on a long-term basis.

## Hepatorenal syndrome

Hepatorenal syndrome (HRS) is a functional renal failure associated with decompensated liver cirrhosis and it can be subclassified as HRS type 1 if the progression of renal failure is very rapid and type 2 if renal failure is more chronic[31]. TIPS is a logical approach to correct the systemic hypovolemia by shunting the increased splanchnic blood flow into the general circulation; this in turn may deactivate the compensatory vasoconstriction, particularly at the cortical glomerular level. On the other hand, TIPS creation might also cause a deterioration in liver function. HRS has been reversed in some patients with HRS type 1 or 2[43,44]; however, TIPS placement must be considered a bridge to liver transplantation always required in these very sick patients.

## Other indications

Hepatopulmonary syndrome is characterized by severe hypoxemia related to the presence of intrapulmonary arteriovenous shunts. Its severity does not always parallel the degree of liver failure and it has been shown that liver transplantation can reverse hypoxemia. TIPS can improve this syndrome, as reported recently[45]. Its efficacy might be related to the relief of portal hypertension which could result in a decrease of nitric oxide production by the endothelial cells of the portal vasculature. It can be used in selected cases as a bridge to liver transplantation.

It has also been suggested that performing a TIPS preoperatively could prevent operative complications associated with abdominal surgery in cirrhotic patients. One recent uncontrolled series showed encouraging results[46]; however a retrospective study comparing postoperative evolution after abdominal surgery in cirrhotic patients with or without preoperative TIPS did not provide evidence that this approach is beneficial, in terms of postoperative morbidity or mortality[47].

## FUTURE ADVANCES

The high rate of stent stenosis during follow-up is related to neointimal proliferation inside the stent[48]. It has been hypothesized that covering the stent with synthetic membranes such as polytetrafluoroethylene (PTFE) could block this phenomenon, and can allow the maintenance of long-term patency of the shunt (Figure 1). A recent controlled trial compared the clinical outcome in cirrhotic patients treated with either PTFE-coated stents or uncovered stents[49]. The actuarial rate of primary patency at 2 years was 80.2% when PTFE-coated stents were used as compared to 18.6% with

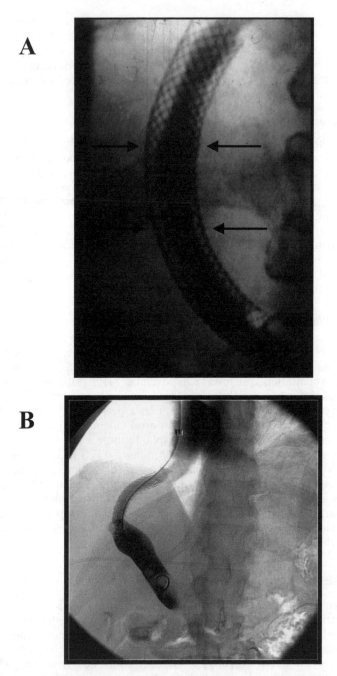

**Figure 1.** Portography 2 years after TIPS placement: severe stenosis developed in an uncovered stent (**A**, arrows) but pseudointimal hyperplasia was not observed in a PTFE-covered stent (**B**)

uncovered stents. This improvement in shunt function translated in a significant decrease of clinical events related to shunt dysfunction such as variceal rebleeding or ascites recurrence. If these exciting results are confirmed in the future, the monitoring of shunt function will become much easier, the need for vascular interventions much lower and a marked decrease in costs of the procedure will ensue.

## CONCLUSIONS

Fifteen years after the introduction of TIPS as a new method of treatment of complications of portal hypertension, the exact role of this procedure is now defined more precisely. Even if it has not markedly improved the prognosis of cirrhotic patients, this treatment probably has a major impact on quality of life and/or on cost-effectiveness, which must be evaluated as main endpoints in future clinical trials. In addition, its use as a bridge to liver transplantation will become more popular given the increasing waiting time on the transplant list.

### References

1. Boyer TD. Transjugular intrahepatic portosystemic shunt: current status. Gastroenterology. 2003;124:1700–10.
2. Rosado B, Kamath KP. Transjugular intrahepatic portosystemic shunts: an update. Liver Transplant. 2003;9:207–17.
3. Richter GM, Palmaz JC, Noldge G et al. The transjugular intrahepatic portosystemic stent-shunt. A new nonsurgical percutaneous method. Radiologe. 1989;29:406–11.
4. Radosevich PM, Ring EJ, Laberge JM et al. Transjugular intrahepatic portosystemic shunts in patients with portal vein occlusion. Radiology. 1993;186:523–27.
5. Freedman AM, Sanyal AJ, Tisnado J et al. Complications of transjugular intrahepatic portosystemic shunt: a comprehensive review. Radiographics. 1993;13:1185–210.
6. Spahr L, Sahai A, Lahaie R et al. Transient healing of a TIPS-induced biliovenous fistula by a PTFE-covered stent graft. Dig Dis Sci. 1996;41:2229–32.
7. Pomier-Layrargues G. TIPS and hepatic encephalopathy. Semin Liver Dis. 1996;16:315–20.
8. Casado M, Bosch J, Garcia-Pagan J et al. Clinical events after transjugular intrahepatic portosystemic shunt: correlation with hemodynamic findings. Gastroenterology. 1998;114: 1296–303.
9. Lafortune M, Martinet JP, Denys A et al. Short- and long-term hemodynamic effects of transjugular intrahepatic portosystemic shunts: a Doppler/manometric correlative study. Am J Roentgenol. 1995;164:997–1002.
10. Hassoun Z, Pomier-Layrargues G. Transjugular intrahepatic portosystemic shunt in the treatment of portal hypertension. J Gastroenterol Hepatol. 2004;16:1–4.
11. Groupe d'Étude des Anastomoses Intrahépatiques. Sclerotherapy plus propranolol in the prevention of variceal bleeding: preliminary results of a multicenter randomized trial. Hepatology. 1995;22:299 (abstract).
12. Cabrera J, Maynar M, Granados R et al. Transjugular intrahepatic portosystemic shunt versus sclerotherapy in the elective treatment of variceal hemorrhage. Gastroenterology. 1996;110:832–9.
13. Rössle M, Deibert P, Haag K et al. Randomized trial of transjugular intrahepatic portosystemic shunt versus endoscopy plus propranolol in prevention of variceal rebleeding. Lancet. 1997;349:1043–9.
14. Sanyal AJ, Freeman AM, Luketic VA et al. Transjugular intrahepatic portosystemic shunts compared with endoscopic sclerotherapy for the prevention of recurrent variceal hemorrhage. A randomized controlled trial. Ann Intern Med. 1997;126:849–57.

15. Sauer P, Theilman L, Stremmel W, Benz C, Richter GM, Stiehl A. Transjugular intrahepatic portosystemic stent shunt versus sclerotherapy + propranolol for variceal rebleeding. Gastroenterology. 1997;113:1623–31.
16. Jalan R, Forrest HE, Stanley AJ et al. A randomized trial comparing transjugular intrahepatic portosystemic stent-shunt with variceal band ligation in the prevention of rebleeding from oesophageal varices. Hepatology. 1997;26:1115–22.
17. Merli M, Salerno F, Riggio O et al. Transjugular intrahepatic portosystemic shunt versus endoscopic sclerotherapy for the prevention of variceal bleeding in cirrhosis: a randomized multicenter trial. Hepatology. 1998;27:48–53.
18. Garcia-Villareal L, Martinez-LaGares K, Sierra A et al. Transjugular intrahepatic portosystemic shunt versus endoscopic sclerotherapy for the prevention of variceal rebleeding after recent variceal hemorrhage. Hepatology. 1999;29:27–32.
19. Cello JP, Ring EJ, Olcott EW et al. Endoscopic sclerotherapy compared with percutaneous transjugular intrahepatic portosystemic shunt after initial sclerotherapy in patients with acute variceal hemorrhage. A randomized, controlled trial. Ann Intern Med. 1997;126: 858–65.
20. Gulberg V, Schepke M, Geigenberger G et al. Transjugular intrahepatic portosystemic shunting is not superior to endoscopic variceal band ligation for prevention of variceal rebleeding in cirrhotic patients: a randomized clinical trial. Scand J Gastroenterol. 2002;37:338–43.
21. Escorsell A, Banares R, Garcia-Pagan JC et al. TIPS versus drug therapy in preventing variceal rebleeding in advanced cirrhosis: a randomized controlled trial. Hepatology. 2002;35:385–92.
22. Pomier-Layrargues G, Villeneuve JP, Deschenes M et al. Transjugular intrahepatic portosystemic shunt (TIPS) versus endoscopic variceal ligation in the prevention of variceal rebleeding in patients with cirrhosis: a randomised trial. Gut. 2001;48:390–6.
23. Papatheodoridis GV, Goulis J, Leandro G, Patch D, Burroughs AK. Transjugular intrahepatic portosystemic shunt compared with endoscopic treatment for prevention of variceal rebleeding: a meta-analysis. Hepatology. 1999;30:612–22.
24. Azoulay D, Castaing D, Majno P et al. Salvage transjugular intrahepatic portosystemic shunt for uncontrolled variceal bleeding in patients with decompensated cirrhosis. J Hepatol. 2001;35:590–7.
25. Sarin SK, Lahoti D, Saxena SP, Murthi NS, Makwane UK. Prevalence, classification and natural history of gastric varices: a long-term follow-up study in 568 portal hypertensive patients. Hepatology. 1992;16:1343–9.
26. Barange K, Peron JM, Imani K et al. Transjugular intrahepatic portosystemic shunt in the treatment of refractory bleeding from ruptured gastric varices. Hepatology. 1999;30:1139–43.
27. Spahr L, Dufresne MP, Bui BT et al. Efficacy of TIPS in the prevention of rebleeding from oesophageal and fundal varices. A comparative study. Hepatology. 1995;22:296 (abstract).
28. Shibata D, Brophy DP, Gordon FD, Anastopoulos HT, Sentovich SM, Bleday R. Transjugular intrahepatic portosystemic shunt for treatment of bleeding ectopic varices with portal hypertension. Dis Colon Rectum. 1999;42:1581–5.
29. Spahr L, Villeneuve JP, Dufresne MP et al. Gastric antral vascular ectasia in cirrhotic patients: absence of relation with portal hypertension. Gut. 1999;44:739–42.
30. Kamath PS, Lacerda M, Ahlquist DA, McKusick MA, Andrews JC, Nagorney DA. Gastric mucosal response to intrahepatic shunting in patients with cirrhosis. Gastroenterology. 2000;118:905–11.
31. Arroyo V, Gines P, Gerbes AL et al. Definition and diagnostic criteria of refractory ascites and hepatorenal syndrome in cirrhosis. Hepatology. 1996;23:164–76.
32. Martinet JP, Legault L, Roy L et al. Treatment of refractory ascites using transjugular intrahepatic portosystemic shunt (TIPS): a caution. Dig Dis Sci. 1997;42:161–6.
33. Wong F, Sniderman K, Liu P, Allidina Y, Sherman M, Blendis L. Transjugular intrahepatic portosystemic stent shunt: effects on hemodynamics and sodium homeostasis in cirrhosis and refractory ascites. Ann Intern Med. 1995;122:816–22.
34. Lebrec D, Giuily N, Hadengue A et al. Transjugular intrahepatic portosystemic shunts: comparison with paracentesis in patients with cirrhosis and refractory ascites: a randomized trial. French group of Clinicians and a Group of Biologists. J Hepatol. 1996;25:135–44.
35. Rossle M, Ochs A, Gulberg V et al. A comparison of paracentesis and transjugular intrahepatic portosystemic shunting in patients with ascites. N Engl J Med. 2000;342:1701–7.

36. Gines P, Uriz J, Calahorra B et al. Transjugular intrahepatic portosystemic shunting versus paracentesis plus albumin for refractory ascites in cirrhosis. Gastroenterology. 2002; 123:1839–47.
37. Sanyal AJ, Genning C, Reddy KR et al. The North American Study for the Treatment of Refractory Ascites. Gastroenterology. 2003;124:634–41.
38. Deschenes M, Dufresne MP, Bui B et al. Predictors of clinical response to transjugular intrahepatic portosystemic shunt (TIPS) in cirrhotic patients with refractory ascites. Am J Gastroenterol. 1999;94:1361–5.
39. Gordon FD, Anastopoulos HT, Crenshaw W et al. The successful treatment of symptomatic, refractory hepatic hydrothorax with transjugular intrahepatic portosystemic shunt. Hepatology. 1997;25:1366–9.
40. Jeffries MA, Kazanijian S, Wilson M, Punch J, Fontana RJ. Transjugular intrahepatic portosystemic shunts and liver transplantation in patients with refractory hepatic hydrothorax. Liver Transplant Surg. 1998;4:416–23.
41. Perello A, Garcia-Pagan JC, Gilabert R et al. TIPS is a useful long-term derivative therapy for patients with Budd–Chiari syndrome uncontrolled by medical therapy. Hepatology. 2002;35:132–9.
42. Mancuso A, Fung K, Mela M et al. TIPS for acute and chronic Budd–Chiari syndrome: a single-centre experience. J Hepatol. 2003;38:751–4.
43. Spahr L, Fenyves D, Nguyen VV et al. Improvement of hepatorenal syndrome by transjugular intrahepatic portosystemic shunt. Am J Gastroenterol. 1995;90:1169–70.
44. Guevara M, Gines P, Bandi JC et al. Transjugular intrahepatic portosystemic shunt in hepatorenal syndrome: effects on renal function and vasoactive systems. Hepatology. 1998;28:416–22.
45. Lasch HM, Fried MW, Zacks SL et al. Use of transjugular intrahepatic portosystemic shunt as a bridge to liver transplantation in a patient with severe hepatopulmonary syndrome. Liver Transplant. 2001;7:147–9.
46. Azoulay D, Buabse F, Damiano I et al. Neoadjuvant transjugular intrahepatic portosystemic shunt: a solution for extra-hepatic abdominal operation in cirrhotic patients with severe portal hypertension. J Am Coll Surg. 2001;193:46–51.
47. Vinet E, Perreault P, Bouchard L et al. Transjugular intrahepatic portosystemic shunt (TIPS) before surgery in cirrhotic patients: a retrospective comparative study. Gastroenterology. 2003;124:1411 (abstract).
48. Sanyal AJ, Contos MJ, Yager D, Zhu YN, Willey A, Graham MF. Development of pseudointima and stenosis after transjugular intrahepatic portosystemic shunts: characterization of cell phenotype and function. Hepatology. 1998;28:22–32.
49. Bureau C, Garcia-Pagan JC, Otal P et al. Improved clinical outcome using polytetrafluoroethylene coated stents for TIPS: results of a randomized study. Gastroenterology. 2004; 126:469–75.

# Section VII
# Present therapy

# 23
# Prevention of first variceal bleeding: drugs

DIDIER LEBREC

## INTRODUCTION

The goal of prophylactic therapy is the prevention of a first episode of bleeding and bleeding-related mortality. Preventive therapy began more than 30 years ago with surgical portacaval shunts, resulting in a significant reduction in variceal bleeding but also a significantly greater risk of hepatic encephalopathy and mortality[1]; therefore this surgical option has been considered unsuitable. Since this period progress has been made in identifying patients with a high risk of bleeding, and various pharmacologic and endoscopic therapies have been proposed to reduce the risk of bleeding and death[2].

This present review of the pharmacologic prevention of first bleeding summarizes firmly established approaches, and discusses approaches which are being studied.

## RISK FACTORS OF FIRST VARICEAL BLEEDING

Variceal bleeding may occur in patients with portal hypertension who develop portosystemic shunts and esophageal varices, but the exact mechanisms of the variceal rupture have not been determined. The risk of developing esophageal varices is approximately 90% at 10 years in patients with cirrhosis. Among these patients 50% bleed and 30–40% of them die within 42 days after admission. Prospective studies have shown that certain factors are associated with the risk of the first gastrointestinal hemorrhage in patients with cirrhosis, and thus may be used to identify candidates for prophylactic treatment. In one study the authors evaluated a prognostic index of bleeding ranging from 6% to 76% at 1 year, based on various clinical and endoscopic variables[3]. They revealed that the severity of cirrhosis, the size of esophageal varices and the presence of red wall markings were the three most important factors. In a second prospective study the authors demonstrated the significance of variceal pressure measurements for the prediction of a first episode of variceal bleeding in patients with cirrhosis and large esophageal varices followed for 1 year[4]. In this study the incidence of bleeding was less than 10% in patients with variceal pressure less than 15 mmHg, and more than 70% in patients with variceal pressure greater than 16 mmHg. In contrast, the values for the hepatic venous pressure gradient were not a predictive factor when it was 12 mmHg or more.

## PREVENTION OF THE DEVELOPMENT OF LARGE VARICES AND BLEEDING

Patients with cirrhosis and portal hypertension should undergo esophago-gastric endoscopic examination to determine the presence, absence and signs of esophageal varices. When varices are small or absent the risk of bleeding is low, probably less than 10% at 2 years.

In patients without or with small esophageal varices, beta-adrenergic antagonist administration has been tested to prevent the occurrence of large varices and thus variceal bleeding, since the drug limits the development of portosystemic shunts in portal hypertensive rats[5]. The results of one published trial show no significant difference between the two groups for the development of large varices and variceal bleeding (beta-blockers vs placebo) at 2 years[6]. The proportion of patients with large varices was 31% in the propranolol group and 14% in the placebo group. Less than 5% of patients bled in both groups. Preliminary results of a multicenter trial found similar results in patients without esophageal varices[7]. These findings suggest that beta-blocker administration cannot be recommended for the prevention of the development of large esophageal varices in patients with cirrhosis. In unselected patients with chronic liver diseases treated with beta-blockers or placebo, similar results of the occurrence of variceal bleeding and survival rate have been observed[8]. In contrast, preliminary results of a trial showed that nadolol administration may prevent the aggravation of esophageal varices in patients with cirrhosis and small esophageal varices, and thus suggested that nadolol may prevent variceal bleeding in these selected patients[9]. Nevertheless, an endoscopic examination should be performed every year in patients with small esophageal varices, and every 2 or 3 years in patients with no varices, to determine the development of large varices.

## PREVENTION OF THE FIRST VARICEAL BLEEDING

### Beta-adrenergic antagonists

In patients with small esophageal varices beta-blockers may reduce the risk of first variceal hemorrhage. In three trials comparing beta-blockers to placebo approximately 20% of patients had small esophageal varices. In patients in the placebo group the risk of bleeding was low (less than 10%), but it was lower in patients treated with beta-blockers; the difference was, however, not significantly different between the two groups, indicating that further clinical studies are needed.

In patients with large esophageal varices the results of nine controlled studies and three meta-analyses indicate that beta-blockers, which decrease portal pressure, significantly reduce the risk of first hemorrhage and significantly improve survival rate[1,10,11]. In these trials, according to the Child–Pugh classification, most patients were in good condition and the proportion of Child–Pugh C patients ranged from 0% to 46%. The cause of cirrhosis was chronic alcohol intoxication in more than 70% of the patients. Seven studies used standard or long-acting propranolol administered in doses that decreased the heart rate by approximately 25% (40–400 mg/day) in two studies another non-selective beta-blocker, nadolol, was used at doses ranging from 40–200 mg/day. At 2 years the beta-blockers significantly reduced the relative risk of the first episode of bleeding by approximately 50% compared to a placebo. Beta-blockers significantly reduced mortality by 20%. These results were observed whatever the cause and severity of cirrhosis; the efficacy was more marked in patients with liver dysfunction, or in patients with ascites, than in patients in good condition or without ascites[10]. Beta-blockers were well tolerated. Side-effects occurred in some patients (3–30%) who received beta-blockers, and the use of these drugs was discontinued in approximately 5% of the patients. Treatment should be continued for life, as in patients treated for arterial hypertension, since it has been observed that patients who discontinue beta-blockers experience increased mortality compared with an untreated population[12].

The prevention of first bleeding episode for gastric or ectopic varices in patients with cirrhosis, and the prevention of variceal bleeding in patients with extrahepatic portal hypertension, have not been evaluated. In these patients beta-blockers may be used, since they reduce portal pressure. Prospective studies are, however, needed in these patients.

## Isosorbide mononitrates

It has been shown that nitrate administration decreases portal pressure and may further decrease the hepatic venous pressure gradient in patients receiving beta-blockers. Three trials have compared the efficacy of isosorbide mononitrate alone versus beta-blocker alone in the prevention of a first bleeding episode in patients with cirrhosis. In one trial isosorbide-5-mononitrate alone was found to be a safe and alternative treatment to propranolol in the prevention of a first episode of bleeding, since bleeding rates were not significantly different between the two groups at 6 years[13]. At 5 years, however, the mortality rate in patients older than 50 receiving nitrates was significantly greater (66%) than in those receiving propranolol (47%). The results of a second trial performed in patients with cirrhosis confirmed the lack of difference on the prevention of first bleeding between isosorbide mononitrate and propranolol[14], and a third study performed in patients with cirrhosis and ascites showed that isosorbide-5-mononitrate was less effective with more side-effects than nadolol[15].

Isosorbide mononitrate alone has also been compared to placebo in the prevention of first variceal bleeding in patients with varices and contraindications or intolerance to beta-blockers[16]. There were no significant differences in the risk of bleeding at 2 years between the two groups. Survival rate and side-effects were similar in the two groups.

These trials suggest that nitrates alone must not be prescribed for the prevention of a first bleeding episode in patients with cirrhosis.

## Beta-adrenergic antagonists plus isosorbide mononitrates

The combination of beta-blockers and nitrates has also been compared with beta-blockers alone in three studies. A first study showed that the combination was significantly more effective than nadolol alone for the risk of a first bleeding episode; the bleeding rate at 7 years was 12% in the combined therapy and 29% in the nadolol group[17]. Two other studies were double-blind and placebo-controlled[18,19]. In one published study, in which 349 patients were randomized, the results found no significant difference in the 2-year actuarial probability of variceal bleeding between the two groups[18]. Survival was also similar, but adverse events were significantly more frequent in the propranolol plus isosorbide-5-mononitrate group than in the propranolol group. Preliminary results of the third trial showed a significantly lower risk of bleeding in the combined group than in the nadolol group, with a similar mortality rate[19]. Side-effects were, however, significantly more frequent in the nadolol and isosorbide mononitrate group than in the nadolol–placebo group.

The meta-analyses of these three trials showed that the bleeding rate was 15% in the beta-blocker group and 10% in the combination group, but there was no significant difference between the two groups[20]. The mortality rate was approximately 10% in both groups. In contrast, the occurrence of side-effects was significantly more frequent with the combination therapy. These results indicate that further clinical studies are needed.

## Beta-adrenergic antagonist plus spironolactone

In patients with cirrhosis it has been shown that spironolactone administration decreases portal pressure by reducing the increase in plasma volume. Thus, a trial has compared the combination of spironolactone and nadolol vs nadolol alone in the prevention of first bleeding in patients with cirrhosis without ascites[21]. The results did not show any significant difference in the appearance of variceal bleeding and ascites between the two groups at 2 years. The cumulative probability of survival was also not significantly different between the two groups.

## HEMODYNAMIC MONITORING OF TREATMENT RESPONSE

A significant sustained decrease in heart rate – approximately 20% for 24 h – is the best hemodynamic control of a correct systemic beta-adrenergic blockade. Similarly, the measurement of a significantly decreased cardiac output may predict the efficacy of beta-blockers. However, no firm relationships have been found between the decrease in heart rate or cardiac output and the occurrence of a first episode of variceal bleeding in patients with cirrhosis receiving beta-blockers.

Results of the measurement of the hepatic venous pressure gradient to predict the response of the pharmacologic prevention of the first episode of bleeding remain unclear[22]. The relationship between the hemodynamic response (decrease in the hepatic venous pressure gradient) and clinical response (variceal bleeding) is complex, since hepatic venous pressure gradient values are not directly related to the risk of bleeding and depend on many factors, including portal pressure, sinusoidal pressure, portal blood flow, hepatic arterial blood flow, and hepatic vascular resistance. Nevertheless, certain hemodynamic studies have shown that the bleeding or rebleeding risk is low in patients in whom the hepatic venous pressure gradient decreases by more than 20%[23,24], while earlier studies of the prevention of rebleeding do not support these results[25,26]. A decrease in heart rate of more than 20%, i.e. approximately 4 mmHg, is uncommon, but may predict the efficacy of the pharmacologic treatment. A decrease in the hepatic venous pressure gradient to below 12 mmHg seems to guarantee the prevention of bleeding, but it may occur only in patients with a gradient of 13 or 14 mmHg, a value which rarely occurs in patients with cirrhosis and varices. Accordingly, more hemodynamic results are needed before the routine clinical use of the hepatic venous pressure gradient measurement can be recommended; on the other hand this evaluation remains very important for the pharmacologic study of portal hypertension.

## CONCLUSION

For the prevention of the development of large varices and bleeding, beta-blockers cannot be recommended, but further studies are needed.

For the prevention of first bleeding in patients with medium or large varices, beta-blockers must be prescribed; nitrates alone must not be prescribed and the combination of beta-blockers and nitrates or spironolactone cannot be recommended but more trials are needed.

New types of drugs or combinations of drugs should be tested.

Finally, new ideas, hypotheses, and approaches are needed to further our understanding of the mechanisms of variceal bleeding and its treatment.

## References

1. Pagliaro L, Burroughs AK, Sorensen TI, Lebrec D, Morabito A, D'Amico G. Therapeutic controversies and randomised controlled trials (RCTs): prevention of bleeding and rebleeding in cirrhosis. Gastroenterol Int. 1989;2:71–84.
2. De Franchis R. Updating consensus in portal hypertension: report of the Baveno III consensus workshop on definitions, methodology and therapeutic strategies in portal hypertension. J Hepatol. 2000;33:846–52.
3. The North Italian Endoscopic Club for the Study and Treatment of Esophageal Varices. Prediction of the first variceal hemorrhage in patients with cirrhosis of the liver and esophageal varices. A prospective multicenter study. N Engl J Med. 1988;319:983–9.
4. Nevens F, Bustami R, Scheys I, Lesaffre E, Fevery J. Variceal pressure is a factor predicting the risk of a first variceal bleeding: a prospective cohort study in cirrhotic patients. Hepatology. 1998;27:15–19.
5. Lin HC, Soubrane O, Cailmail S, Lebrec D. Early chronic administration of propranolol reduces the severity of portal hypertension and portal–systemic shunts in conscious portal vein stenosed rats. J Hepatol. 1991;3:213–19.
6. Calès P, Oberti F, Payen JL et al. and the French-Speaking Club for the Study of Portal Hypertension. Lack of effect of propranolol in the prevention of large oesophageal varices in patients with cirrhosis: a randomized trial. Eur J Gastroenterol Hepatol. 1999;11:741–5.

7. Groszmann RJ, Garcia-Tsao G, Makuch R et al. Multicenter randomized placebo-controlled trial of non-selective beta-blockers in the prevention of the complications of portal hypertension: final results and identification of a predictive factor. Hepatology. 2003;38(Suppl. 1):206A.
8. Plevris JN, Elliot R, Mills PR et al. Effect of propranolol on prevention of first variceal bleed and survival in patients with chronic liver disease. Aliment Pharmacol Ther. 1994;8:63–70.
9. Merkel C, Marin R, Angeli P et al. Beta-blockers in the prevention of aggravation of esophageal varices in patients with cirrhosis and small varices: a placebo-controlled clinical trial. Hepatology. 2003;38(Suppl. 1):217A.
10. Poynard T, Calès P, Pasta L et al. and the Franco-Italian Multicenter Study Group. Beta-adrenergic-antagonist drugs in the prevention of gastrointestinal bleeding in patients with cirrhosis and esophageal varices. N Engl J Med. 1991;324:1532–8.
11. Hayes PC, Davis JM, Lewis JA, Bouchier IA. Meta-analysis of value of propranolol in prevention of variceal haemorrhage. Lancet. 1990;336:153–6.
12. Abraczinskas DR, Ookubo R, Grace ND et al. Propranolol for the prevention of first esophageal variceal hemorrhage: a lifetime commitment. Hepatology. 2001;34:1096–102.
13. Angelico M, Carli L, Piat C, Gentile S, Capocaccia L. Effects of isosorbide-5-mononitrate compared with propranolol on first bleeding and long-term survival in cirrhosis. Gastroenterology. 1997;113:1632–9.
14. Lui HF, Stanley AJ, Forrest EH et al. Primary prophylaxis of variceal hemorrhage: a randomized controlled trial comparing band ligation, propranolol, and isosorbide mononitrate. Gastroenterology. 2002;123:735–44.
15. Borroni G, Salerno F, Cazzaniga M et al. Nadolol is superior to isosorbide mononitrate for the prevention of the first variceal bleeding in cirrhotic patients with ascites. J Hepatol. 2002;37:315–21.
16. Garcia-Pagan JC, Villanueva C, Vila MC et al. and Members of the Move Group. Isosorbide mononitrate in the prevention of first variceal bleed in patients who cannot receive beta-blockers. Gastroenterology. 2001;121:908–14.
17. Merkel C, Marin R, Sacerdoti D et al. and the Gruppo Triveneto per l'Ipertensione portale (GTIP). Long-term results of a clinical trial of nadolol with or without isosorbide mononitrate for primary prophylaxis of variceal bleeding in cirrhosis. Hepatology. 2000;31:324–9.
18. Garcia-Pagan JC, Morillas R, Banares R et al. and the Spanish Variceal Bleeding Study Group. Propranolol plus placebo versus propranolol plus isosorbide-5-mononitrate in the prevention of a first variceal bleed: a double-blind RCT. Hepatology. 2003;37:1260–6.
19. Pietrosi G, D'Amico G, Pasta L et al. Isosorbide mononitrate with nadolol compared to nadolol alone for prevention of first bleeding in cirrhosis, a double-blind placebo-controlled randomised trial. J Hepatol. 1999;30(Suppl. 1):66A.
20. D'Amico G, Pagliaro L, Bosch J. Pharmacological treatment of portal hypertension: an evidence-based approach. Semin Liver Dis. 1999;19:475–505.
21. Abecasis R, Kravetz D, Fassio E et al. Nadolol plus spironolactone in the prophylaxis of first variceal bleed in nonascitic cirrhotic patients: a preliminary study. Hepatology. 2003;37:359–65.
22. Sanyal A. Hepatic venous pressure gradient: to measure or not to measure, that is the question. Hepatology. 2000;32:1175–6.
23. Groszmann RJ, Bosch J, Grace ND et al. Hemodynamic events in a prospective randomized trial of propranolol versus placebo in the prevention of a first variceal hemorrhage. Gastroenterology. 1990;99:1401–7.
24. Merkel C, Bolognesi M, Sacerdoti D et al. The hemodynamic response to medical treatment of portal hypertension as a predictor of clinical effectiveness in the primary prophylaxis of variceal bleeding in cirrhosis. Hepatology. 2000;32:930–4.
25. Valla D, Jiron MI, Poynard T, Braillon A, Lebrec D. Failure of haemodynamic measurements to predict recurrent gastrointestinal bleeding in cirrhotic patients receiving propranolol. J Hepatol. 1987;5:144–8.
26. McCormick PA, Patch D, Greenslade L, Chin J, McIntyre N, Burroughs AK. Clinical vs. haemodynamic response to drugs in portal hypertension. J Hepatol. 1998;28:1015–19.

# 24
# Prevention of first variceal bleeding: endoscopy

**MICHAEL SCHEPKE and TILMAN SAUERBRUCH**

## INTRODUCTION

Although the mortality due to first variceal bleeding has decreased during recent decades[1], intestinal hemorrhage is still one of the leading causes of death in patients with cirrhosis. It occurs in 30% of patients with cirrhosis, with each bleeding episode bearing a mortality risk of 30–50%[1]. Therefore, high-risk patients – commonly defined by the presence of esophageal varices with a diameter of at least 5 mm – should receive prophylactic treatment[2,3]. The risk of bleeding in these patients amounts to around 40% within 2 years after diagnosis of varices[4].

Portosystemic shunts, drugs and endoscopic measures have been evaluated for primary prophylaxis of variceal bleeding. Since early trials showed an excess encephalopathy rate and mortality of operated patients compared to untreated controls, open shunts have been abandoned[4]. With respect to drug treatment, non-selective beta-blockers (propranolol, nadolol) have proven effective in numerous trials[4,5]; these drugs reduce the bleeding risk by nearly 50%. The drugs are still considered as standard treatment[3,6]; however, drug treatment with beta-blockers carries disadvantages, most importantly the highly variable and unpredictable effect on portal hemodynamics: 30–40% of patients will not achieve a sufficient reduction of portal pressure to prevent bleeding[7–9]. Furthermore, contraindications and side-effects are common[10–12] and may require withdrawal which re-increases the risk of bleeding[13].

## ENDOSCOPIC INJECTION SCLEROTHERAPY

Repeated endoscopic injection of sclerosing agents such as polidocanol leads to obliteration and eradication of esophageal varices, and has been shown to be an effective technique, both for hemostasis of acute variceal bleeding and for the prevention of variceal rebleeding[4]. Thus, attempts have been made to apply this procedure for primary prevention of variceal bleeding.

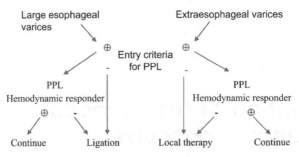

**Figure 1.** Algorithm for prophylaxis of first variceal bleeding (PPL = propranolol)

Although early trials – comparing endoscopic sclerotherapy with non-active treatment in patients with a high baseline bleeding risk – suggested favorable results, this method is no longer regarded as a primary option for the prevention of first bleeding: complications have been observed in approximately 20% of patients[14], including severe adverse events such as ulcers, bleeding, pleural effusions and esophageal perforation. With respect to efficacy there is a marked heterogeneity among the sclerotherapy trials: favorable results have been reported in trials with high bleeding rates in the untreated controls, whereas particularly those trials with the highest number of patients demonstrated an excess bleeding and mortality rate in the sclerotherapy patients[4]. Thus, endoscopic injection sclerotherapy is no longer advised for the primary prophylaxis of variceal bleeding.

## ENDOSCOPIC VARICEAL BANDING LIGATION

It is widely accepted that banding ligation is nowadays the endoscopic method of choice for the elective treatment of esophageal varices[3]. Single studies comparing sclerotherapy and banding ligation for rebleeding prophylaxis, as well as a meta-analysis from these studies, have convincingly shown that ligation is associated with fewer side-effects and eradicates varices more rapidly[15]. Probably this method is also advantageous with respect to efficacy of rebleeding prophylaxis. These favorable results prompted trials on the role of endoscopic banding ligation for the primary prevention of variceal bleeding.

According to the results from the trials comparing variceal band ligation (VBL) with non-active treatment[16–18], which are more homogeneous than the trials investigating endoscopic sclerotherapy for primary prophylaxis, and the recent meta-analysis including 601 patients in five trials[19], it can be concluded that ligation is effective in patients with high-risk varices. Ligation reduces not only the risk of first bleed (number needed to treat, NNT (CI): 4 (3–6) but also – according to the meta-analysis – bleeding-related mortality (NNT (CI): 7 (5–11)) and overall mortality (NNT 5 (4–9))[19]. However, since in these trials control patients did not receive the standard treatment for primary prophylaxis (beta-blockers), they are of limited value. Nitrates as monotherapy or combined with propranolol[6] have failed to prove superiority over propranolol alone, which is still the adequate control arm for any trial on primary prophylaxis of variceal bleeding. Thus, banding ligation has to be compared with beta-blockers.

To date four randomized studies investigating ligation for the primary prophylaxis of variceal bleeding in comparison to propranolol have been published[10,20,21], or will shortly be published[12]. In addition, preliminary results of a fifth small study have been reported[22]. The first study on this topic, a single-center trial[20], demonstrated a significant benefit of banding ligation with an actuarial bleeding risk of 15% at 18 months compared to 40% in the propranolol group. However, this unexpectedly high bleeding incidence in the control group which, in fact, is similar to the bleeding rate in untreated controls reported by the same authors a few years earlier[16], prompted criticism concerning compliance and propranolol dosage in that trial. The second study on primary prevention of variceal bleeding, the Scottish multicenter trial[10], showed a trend in favor of banding ligation (bleeding rate at 2 years was 6% vs 19% in the propranolol group). However, possibly due to a type 2 error (only 44 patients ligated in that study), this difference was not statistically significant. Furthermore, in the Scottish trial ligation has been performed only at highly specialized endoscopic units. It may therefore be difficult to translate these results into everyday clinical practice. The largest trial comparing ligation and propranolol for primary prophylaxis of variceal bleeding, the German multicenter study[12], included 27 centers and therefore provided rather robust data: that study found no differences between banding ligation and propranolol with respect to actuarial risks of first bleeding ($20.0 \pm 4.8\%$ for ligation and $17.6 \pm 4.6\%$ for propranolol) and mortality at 2 years. These results are very similar to those from a very recently puplished single-center trial from Taiwan[21]. Taken together, although ligation is clearly effective in preventing a first variceal hemorrhage, it is questionable whether this method really is superior to the therapeutic standard, i.e. unselective beta-blockers.

Since there is no or only a marginal difference between banding ligation and propranolol with respect to efficacy of bleeding prophylaxis, the decision as to which method should be applied depends on issues such as complications, costs and treatment tolerability. Side-effects are quite common under beta-blocker treatment (up to 70%[12]). However, these side-effects are usually mild and resolve after dosage reduction[12]. Side-effects that persist after dosage reduction, and therefore require drug withdrawal, are reported in approximately 15% of patients[12]. Severe, life-threatening adverse events do not occur in a relevant percentage under beta-blocker treatment, provided primary contraindications are respected. In contrast, banding ligation may be associated with a treatment-related mortality due to fatal bleeding from ligation ulcers which was reported in two of 75 patients (2.6%) in the German trial[12]. Treatment tolerability was also assessed in the German trial, and tended to be more favorable in the ligation group (difference not significant). With respect to costs, propranolol is clearly more cost-effective: it has been calculated that the cost for the initial endoscopic eradication of varices (not including costs for surveillance endoscopies and re-ligation) is nearly equivalent to the cost for 6 years of propranolol treatment[12].

Extraesophageal varices (e.g. in the stomach or the duodenum) may be successfully treated by propranolol, but not using ligation. By contrast, portal hypertensive gastropathy may develop or be aggravated following ligation[23]. Nevertheless, these sources of hemorrhage are rarely causes of overt bleeding (less than 5% of patients with concomitant esophageal varices).

Recurrent varices occur more often after ligation (50–60% within 1 year[12,24]) than after sclerotherapy (20–30%[24]); they are one reason for the necessity of a regular endoscopic follow-up in patients undergoing prophylactic ligation. If the recurrent varices are large enough they should be ligated – although this is not evidence-based. Whether sclerotherapy of small recurrent varices is protective, and should be performed, is not known.

## SUMMARY

What is the place for banding ligation in primary prophylaxis of variceal bleeding? Assuming an equivalent efficacy of banding and propranolol, banding ligation can certainly be offered to patients non-compliant to propranolol (around 10%), as well as to patients with large varices in whom severe side-effects or contraindications preclude the use of propranolol (around 20% of patients), although this has been questioned by a very recent abstract (J Hepatol. 2004;40:S73–4). Furthermore, prophylactic ligation might be considered for patients who show no adequate reduction of the portal pressure gradient to propranolol (40% according to the literature). Thus, although we still consider propranolol to be the first-choice treatment, more than 50% of patients may be candidates for prophylactic banding ligation (Figure 1).

## References

1. McCormick PA, O'Keefe C. Improving prognosis following a first variceal haemorrhage over four decades. Gut. 2001;49:482–5.
2. De Franchis R, editor. Portal Hypertension. III. Proceedings of the third Baveno international consensus workshop on definitions, methodology and therapeutic strategies. Oxford: Blackwell Science, 2001.
3. Garcia-Tsao G. Current management of the complications of cirrhosis and portal hypertension: variceal hemorrhage, ascites and spontaneous bacterial peritonitis. Gastroenterology. 2001;120:726–48.
4. D'Amico G, Pagliaro L, Bosch J. The treatment of portal hypertension: a meta-analytic review. Hepatology. 1995;22:332–54.
5. Poynard T, Cales P, Pasta L et al. Beta-adrenergic-antagonist drugs in the prevention of gastrointestinal bleeding in patients with cirrhosis and esophageal varices. N Engl J Med. 1991;324:1532–8.
6. Garcia-Pagan JC, Morillas R, Banares R et al. Propranolol plus placebo versus propranolol plus isosorbide-5-mononitrate in the prevention of a first variceal bleed: a double-blind RCT. Hepatology. 2003;37:1260–6.
7. Bosch J, Mastai R, Kravetz D et al. Effects of propranolol on azygos blood flow and hepatic and systemic hemodynamics in cirrhosis. Hepatology. 1984;4:1200–5.
8. Garcia-Tsao G, Grace ND, Groszmann RJ et al. Short-term effects of propranolol on portal venous pressure. Hepatology. 1986;6:101–6.

9. Vorobioff J, Picabea E, Villavicencio R et al. Acute and chronic hemodynamic effects of propranolol in unselected cirrhotic patients. Hepatology. 1987;7:648–53.
10. Lui HF, Stanley AJ, Forrest EW et al. Primary prophylaxis of variceal hemorrhage: a randomized controlled trial comparing band ligation, propranolol, and isosorbide mononitrate. Gastroenterology. 2002;123:735–44.
11. D'Amico G, Pagliaro L, Bosch J. Pharmacological treatment of portal hypertension: an evidence-based approach. Semin Liver Dis. 1999;19:475–505.
12. Schepke M, Kleber G, Nürnberg D et al. Ligation versus propranolol for the primary prophylaxis of variceal bleeding in cirrhosis. Hepatology. 2004 (In press).
13. Abraczinskas D, Ookubo R, Grace N et al. Propranolol for the prevention of first variceal bleeding: a lifetime commitment? Hepatology. 2001;34:1096–102.
14. Sauerbruch T, Wotzka R, Köpcke W et al. Prophylactic sclerotherapy before the first episode of variceal hemorrhage in patients with cirrhosis. N Engl J Med. 1988;319:8–15.
15. Laine L, Cook D. Endoscopic ligation compared with sclerotherapy for the treatment of esophageal variceal bleeding. A meta-analysis. Ann Intern Med. 1995;123:280–7.
16. Sarin SK, Guptan R, Jain A, Sundaram K. A randomized controlled trial of endoscopic variceal band ligation for primary prophylaxis of variceal bleeding. Eur J Gastroenterol Hepatol. 1996;4:337–42.
17. Lay CS, Tsai Y, Teg C et al. Endoscopic variceal ligation in prophylaxis of first variceal bleeding in cirrhotic patients with high-risk esophageal varices. Hepatology. 1997;25: 1346–50.
18. Lo GH, Lai KH, Cheng JS, Lin CK, Hsu PI, Chiang HAT. Prophylactic banding ligation of high risk esophageal varices in patients with cirrhosis: a prospective, randomized trial. J Hepatol. 1999;31:451–6.
19. Imperiale T, Chalasani N. A meta-analysis of endoscopic variceal ligation for primary prophylaxis of esophageal variceal bleeding. Hepatology. 2001;33:802–7.
20. Sarin SK, Lamba G, Kumar M, Misra A, Murthy N. Comparison of endoscopic ligation and propranolol for the primary prevention of variceal bleeding. N Engl J Med. 1999;340:988–93.
21. Lo GH, Chen W, Chen M et al. Endoscopic ligation versus nadolol in the prevention of first variceal bleeding in patients with cirrhosis. Gastrointest Endosc. 2004;59:333–8.
22. De BK, Goshal U, Das T, Santra A, Biswas P. Endoscopic variceal ligation for primary prophylaxis of oesophageal variceal bleeding: preliminary report of a randomized controlled trial. J Gastroenterol Hepatol. 1999;14:220–4.
23. Lo GH, Lai KH, Cheng JS et al. The effects of endoscopic variceal ligation and propranolol on portal hypertensive gastropathy: a prospective, controlled trial. Gastrointest Endosc. 2001;53:579–84.
24. De la Pena J, Rivero M, Sanchez E, Fabrega E, Crespo J, Pons-Romero F. Variceal ligation compared with endoscopic sclerotherapy for variceal hemorrhage: prospective randomized trial. Gastrointest Endosc. 1999;49:417–23.

# 25
# Treatment of acute variceal bleeding: general management and prevention of infections

GUADALUPE GARCIA-TSAO

## INTRODUCTION

Ruptured esophageal varices cause 60–80% of all upper gastrointestinal bleeding episodes in cirrhosis. Variceal bleeding ceases spontaneously in 40–50% of patients; however, a small percentage of patients ($\sim 5\%$) die from uncontrolled bleeding. Even in patients in whom bleeding stops, rebleeding occurs within the first 6 weeks in $\sim 20\%$. A poor outcome, either failure to control bleeding, early recurrent bleeding or death, occurs in 15–30% of cases. Several factors predictive of a poor outcome have been identified in various studies. Some of them, such as hypovolemia, renal dysfunction and bacterial infection, apply to cirrhotic patients with any gastrointestinal hemorrhage, independent of etiology. Other predictive factors, such as active variceal bleeding at the time of diagnostic endoscopy and an hepatic venous pressure gradient $> 20\,\mathrm{mmHg}$, apply to cirrhotic patients with variceal hemorrhage and are factors that can be prevented or treated by using pharmacologic or other portal pressure-reducing methods. A third group of predictive factors are intrinsic to the cirrhotic patient, as is the case of an alcoholic etiology of cirrhosis, the degree of liver dysfunction (albumin, bilirubin levels and the presence of hepatic encephalopathy) and the presence of hepatocellular carcinoma.

General management of variceal bleeding (and of any gastrointestinal hemorrhage in patients with cirrhosis) should be aimed at correcting or, better still, at preventing hypovolemia, renal dysfunction and bacterial infections, factors that are predictive of a poor outcome in these patients.

## CORRECTING HYPOVOLEMIA

Renal failure has been shown to occur more frequently in hospitalized cirrhotic patients with gastrointestinal hemorrhage than in non-cirrhotic patients with gastrointestinal hemorrhage[1]. In a retrospective study that included 175 episodes of gastrointestinal hemorrhage in patients with cirrhosis (82% variceal), hypovolemia and a poor liver function were the only two factors independently predictive of renal failure. Additionally, this study showed that the only two independent predictors of in-hospital mortality were the presence of hypovolemic shock and renal failure[1]. While in-hospital mortality was only 3% (4/147) in patients without either of these factors, it was 67% (8/12) in patients with both of them[1]; therefore avoidance of hypovolemia and maintenance of hemodynamic stability are particularly important in these patients.

## RESTITUTION OF LOST BLOOD

Blood volume replacement should be initiated as soon as possible; however, overtransfusion should be avoided, not only because of the risks inherent with blood transfusion, but also because experimental studies performed in portal hypertensive animals have shown that, while restitution of 100% of extracted blood returns mean arterial pressure to baseline levels, it leads to a rebound increase in portal pressure that could lead to rebleeding[2]. Further experimental studies in cirrhotic rats show that 100% blood volume restitution leads to greater rebleeding (and therefore a greater fall in hematocrit) as well as 100% mortality, while restitution of 50% of blood lost carries the best prognosis[3]; therefore, transfusions of packed red blood cells in the cirrhotic patient with gastrointestinal hemorrhage should be aimed at maintaining the hematocrit between 25% and 30%.

## PREVENTION OF INFECTIONS

### Bacterial infections in cirrhosis

Bacterial infections are a well-described complication of cirrhosis. Recent large prospective series, performed in consecutively admitted cirrhotic patients, report bacterial infection rates (either at the time of admission or during hospitalization) of 32% (507 of 1567 admissions)[4] and 34% (139 of 405 admissions)[5]. These figures clearly contrast with the hospital-acquired infection rate in the general hospital population reported to be between 5% and 7%.

### Factors predictive of infection in cirrhotic patients

Two factors play an important role in the development of bacterial infection in cirrhotic patients: the severity of the liver disease and admission for gastrointestinal hemorrhage. Patients with decompensated cirrhosis have been consistently shown in retrospective studies to develop infections at a higher rate compared to compensated cirrhotics[6-8]. The prospective study by Bernard et al. demonstrated that patients who develop infections had a significantly higher Child–Pugh score, higher serum bilirubin levels and a lower serum albumin on admission than those who did not develop a bacterial infection[9].

In prospective studies, summarized in Table 1[9-15], the incidence of bacterial infections in cirrhotic patients hospitalized with gastrointestinal hemorrhage is 44% (greater than the 32–34% infection rate in hospitalized cirrhotic patients at large), with lower incidences in patients with a good liver function[13] and a higher infection rate in Child C cirrhotic patients[12]. In a prospective study, admission for gastrointestinal bleeding and a low serum albumin were identified as the only two variables independently associated with the development of a bacterial infection[16].

## Sources and etiology of infection in cirrhotics with gastrointestinal hemorrhage

In prospective series (Table 1) the most common infections in cirrhotics with gastrointestinal hemorrhage are spontaneous bacterial peritonitis (SBP) and/or spontaneous bacteremia, followed by urinary tract infections and pneumonia. Although approximately half the organisms isolated (120/222 or 54%) are aerobic Gram-negative, in studies in which SBP/bacteremia are the predominant infections[10,14], the most frequently isolated microorganisms are Gram-negative ($\sim 75\%$), while infections by Gram-positive organisms predominate in series in which pneumonia is the most common infection[12,15].

## Consequences of infection in patients with gastrointestinal hemorrhage

In prospective series of cirrhotic patients admitted with gastrointestinal hemorrhage (Table 1), mortality has ranged between 9% (in low-risk patients) and 48%, with an overall mortality of 23% (129/552). Studies that have compared mortality in infected vs non-infected patients uniformly show that patients who develop an infection have a significantly higher mortality rate[6,8,17]. Although this higher mortality may be related to the predisposition of patients with more severe liver disease to develop infections, a recent study, performed in 405 consecutively hospitalized cirrhotic patients, identified Child C and the occurrence of bacterial infection as independent predictors of mortality[18].

Besides a higher mortality, another consequence of infection is a higher rate of variceal rebleeding. The first study to suggest this association was the one by Bernard et al., that showed that, while recurrent variceal hemorrhage occurred in 10/23 (43%) patients who developed a bacterial infection, it occurred only in 4/41 (10%) of non-infected patients[9]. On multivariate analysis the only factor independently predictive of rebleeding was the presence of a bacterial infection. In another study, of 163 patients admitted with gastrointestinal hemorrhage, the incidence of bacterial infections was significantly higher in those who developed failure to control bleeding (defined as the initial failure to control bleeding or the occurrence of early rebleeding)[15].

Endotoxins and cytokines resulting from infection may induce hematologic abnormalities, including platelet dysfunction and activation of coagulation and fibrinolytic systems. A recent study that assessed the entire clotting process by measuring routine hemostasis tests and thromboelastography

**Table 1.** Prospective series of infections in cirrhotic patients admitted for gastrointestinal hemorrhage not placed on antibiotic prophylaxis

| Main author and year | n | Ascites (%) | Child C (%) | Developed infection | SBP/SB (%) | UTI (%) | Pneumonia (%) | Gram-negative organisms (%) |
|---|---|---|---|---|---|---|---|---|
| Rimola (1985)[10] | 72* | 36% | NR | 25 (35%) | 60 | 36 | 16 | 75 |
| Soriano (1992)[11] | 59* | 24 | 22 | 22 (37%) | 38 | 42 | 15 | 56 |
| Blaise (1994)[12] | 45* | 38 | 80 | 30 (67%) | 26 | 26 | 47 | 35 |
| Bernard (1995)[9] | 64 | 47 | 52 | 23 (36%) | 43 | 17 | 19 | NR |
| Pauwels (1996)[13] | 55 | 14 | None | 8 (14%) | 70 } | 13 | 13 | NR |
| Pauwels (1996)[13] | 34* | 38 | 71 | 16 (47%) | | | | |
| Hsieh (1998)[14] | 60* | 50 | 38 | 27 (45%) | 59 | 30 | 8 | 76 |
| Goulis (1998)[15] | 163 | 50% | 44 | 91 (56%) | 36 | 19 | 43 | 50 |
| Total | 552 | | | 242 (44%) | 48 | 23 | 23 | 54 |

*Untreated or placebo-treated control group of a randomized study.
NR = not reported.
SB = spontaneous bacteremia.
SBP = spontaneous bacterial peritonitis.

(TEG) demonstrated that, with the development of infection, there is a significant alteration in prothrombin time, INR, PTT and all TEG parameters[19]. This alteration improved in patients in whom infection resolved, and was not observed in cirrhotic patients who did not develop infection. Infection may therefore have a role in the bleeding diathesis of cirrhosis, and may contribute to variceal rebleeding. As hypothesized recently, bacterial infection and endotoxemia may also exert their effect through the synthesis of endothelin and nitric oxide, that may further alter the hemodynamics of patients with cirrhosis and further alter platelet aggregation, leading to variceal hemorrhage[20,21].

## Prevention of infections in cirrhotic patients with gastrointestinal hemorrhage

Since infections are associated with a higher mortality and a higher rebleeding rate in cirrhotics admitted with gastrointestinal hemorrhage, it would appear logical to prevent the occurrence of these infections through the use of antibiotics.

Five randomized controlled trials have evaluated the use of antibiotics in preventing bacterial infections in cirrhotic patients admitted for gastrointestinal hemorrhage, and are summarized in Table 2. Two of them utilized oral non-absorbable or poorly absorbable antibiotics[10,11] and three used systemic antibiotics (intravenous administration and/or oral administration of widely bioavailable antibiotics)[12–14]. One included randomized patients who were Child C and/or had had recurrence of variceal hemorrhage[13]. Only one of them was placebo-controlled and 40% of patients included in this study had hepatocellular carcinoma[14].

In each of these studies the incidence of bacterial infections was lower in the group treated with antibiotics with an overall incidence of 13% (Table 2). This percentage is markedly lower than the 44% rate in untreated patients. In each study there was also a trend for lower in-hospital mortality in patients treated with antibiotics.

A meta-analysis of these five trials shows that short-term antibiotic prophylaxis not only resulted in a significant decrease in the incidence of infections, including SBP, but was also associated with a significant reduction in mortality[22]. Sensitivity analysis did not demonstrate any differences between antibiotics administered by mouth and trials in which antibiotics were administered intravenously. Based on these studies the use of short-term antibiotic prophylaxis in cirrhotic patients admitted with gastrointestinal hemorrhage is considered mandatory[23].

In the above-mentioned studies variceal rebleeding was not one of the endpoints. A recent randomized trial analyzed the effect of ofloxacin (200 mg intravenously b.i.d. for 2 days followed by oral ofloxacin 200 mg b.i.d. for 5 days) vs on-demand antibiotics (i.e. antibiotics were administered if and when an infection developed) in preventing variceal rebleeding[24]. The incidence of bacterial infections was lower in patients receiving antibiotic prophylaxis (2/59 or 3% vs 16/61 or 26%). Importantly, early rebleeding (within the first 15 days) was significantly lower in patients randomized to antibiotic prophylaxis (5/59 or 8% vs 23/61 or 38%). On multivariable analysis,

**Table 2.** Randomized controlled trials of prophylactic antibiotics in cirrhotic patients admitted with gastrointestinal hemorrhage

| Main author and year | n | Antibiotic | Duration | Developed infection | | In-hospital mortality | |
|---|---|---|---|---|---|---|---|
| | | | | Control | Antibiotic | Control | Antibiotic |
| Rimola (1985)[10] | 140 | Genta/vanco/nystat or neomycin/colistin/nystat* | 2 days after bleeding stopped | 25/72 (35%) | 11/68 (16%) | 23/72 (32%) | 18/68 (26%) |
| Soriano (1992)[11] | 119 | Oral norfloxacin* | 7 days | 22/59 (37%) | 6/60 (10%) | 7/59 (12%) | 4/60 (7%) |
| Blaise (1994)[12] | 91 | Ofloxacin intravenous then oral | 10 days | 30/45 (67%) | 9/46 (20%) | 16/45 (36%) | 11/46 (25%) |
| Pauwels (1996)[13] | 64 | Amoxi/clavulanic + ciprofloxacin | 3 days after bleeding stopped | 16/34 (47%) | 2/30 (7%) | 8/34 (24%) | 4/30 (13%) |
| Hsieh (1998)[14] | 120 | Oral ciprofloxacin | 7 days | 27/60 (45%) | 6/60 (10%) | 18/60 (30%) | 13/60 (22%) |
| Total | | | | 120/270 (44%) | 34/264 (13%) | 72/270 (27%) | 50/264 (19%) |

*Selective intestinal decontamination.

238

bacterial infection and the presence of hepatocellular carcinoma were independent determinants of rebleeding.

## Recommended prophylaxis

The theory behind the development of spontaneous bacterial infections in cirrhosis, particularly those due to Gram-negative organisms, is that gut bacteria translocate to extraintestinal sites. Bacterial translocation has been shown to occur in experimental and human cirrhosis, particularly in cirrhosis with ascites[25,26]; therefore, the most rational prophylaxis is that aimed at eliminating Gram-negative bacteria in the gut by the use of non- or poorly-absorbable antibiotics (selective intestinal decontamination or SID). The two randomized controlled trials that analyzed the effect of short-term SID in preventing infections in cirrhotic patients with gastrointestinal hemorrhage showed a significant reduction in infection rate and in mortality with SID[10,11] (Table 2). One of these studies used two combinations of oral, nonabsorbable antibiotics: gentamycin (200 mg)/vancomycin (500 mg)/nystatin (1 M units) every 6 h or neomycin (1 g)/colistin (1.5 MU)/nystatin (1 MU) every 6 h[10], while the other study used oral norfloxacin, a poorly absorbed quinolone, at a dose of 400 mg twice a day[11].

Given its lower cost, and simpler administration, the preferred antibiotic is norfloxacin administered orally at a dose of 400 mg twice a day for 7 days[23]. In patients in whom it cannot be administered by mouth or by nasogastric tube, quinolones (ciprofloxacin, levofloxacin) can be administered intravenously until re-establishment of the oral route.

## References

1. Cardenas A, Gines P, Uriz J et al. Renal failure after upper gastrointestinal bleeding in cirrhosis: incidence, clinical course, predictive factors, and short-term prognosis. Hepatology. 2001;34:671–6.
2. Kravetz D, Sikuler E, Groszmann RJ. Splanchnic and systemic hemodynamics in portal hypertensive rats during hemorrhage and blood volume restitution. Gastroenterology. 1986;90:1232–40.
3. Castaneda B, Morales J, Lionetti R et al. Effects of blood volume restitution following a portal hypertensive-related bleeding in anesthetized cirrhotic rats. Hepatology. 2001;33:821–5.
4. Fernandez J, Navasa M, Gomez J et al. Bacterial infections in cirrhosis: epidemiological changes with invasive procedures and norfloxacin prophylaxis. Hepatology. 2002;35:140–8.
5. Borzio M, Salerno F, Piantoni L et al. Bacterial infection in patients with advanced cirrhosis: a multicentre prospective study. Dig Liver Dis. 2001;33:41–8.
6. Bleichner G, Boulanger R, Squara P et al. Frequency of infections in cirrhotic patients presenting with acute gastrointestinal hemorrhage. Br J Surg. 1986;73:724–6.
7. Yoshida H, Hamada T, Inuzuka S et al. Bacterial infection in cirrhosis, with and without hepatocellular carcinoma. Am J Gastroenterol. 1993;88:2067–71.
8. Caly WR, Strauss E. A prospective study of bacterial infections in patients with cirrhosis. J Hepatol. 1993;18:353–8.
9. Bernard B, Cadranel JF, Valla D et al. Prognostic significance of bacterial infection in bleeding cirrhotic patients: A prospective study. Gastroenterology. 1995;108:1828–34.
10. Rimola A, Bory F, Teres J et al. Oral, nonabsorbable antibiotics prevent infection in cirrhotics with gastrointestinal hemorrhage. Hepatology. 1985;5:463–7.
11. Soriano G, Guarner C, Tomas A et al. Norfloxacin prevents bacterial infection in cirrhotics with gastrointestinal hemorrhage. Gastroenterology. 1992;103:1267–72.

12. Blaise M, Pateron D, Trinchet C et al. Systemic antibiotic therapy prevents bacterial infection in cirrhotic patients with gastrointestinal hemorrhage. Hepatology. 1994;20:34–8.
13. Pauwels A, Mostefa-Kara N, Debenes B et al. Systemic antibiotic prophylaxis after gastrointestinal hemorrhage in cirrhotic patients with a high risk of infection. Hepatology. 1996;24:802–6.
14. Hsieh WJ, Lin HC, Hwang SJ et al. The effect of ciprofloxacin in the prevention of bacterial infection in patients with cirrhosis after upper gastrointestinal bleeding. Am J Gastroenterol. 1998;93:962–6.
15. Goulis J, Armonis A, Patch D et al. Bacterial infection is independently associated with failure to control bleeding in cirrhotic patients with gastrointestinal hemorrhage. Hepatology. 1998;27:1207–12.
16. Deschenes M, Villeneuve JP. Risk factors for the development of bacterial infections in hospitalized patients with cirrhosis. Am J Gastroenterol. 1999;94:2193–7.
17. Rimola A, Bory F, Planas R et al. Infecciones bacterianas agudas en la cirrosis hepatica. Gastroenterol Hepatol. 1981;4:453–8.
18. Borzio M, Salerno F, Piantoni L et al. Bacterial infection in patients with advanced cirrhosis: a multicentre prospective study. Dig Liver Dis. 2001;33:41–8.
19. Papatheodoridis GV, Patch D, Webster JM et al. Infection and hemostasis in decompensated cirrhosis: a prospective study using thromboelastography. Hepatology. 1999;29: 1085–90.
20. Wiest R, Das S, Cadelina G et al. Bacterial translocation to lymph nodes of cirrhotic rats stimulates eNOS-derived NO production and impairs mesenteric vascular contractility. J Clin Invest. 1999;104: 1223–33.
21. Goulis J, Patch D, Burroughs AK. Bacterial infection in the pathogenesis of variceal bleeding. Lancet. 1999;353:139–42.
22. Bernard B, Grange JD, Khac EN et al. Antibiotic prophylaxis for the prevention of bacterial infections in cirrhotic patients with gastrointestinal bleeding: a meta-analysis. Hepatology. 1999;29:1655–61.
23. Rimola A, Garcia-Tsao G, Navasa M et al. Diagnosis, treatment and prophylaxis of spontaneous bacterial peritonitis: a consensus document. J Hepatol. 2000;32:142–53.
24. Hou MC, Lin HC, Liu TT et al. Antibiotic prophylaxis after endoscopic therapy prevents rebleeding in acute variceal hemorrhage: a randomized trial. Hepatology. 2004;39:746–53.
25. Garcia-Tsao G, Lee FY, Barden GE et al. Bacterial translocation to mesenteric lymph nodes is increased in cirrhotic rats with ascites. Gastroenterology. 1995;108:1835–41.
26. Cirera I, Bauer TM, Navasa M et al. Bacterial translocation of enteric organisms in patients with cirrhosis. J Hepatol. 2001;34:32–7.

# 26
# Hemostatic treatments

## ROBERTO DE FRANCHIS

### INTRODUCTION

Treatment of acute variceal bleeding should aim both at controlling bleeding and at preventing early rebleeding, which is particularly common within the first week and is associated with increased mortality[1].

Over the years pharmacologic therapy with vasoactive drugs (terlipressin, somatostatin, octreotide)[2], endoscopic therapy (sclerotherapy and band ligation)[3] and the combination of these two treatment modalities has been used to control bleeding and prevent early rebleeding[3].

Recently, possible new approaches, such as tailoring the dose of vasoactive drugs according to the presence or absence of active bleeding at endoscopy[4], and the correction of coagulation defects in patients with more severe liver dysfunction[5], have been proposed.

This chapter will discuss the established therapies and the possible new approaches to the treatment of acute variceal bleeding.

### VASOACTIVE DRUGS

The use of vasoactive drugs to control variceal hemorrhage in cirrhotic patients was first introduced in clinical practice in 1962[6]. Vasopressin was the first vasoactive agent studied, because of its ability to induce splanchnic vasoconstriction, followed by a reduction of portal venous inflow and portal pressure. However, vasopressin has been practically abandoned, because it frequently induces severe side-effects such as myocardial ischemia or infarction, cardiac arrhythmias, ischemia of the limbs or the mesenteric axis and cerebrovascular accidents. In the following decades research was aimed at developing more effective and safer drugs, and several clinical trials have been performed to determine the most appropriate drug to use, and the best treatment protocol for each agent.

Glypressin or terlipressin is a synthetic analog of lysine-vasopressin, with an immediate vasoconstricting effect followed by a delayed effect caused by the slow transformation of glypressin into vasopressin *in vivo*, due to the enzymatic cleavage of the triglycyl residues[7]. Compared with vasopressin,

**Table 1.**  Randomized controlled trials comparing somatostatin, glypressin and octreotide

| Reference | Treatment | No. of patients | Efficacy (%) | Mortality (%) |
|---|---|---|---|---|
| *Somatostatin vs glypressin* | | | | |
| Walker et al. 1992[13] | Glypressin/somatostatin | 25/25 | 80/68 | 16/24 |
| Pauwels et al. 1994[14] | Glypressin/somatostatin | 17/18 | 59/78 | 35/39 |
| Walker et al. 1996[15] | Glypressin/somatostatin | 53/53 | 83/72 | 21/21 |
| Feu et al. 1996[16] | Glypressin/somatostatin | 80/81 | 80/84 | 20/17 |
| Summary data | Glypressin/somatostatin | 175/177 | 79/79 | 20/20 |
| *Octreotide vs glypressin* | | | | |
| Silvain et al. 1993[17] | Glypressin + N/octreotide | 41/46 | 46/57 | 27/22 |
| Pedretti et al. 1994[18] | Glypressin/octreotide | 30/30 | 53/77 | 13/10 |
| Summary data | Glypressin ± N/octreotide | 71/76 | 49/65 | 21/17 |

glypressin has a prolonged biological activity, which allows administration of the drug by intravenous boluses every 4–6 h, and is associated with significantly lower complication rates.

Somatostatin is a naturally occurring tetradecapeptide hormone that is used to treat variceal hemorrhage because it reduces portal pressure and portocollateral blood flow, but is devoid of the systemic effects of vasopressin[8].

Octreotide is a synthetic octapeptide that, by virtue of a shared four amino acid segment, has similar pharmacologic activity with longer duration of action in comparison to somatostatin.

In randomized controlled trials terlipressin was significantly better than placebo for bleeding control and survival[9]. When compared with vasopressin, terlipressin was equivalent for bleeding control and survival, but showed significantly fewer side-effects[2]. As far as somatostatin is concerned, a 5-day infusion of this drug significantly increased bleeding control[10] in comparison with placebo. Meta-analysis of trials comparing somatostatin with vasopressin and terlipressin[2,9] shows similar efficacy of the three drugs, while somatostatin has a significantly better safety profile in comparison with vasopressin. Data concerning octreotide are less abundant. In the only available placebo-controlled study, published only in abstract form[11], octreotide was not superior to placebo in controlling bleeding and in preventing early rebleeding. When compared with balloon tamponade, octreotide was less effective in controlling bleeding, but was significantly better for survival[12]. In the studies which have compared octreotide with vasopressin and with terlipressin[9], octreotide was somewhat better than the alternative drug for bleeding control, with the difference barely missing statistical significance, while there was no difference in mortality. Table 1 shows the studies comparing somatostatin[13–16] and octreotide[17,18] with glypressin.

## ENDOSCOPIC THERAPY

Sclerotherapy has been compared with balloon tamponade, with vasopressin ± balloon tamponade, with terlipressin, with somatostatin and

**Table 2.** Randomized controlled trials comparing rubber-band ligation (EBL) with sclerotherapy (EVS) for acute variceal bleeding

| Reference | No. of patients EBL/EVS | Failure (%) | Mortality (%) |
|---|---|---|---|
| Stiegmann et al. 1992[20] | 14/13 | 14/23 | n.a. |
| Laine et al. 1993[21] | 9/9 | 11/11 | n.a. |
| Gimson et al. 1993[22] | 21/23 | 10/ 9 | n.a. |
| Jensen et al. 1993[23] | 14/11 | 20/0 | n.a. |
| Lo et al. 1995[24] | 18/15 | 6/20 | n.a. |
| Hou et al. 1995[25] | 20/16 | 0/12 | n.a. |
| Fakhry et al. 1995[26] | 10/12 | 10/8 | 10/8 |
| Sarin et al. 1997[27] | 5/7 | 20/14 | n.a. |
| Lo et al. 1997[28] | 37/34 | 3/24 | 19/38 |
| Pooled data | 148/140 | 4/19 | 17/30 |
| POR (95% CI) | | 0.56 (0.27–1.14) | n.a. |

with octreotide[5]. A recent meta-analysis of studies comparing sclerotherapy with vasoactive drugs[19] has shown that the two treatment modalities are equivalent for bleeding control and survival, while the incidence of adverse events is significantly higher with sclerotherapy.

Nine randomized controlled trials[20-28] comparing sclerotherapy with rubber-band ligation give separate data for acutely bleeding patients (Table 2). Meta-analysis of these studies[3] shows that the difference in control of bleeding is not statistically significant (POR for failure to control bleeding 0.56; 95% CI 0.27–1.14) Mortality figures are available from two studies only[26,28], both showing no difference between treatments. From these results, sclerotherapy and band ligation appear to be equally effective in the emergency situation. However, the number of patients on which this conclusion is based is small.

## COMBINATION OF VASOACTIVE + ENDOSCOPIC TREATMENT

Treatment regimens combining the use of a vasoactive drug (terlipressin, somatostatin or its analogs octreotide or vapreotide) with endoscopic therapy (sclerotherapy or band ligation) have received a great deal of attention in recent years. Between 1995 and 2001, 10 studies[29-38], including a total of 1359 patients, have compared combined treatments with endoscopic treatments alone. Meta-analysis of these trials shows that pharmacologic + endoscopic treatment is more effective than endoscopic therapy alone in controlling acute bleeding and preventing 5-days rebleeding (control of acute bleeding: combination 90%; endoscopic treatment alone 76%; relative risk reduction 16%; absolute risk reduction 14% (95% CI + 4% to + 23%), NNT = 7; 5-days prevention of rebleeding: combination 72%; endoscopic treatment alone 59%; relative risk reduction 18%; absolute risk reduction 13% (95% CI −8% to −17%); NNT = 7.7). There was no difference in 5-day and 42-day mortality figures (combination 7%; endoscopic treatment alone 9% at 5 days; 22% and 27% respectively at 42 days) (Table 3 and Figure 1).

**Table 3.** Randomized controlled trials: comparison between endoscopic treatments alone and in combination with pharmacologic therapy

| Reference | Treatment | No. of patients | Failure (%) C/A | Mortality (%) C/A |
|---|---|---|---|---|
| Levacher et al. 1995[29] | Placebo + sclerotherapy vs terlipressin + nitroglycerin + sclerotherapy | 43/41 | 47/71 | 42/20 |
| Besson et al. 1995[30] | Sclerotherapy vs sclerotherapy + i.v. octreotide | 101/98 | 71/87[a] | 10/7[b] |
| Sung et al. 1995[31] | Ligation vs ligation + i.v. octreotide | 47/47 | 94/96[c] 62/91[d] | 19/9[e] |
| Signorelli et al.*1996[32] | Sclerotherapy vs sclerotherapy + somatostatin | 30/33 | 62/81 | 15/13 |
| | Sclerotherapy vs sclerotherapy + s.c. octreotide | 30/31 | 62/75 | 15/15 |
| Brunati et al.*1996[33] | Sclerotherapy vs sclerotherapy + s.c. octreotide | 27/28 | 60/80[g] | 15/13[b] |
| | Sclerotherapy vs sclerotherapy + terlipressin | 27/28 | 60/75[g] | 13/13[b] |
| Burroughs* 1996[34] | Placebo vs. octreotide | 137/123 | 31/32[f] | 27/22 |
| Signorelli et al.*1997[35] | Sclerotherapy vs sclerotherapy + octreotide | 42/44 | 71/84 | n.a. |
| Avgerinos et al. 1997[36] | Sclerotherapy vs sclerotherapy + somatostatin | 104/101 | 45/65[f] | 7/3[b] |
| Zuberi and Baloch 2000[37] | Sclerotherapy vs sclerotherapy + i.v. octreotide | 35/35 | 86/94 | 3/3 |
| Calés et al. 2001[38] | Placebo + sclerotherapy vs vapreotide + sclerotherapy | 93/91 | 50/66[f] | 21/14 |
| Summary data | Sclerotherapy vs sclerotherapy + drugs | 659/700 | 76/90[†] | 9/7[¶] |
| | | | 59/72[‡] | 27/22[||] |

*Available only in abstract form.
[†]24 h bleeding control, five trials.
[‡]5 days bleeding control, 10 trials.
[¶]5 days mortality, seven trials.
[||]42 days mortality, six trials.

[a]5-day survival without rebleeding; [b]5-day mortality; [c]initial hemostasis; [d]percent patients without rebleeding at 2 days; [e]in-hospital mortality; [f]percent patients without treatment failure at 5 days; [g]Control of acute bleeding at 5 days.

The combination of emergency sclerotherapy plus somatostatin or octreotide infusion has been compared with somatostatin or octreotide alone in two trials[39,40]. In both trials the combined treatment was more effective than drug treatment alone in controlling bleeding and preventing early rebleeding, although statistical significance was reached only in the first one. It thus appears that the combination of endoscopic and pharmacologic treatment can control bleeding in about 90% of patients and prevent early rebleeding in about 80%[41]. Accordingly, the current recommendations[42] are that, in suspected variceal bleeding, vasoactive drugs should be started as soon as possible, before diagnostic endoscopy; and that endoscopic therapy should be performed even if there is no active bleeding at endoscopy, especially in

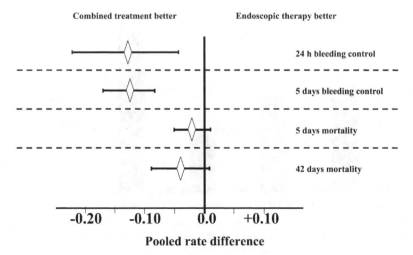

**Figure 1.** Meta-analysis of treatments for acute variceal bleeding: combined pharmacologic + endoscopic treatments vs endoscopic treatments alone

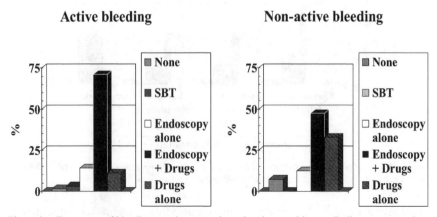

**Figure 2.** Treatment of bleeding esophagogastric varices in a multicenter Italian survey: active vs non-active bleeding at endoscopy[43]

high-risk patients. In acute bleeding, either ligation or endoscopic sclerotherapy can be used. Drug therapy may be maintained for up to 5 days to prevent early rebleeding[42]. A recent survey has shown that the combination of vasoactive drugs and endoscopic therapy is widely adopted in the routine management of variceal bleeders[43] (Figure 2).

A still-open question is whether it is really necessary to perform endoscopic therapy if there is no active bleeding at endoscopy and the patient is receiving vasoactive treatment. In this respect the existing data are controversial: Escorsell et al.[44] have shown that somatostatin infusion and sclerotherapy are equivalent in preventing early rebleeding (Figure 3), while according to

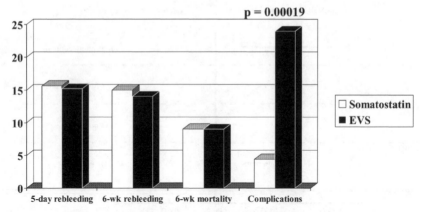

**Figure 3.** Randomized controlled trial of sclerotherapy vs somatostatin infusion in the prevention of early rebleeding following acute variceal hemorrhage in patients with cirrhosis[44]

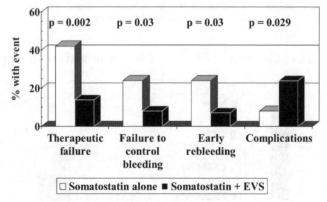

**Figure 4.** Randomized controlled trial comparing somatostatin alone or combined with emergency sclerotherapy in the treatment of acute esophageal variceal bleeding[39]

Villanueva et al.[39] the combination of somatostatin and sclerotherapy is better than somatostatin alone (Figure 4).

## POSSIBLE NEW APPROACHES

A possible means of increasing the efficacy of hemostatic treatments for variceal bleeding could be to tailor the dose of vasoactive drugs according to the presence or absence of active bleeding at endoscopy. To this effect a recent study from Spain[4] compared different schedules of somatostatin administration. In a retrospective analysis of the data, patients actively bleeding at endoscopy treated with a double dose of somatostatin infusion (500 µg/h) had a higher bleeding control rate and even a significantly higher 6-week survival in comparison with patients treated with the standard 250 µg/h dose. Whether the policy of increasing the dose of vasoactive drugs in patients actively bleeding at endoscopy is indeed effective will have to be confirmed in prospective studies.

Another possible approach could be to correct the coagulation defects that are present in the majority of bleeding cirrhotic patients. It has recently been shown that the administration of recombinant activated factor VII (rFVIIa) normalizes prothrombin time in bleeding cirrhotics[45,46]. The potential role of rFVIIa has been evaluated in a multicenter European trial[5], including 245 bleeding cirrhotic patients who were randomized to receive eight doses of rFVIIa,100 µg/kg or placebo in addition to combined endoscopic + pharmacologic treatment. The primary endpoint was a composite including: failure to control bleeding at 24 h, failure to prevent rebleeding between 24 h and 5 days, and death within 5 days. No significant effect was found when analyzing the whole patient population; however, an exploratory analysis showed that, in Child–Pugh B and C variceal bleeders, rFVIIa significantly reduced the occurrence of the primary endpoint (from 23% in patients receiving placebo to 8% in patients receiving rFVIIa, $p = 0.03$), and improved bleeding control at 24 h (from 89% to 100%, $p = 0.03$). These data are encouraging, but require confirmation by studies specifically targeted on the appropriate patients.

## References

1. Ben-Ari Z, Cardin F, McCormick PA, Wannamethee G, Burroughs AK. A predictive model for failure to control bleeding during acute variceal hemorrhage. J Hepatol. 1999;31:443–50.
2. D'Amico G, Pagliaro L, Bosch J. Pharmacologic treatment of portal hypertension: an evidence-based approach. Semin Liver Dis. 1999;19:475–505.
3. de Franchis R, Primignani M. Endoscopic treatments for portal hypertension. Semin Liver Dis. 1999;19:439–55.
4. Moitinho E, Planas R, Bañares R et al. Multicenter randomized controlled trial comparing different schedules of somatostatin in the treatment of acute variceal bleeding. J Hepatol. 2001;35:712–18.
5. Thabut D, de Franchis R, Bendtsen F et al. Efficacy of activated recombinant factor VIII (RFVIIa; Novoseven®) in cirrhotic patients with upper gastrointestinal bleeding: a randomised placebo-controlled double-blind multicenter trial. J Hepatol. 2003;38(Suppl. 2):13 (abstract).
6. Merigan TC, Plotkin GR, Davidson CS. Effect of intravenously administered posterior pituitary extract on hemorrhage from bleeding esophageal varices. N Engl J Med. 1962; 266:134–5.
7. Cort J, Albrecht I, Novakova J, Mulder J, Jost K. Regional and systemic haemodynamic effects of some vasopressins: structural features of the hormone which prolong activity. Eur J Clin Invest. 1975;5:165–75.
8. Bosch J, Kravetz D, Rodes J. Effects of somatostatin on hepatic and systemic hemodynamics in patients with cirrhosis of the liver: comparison with vasopressin. Gastroenterology. 1981;80:518–25.
9. de Franchis R Somatostatin, somatostatin analogues and other vasoactive drugs in the treatment of bleeding oesophageal varices. Dig Liver Dis. 2004;36(Suppl. 1):S93–100.
10. Burroughs A, McCormick P, Hughes M, Sprengers D, D'Heygere F, McIntyre N. Randomized, double-blind, placebo-controlled trial of somatostatin for variceal bleeding. Emergency control and prevention of early variceal rebleeding. Gastroenterology. 1990;99:1388–95.
11. Burroughs AK and the International Octreotide Varices Study Group. Double blind RCT of 5 day octreotide versus placebo, associated with sclerotherapy for trial/failures. AASLD Abstracts. Hepatology. 1996;24:352A (abstract).
12. McKee R. A study of octreotide in oesophageal varices. Digestion. 1990;45:60–5.

13. Walker S, Kreichgauer H, Bode J. Terlipressin vs. somatostatin in bleeding esophageal varices: a controlled double blind study. Hepatology. 1992;15:1023–30.
14. Pauwels A, Florent C, Desaint B, Guivarch P, Van H, Levy VG. Terlipressine et somatostatine dans le traitement des hemorragies par rupture de varices oesophagiennes (Letter). Gastroenterol Clin Biol. 1994;18:388–9.
15. Walker S, Kreigauer HP, Bode JC. Terlipressin versus somatostatin in the treatment of bleeding esophageal varices. Final report of a placebo-controlled, double blind study. Z Gastroenterol. 1996;34:692–8.
16. Feu F, Ruiz Del Arbol L, Banares R, Planas R, Bosch J. Double blind randomized controlled trial comparing terlipressin and somatostatin for acute variceal hemorrhage. Gastroenterology. 1996;111:1291–9.
17. Silvain C, Carpentier S, Sautereau D et al. Terlipressin plus transdermal nitroglycerin vs. octreotide in the control of acute bleeding from esophageal varices: a multicenter randomized trial. Hepatology. 1993;18:61–5.
18. Pedretti G, Elia G, Calzetti C, Magnani G, Fiaccadori F. Octreotide versus terlipressin in the acute variceal hemorrhage in cirrhosis. Emergency control and prevention of early rebleeding. Clin Invest. 1994;72:653–9.
19. D'Amico G, Pietrosi G, Tarantino I, Pagliaro L. Emergency sclerotherapy versus vasoactive drugs for variceal bleeding in cirrhosis: a Cochrane meta-analysis. Gastroenterology. 2003;124:1277–91.
20. Stiegmann GV, Goff JS, Michaletz-Onody PA et al. Endoscopic sclerotherapy as compared with endoscopic ligation for bleeding esophageal varices. N Engl J Med. 1992;326:1527–32.
21. Laine L., El-Newihi HM, Migikowsky B, Sloane R, Garcia F. Endoscopic ligation compared with sclerotherapy for the treatment of bleeding esophageal varices. Ann Intern Med. 1993;119:1–7.
22. Gimson AES, Ramage JK, Panos MZ et al. Randomized trial of variceal banding ligation versus injection sclerotherapy for bleeding esophageal varices. Lancet. 1993;342:391–4.
23. Jensen DM, Kovacs TOG, Randall GM et al. Initial results of a randomized prospective study of emergency banding vs sclerotherapy for bleeding gastric or esophageal varices. Gastrointest Endosc. 1993;39:279 (abstract).
24. Lo GH, Lai KH, Cheng JS et al. A prospective, randomized trial of injection sclerotherapy versus banding ligation in the management of bleeding esophageal varices. Hepatology. 1995;22:466–71.
25. Hou MC, Lin HC, Kuo BIT, Chen CH, Lee FY, Lee SD. Comparison of endoscopic variceal injection sclerotherapy and ligation for the treatment of esophageal variceal hemorrhage: a prospective randomized trial. Hepatology. 1995;21:1517–22.
26. Fakhry S, Omer M, Nouh A et al. Endoscopic sclerotherapy versus endoscopic variceal ligation in the management of bleeding esophageal varices: a preliminary report of a prospective randomized study in schistosomal hepatic fibrosis. Hepatology. 1995;22:251A (abstract).
27. Sarin SK, Goyal A. Jain A, Guptan RC, Murthy MS. Randomized prospective trial of endoscopic sclerotherapy vs variceal ligation for bleeding esophageal varices: influence on gastropathy, gastric varices and recurrences. J Hepatol. 1997;26:826–32.
28. Lo GH, Lai KH, Cheng JS et al. Emergency banding ligation vs. sclerotherapy for the control of active bleeding from esophageal varices. Hepatology. 1997;25:1101–4.
29. Levacher S, Letoumelin PH, Paternon D, Blaise M, Lepandry C, Pourriat JL. Early administration of terlipressin plus glyceryltrinitrate for active upper gastrointestinal hemorrhage in cirrhotic patients. Lancet. 1995;346:865–8.
30. Besson I, Ingrand P, Person B et al. Sclerotherapy with or without octreotide for acute variceal bleeding. N Engl J Med. 1995;333:555–60.
31. Sung JJ, Chung SCS, Yung MY et al. Prospective randomised study of effect of octreotide on rebleeding from esophageal varices after endoscopic ligation. Lancet. 1995;346:1666–9.
32. Signorelli S, Negrini F, Paris B, Bonelli M, Girola M. Sclerotherapy with or without somatostatin or octreotide in the treatment of acute variceal hemorrhage: our experience. Gastroenterology. 1996;110(Suppl.)A1326 (abstract).
33. Brunati S, Ceriani R, Curioni R, Brunelli L, Repaci G, Morini L. Sclerotherapy alone vs. sclerotherapy plus terlipressin vs. sclerotherapy plus octreotide in the treatment of acute variceal hemorrhage. Hepatology. 1996;24(Suppl.l):207A (abstract).

34. Burroughs AK. Double blind RCT of 5 day octreotide versus placebo, associated with sclerotherapy for trial failures. Hepatology. 1996;24(Suppl.):352A (abstract).
35. Signorelli S, Paris B, Negrin F, Bonelli M, Auriemma M. Esophageal varices bleeding: comparison between treatment with sclerotherapy alone vs. sclerotherapy plus octreotide. Hepatology. 1997;26(Suppl.):137A (abstract).
36. Avgerinos A, Nevens F, Raptis S, Fevery J. Early administration of somatostatin and efficacy of sclerotherapy in acute oesophageal variceal bleeds: the European Acute Bleeding Oesophageal Variceal Episodes (ABOVE) randomised trial. Lancet. 1997;350:1495–9.
37. Zuberi BF, Baloch Q. Comparison of endoscopic variceal sclerotherapy alone and in combination with octreotide in controlling acute variceal hemorrhage and early rebleeding in patients with low-risk cirrhosis. Am J Gastroenterol. 2000;95:768–71.
38. Calés P, Masliah C, Bernard B et al. Early administration of vapreotide for variceal bleeding in patients with cirrhosis. N Engl J Med. 2001;344:23–8.
39. Villanueva C, Ortiz J, Sàbat M et al. Somatostatin alone or combined with emergency sclerotherapy in the treatment of acute esophageal variceal bleeding: a prospective randomized trial. Hepatology. 1999;30:384–9.
40. Novella MT, Villanueva C, Ortiz J et al. Octreotide vs. sclerotherapy and octreotide for acute variceal bleeding: a pilot study. Hepatology. 1996;24(Suppl.):207A (abstract).
41. Bañares R, Albillos A, Rincon D et al. Endoscopic treatment versus endoscopic plus pharmacologic treatment for acute variceal bleeding: a meta-analysis. Hepatology. 2002;35:609–15.
42. de Franchis R. Updating consensus in portal hypertension: report of the Baveno III consensus workshop on definitions, methodology and therapeutic strategies in portal hypertension. J Hepatol. 2000;33:846–52.
43. D'Amico G, de Franchis R and a cooperative study group. Upper digestive bleeding in cirrhosis. Post-therapeutic outcome and prognostic indicators. Hepatology. 2003;38:599–612.
44. Escorsell A, Bordas JM, Ruiz del Arbol L et al. Randomized controlled trial of sclerotherapy versus somatostatin infusion in the prevention of early rebleeding following acute variceal hemorrhage in patients with cirrhosis. J Hepatol. 1998;29:779–88.
45. Ejlersen E, Melsen T, Ingerslev J, Andreasen RB, Vilstrup H. Recombinant activated factor VII (rFVIIa) acutely normalizes prothrombin time in patients with cirrhosis during bleeding from oesophageal varices. Scand J Gastroenterol. 2001;36:1081–5.
46. Romero-Castro R, Jimenez-Saenz M, Pellicer-Bautista F et al. Recombinant-activated factor VII as hemostatic therapy in eight cases of severe hemorrhage from esophageal varices. Clin Gastroenterol Hepatol. 2004;2:78–84.

# 27
# Prevention of recurrent portal hypertensive bleeding

NORMAN D. GRACE

## INTRODUCTION

In patients with cirrhosis who have survived an episode of acute variceal hemorrhage, the risk of recurrent bleeding approaches 65–70%, with the highest risk period occurring within 6 weeks of the index bleed[1–3]. The associated mortality for each episode of variceal hemorrhage has improved considerably over the past 20 years, but remains at 15–20%[3,4]. Therefore, treatment to prevent recurrent hemorrhage is mandatory[5]. Although current pharmacologic and/or endoscopic treatment is successful in controlling bleeding in 90% of patients, rebleeding is not uncommon, with an 18% rate reported in a recent study, and a 5-day failure rate of 13%[3]. Therefore treatment to prevent recurrent bleeding should be initiated as soon as the patient is stable.

A plethora of randomized controlled trials (RCT) comparing pharmacologic and endoscopic techniques to no treatment, to each other, and in a variety of combinations for the prevention of recurrent bleeding have been published in the past 30 years. One problem in evaluating these trials has been lack of specific definitions of rebleeding and failure, especially in earlier studies dealing with endoscopic sclerotherapy. In an attempt to bring uniformity to definitions of rebleeding and failure, the Baveno II consensus conference adopted the following definition: "The occurrence of new haematemesis or new melaena after a period of 24 hours or more from the 24 hours point of stable vital signs and HCT/HB following an episode of acute bleeding. Clinically significant rebleeds should be evaluated as a separate end point and all rebleeding regardless of severity should be counted in evaluating rebleeding"[6]. The Baveno III consensus conference further refined the definition as "failure of secondary prevention is a single episode of clinically significant rebleeding from portal hypertensive sources"[7]. An important concept in these definitions is that rebleeding from all sources should be counted irrespective of the therapeutic modality employed. Rebleeding from esophageal varices should be considered as a subgroup of the total rebleeding population.

251

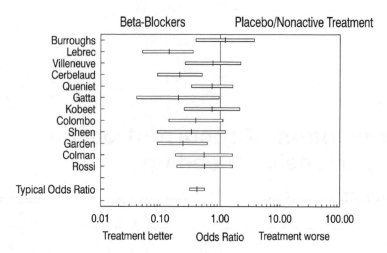

**Figure 1.** Randomized controlled trials of β-blockers vs placebo/non-active treatment for the prevention of rebleeding. The odds ratio for the group is 0.41; 95% confidence interval 0.31–0.55 ($p < 0.0001$)

First-line therapy for prevention of recurrent variceal bleeding includes the use of non-selective β-adrenergic blockers and endoscopic variceal ligation. Combinations of vasoconstrictors and vasodilators may potentiate the portal hemodynamic effect of pharmacologic agents. Also, the combination of a non-selective β-blocker and endoscopic variceal ligation has been reported in a single trial. For patients who fail initial therapy, surgical shunts or TIPS are options for good-risk patients. For patients with significant hepatic decompensation, TIPS or liver transplantation for appropriate candidates are options.

## PHARMACOLOGIC AGENTS TO PREVENT BLEEDING

In 1980 Lebrec et al. first described the use of propranolol, a non-selective β-adrenergic blocker, for the treatment of portal hypertension in patients with cirrhosis[8]. This was followed in 1981 by the publication of the first RCT demonstrating the efficacy of propranolol for the prevention of recurrent hemorrhage, both from esophageal varices and portal hypertensive gastropathy[9]. Since then, a total of 13 RCT comparing either propranolol or nadolol to a placebo or no treatment have been published. A meta-analysis of these trials shows a reduction in the rebleeding rate from 63% in the untreated group to 42% in patients with cirrhosis receiving non-selective β-blockers ($p < 0.0001$)[10,11] (Figure 1). The studies are homogeneous, with all but one showing at least a trend in favor of β-blocker therapy and four clearly reporting a significant benefit. Mortality in these trials was reduced from 27% in the non-treatment group to 20% in patients treated with β-blockers. (Figure 2). Death due to bleeding was significantly reduced with the use of β-blockers[12]. The number needed to treat (NNT) to prevent

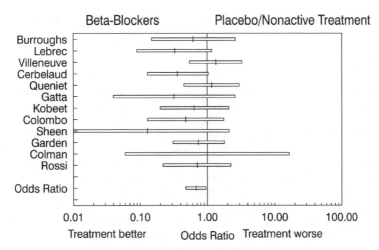

**Figure 2.** Randomized controlled trials of β-blockers vs placebo/non-active treatment; mortality. The odds ratio for the group is 0.68; 95% confidence interval 0.48–0.96 ($p < 0.03$)

an episode of rebleeding was 5 and mortality, 14[10]. The time interval between the index bleed and initiation of therapy in these trials ranged from 12 hours to 21 days. Five of the trials did not include patients with Child–Pugh (CP) class C decompensation while only three trials included at least 20% CP class C patients. In two of the three trials with a significant number of CP class C patients, the absolute risk reduction was less than 10%. Based on the results of these trials, non-selective β-blockers have become standard therapy for prevention of portal hypertensive rebleeding.

From 15% to 20% of patients have contraindications to the use of non-selective β-blockers and an additional 5–15% have significant side-effects requiring withdrawal of treatment. Although there are no published RCT evaluating long-acting nitrates as monotherapy for the prevention of rebleeding, the poor results in RCT evaluating isosorbide-5-mononitrate for prevention of first variceal hemorrhage do not support the use of these agents for prevention of rebleeding. Although a number of pharmacologic agents have been shown to decrease portal pressure in both animal models and acute clinical trials, side-effects of treatment, especially systemic arterial hypotension, have precluded their evaluation in larger RCT.

## ENDOSCOPIC THERAPY TO PREVENT PORTAL HYPERTENSION REBLEEDING

Ten trials, totaling 1259 patients, have compared endoscopic sclerotherapy to conservative treatment. A meta-analysis of these trials shows a significant benefit for prevention of rebleeding, with a 43% rebleeding rate in the sclerotherapy group compared to a 57% rebleeding rate in the control group (OR 0.57, CI 0.45–0.71)[13]. There was also a significant reduction in mortality, from 54% to 46%. Although the nine trials comparing sclerotherapy with non-selective β-blockers showed a slight advantage for prevention of rebleeding, but no survival benefit, the qualitative heterogeneity between trials results ($p = 0.07$) suggests that this perceived difference is not clinically significant[13].

Concerns regarding the complications of sclerotherapy prompted Stiegmann et al.[14,15] to introduce esophageal variceal ligation as a safer and possibly more effective technique. In 13 RCT comparing variceal ligation with sclerotherapy for the prevention of recurrent variceal bleeding, comprising 1091 patients, ligation was clearly superior to sclerotherapy, with a rebleeding rate of 21% for ligation compared to 36% for sclerotherapy (OR 0.46, CI 0.46–0.60)[13]. There was no difference in overall mortality but mortality related to recurrent bleeding was reduced in patients treated with band ligation. In addition, there were fewer sessions required to eradicate varices and fewer complications of treatment. Recurrence of varices was similar for the two endoscopic therapies. As a result of these trials, esophageal variceal ligation has replaced sclerotherapy as the endoscopic treatment of choice for prevention of recurrent variceal bleeding. There are no published trials comparing variceal ligation to non-selective β-blockers as monotherapy for the prevention of variceal rebleeding.

Prevention of recurrent bleeding from gastric varices is problematic, with neither sclerotherapy nor variceal ligation effective, and both associated with significant complications. Endoscopic techniques that may offer benefit are the use of cyanoacrylate glue and endoscopically placed detachable snares, but these techniques have been evaluated more for the control of acute bleeding than the prevention of recurrent bleeding[16].

## COMBINATION THERAPIES: β-BLOCKERS PLUS ISOSORBIDE-5-MONONITRATE VS β-BLOCKERS

The rationale for the combined use of a non-selective β-blocker and a long-acting nitrate is the greater hemodynamic response (HVPG decrease $> 20\%$ or to $< 12$ mmHg) achieved with combination therapy. In an acute study, Garcia-Pagan et al. were able to achieve a significant reduction in HVPG when isosorbide-5-mononitrate was added to propranolol in patients who previously had not responded to propranolol[17]. In a subsequent study, in which HVPG was measured at baseline and 3 months, the combination of propranolol and isosorbide-5-mononitrate achieved a reduction in HVPG $> 20\%$ in 50% of patients compared to 10% for propranolol monotherapy[18]. Larger trials have reported that 36% of patients treated with maximal doses of propranolol will achieve a $> 20\%$ reduction in HVPG[19]. In this study patients achieving a hemodynamic response had a rebleeding rate of 8% compared to 53% for patients unable to reach this hemodynamic endpoint with β-blocker therapy. A more detailed discussion of hemodynamic measurements in the management of portal hypertension can be found in the chapters by Groszmann and Burroughs.

In a trial involving 95 patients, patients randomized to receive propranolol and isosorbide-5-mononitrate to prevent variceal rebleeding achieved a statistically significant lower rebleeding rate at 3 years compared to propranolol monotherapy (45.5% vs 66.1%) that was not achieved in the first 2 years of follow-up[20]. The beneficial effect was more pronounced in patients $\geq 50$ years old. Survival was similar for the two groups. Patients treated with combination therapy had significantly more side-effects of therapy. In contrast, a study published only in abstract found a somewhat higher mortality in patients randomized to receive nadolol plus placebo (32% vs 20%, $p = 0.15$) with no difference in rebleeding and more side-effects in patients on combination therapy[21]. Therefore, the limited available data do not support the use of combination therapy over a β-blocker alone for prevention of recurrent variceal bleeding.

The combination of a non-selective β-blocker and a long-acting nitrate has been compared to endoscopic variceal ligation in three RCT, including 365 patients[22-24]. Villanueva et al. compared nadolol and isosorbide-5-mononitrate to variceal ligation in a trial in which baseline and 3-month measurements of HVPG were obtained in all patients. With a mean follow-up of 24 months they reported significantly less total rebleeding and rebleeding from esophageal varices in patients treated with combination pharmacologic therapy[22]. Although there was a trend toward lower transfusion requirements and death related to bleeding in the pharmacologic treatment group, it did not reach statistical significance, and overall mortality was similar for both treatment groups. In patients achieving a hemodynamic response, defined as a $> 20\%$ decrease in HVPG and/or a decrease in HVPG $< 12$ mmHg, the rebleeding rate was 16% compared to 67% in patients not achieving this hemodynamic goal. Similarly, the rebleeding rate was 14% in patients spontaneously achieving a hemodynamic response in the variceal ligation group, compared to 59% in the patients who had no significant change in HVPG. Patch et al. designed a trial comparing propranolol and isosorbide-5-mononitrate to variceal ligation in which measurements of HVPG were made at baseline and 8–12 weeks after being started on propranolol monotherapy[23]. If the patients did not achieve a hemodynamic response, isosorbide-5-mononitrate was added in a dose of 10–20 mg/day. However, only 50% of patients on propranolol had a repeat measurement of HVPG because death, liver transplantation or the need for TIPS for uncontrolled recurrent bleeding preceded the timing of the second measurement. Nevertheless, five patients achieved an HVPG $< 12$ mm at some point during follow-up, and none of these rebled. Although not statistically significant, there was a trend toward less rebleeding in patients randomized to pharmacologic treatment, with no difference in mortality. A third RCT by Lo et al., comparing nadolol and isosorbide-5-mononitrate with variceal ligation, was a single-center trial in which patients receiving nadolol had a mean dose of 48 mg/day, which is considerably lower than most other RCT evaluating non-selective β-blockers and compares to a mean dose of 96 mg/day in the trial by Villanueva et al.[24]. The 57% rebleeding rate in patients receiving pharmacologic therapy is similar to the 63% rebleeding rate reported in the meta-analysis of β-blocker RCT for patients on placebo or no treatment for prevention of recurrent bleeding[10] Lo et al. report a significant benefit for prevention of rebleeding from esophageal varices in patients receiving variceal ligation (RR 0.45, CI 0.24–0.85),

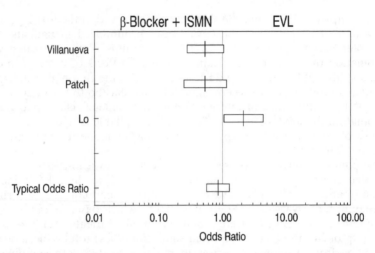

**Figure 3.** Randomized controlled trials of β-blockers plus isosorbide-5-mononitrate vs esophageal variceal ligation for the prevention of rebleeding. The odds ratio for the group is 0.85; 95% confidence interval 0.56–1.28 (n.s.)

although prevention of rebleeding from all sites did not reach statistical significance (38% ligation vs 57% pharmacologic therapy, $p = 0.10$). Despite the success in preventing rebleeding from varices, death occurred in 15 patients randomized to variceal ligation compared to eight on combination pharmacologic therapy ($p = 0.06$). A meta-analysis of these trials shows a trend in favor of pharmacologic therapy, but more data are needed to ascertain whether this perceived benefit will be clinically significant (Figures 3 and 4)[25].

## VARICEAL LIGATION PLUS β-BLOCKERS VS VARICEAL LIGATION

In a single-center, non-blinded RCT, Lo et al. compared esophageal variceal ligation, nadolol and sucralfate to variceal ligation monotherapy for the prevention of recurrent hemorrhage[26]. With a median follow-up of 21 months, 23% of patients receiving triple therapy experienced recurrent bleeding compared to 47% treated with ligation only ($p = 0.005$). Triple therapy was also superior for preventing recurrent variceal hemorrhage and recurrence of esophageal varices after initial ligation therapy. The mortality was 16.7% for patients receiving triple therapy compared to 32.3% for patients treated with ligation ($p = 0.08$). Although this initial trial is promising, additional studies supporting their conclusions are needed before we can consider the combination of endoscopic and pharmacologic therapy as having an advantage over variceal ligation as a single therapy.

## TREATMENT FOR MEDICAL FAILURES

TIPS has become the primary treatment for patients failing medical therapy for the prevention of recurrent variceal bleeding. However, in most of the

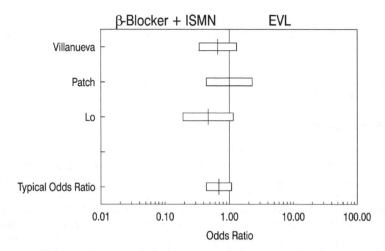

**Figure 4.** Randomized controlled trials of β-blockers vs isosorbide-5-mononitrate vs esophageal variceal ligation; mortality. The odds ratio for the group is 0.69; 95% confidence interval 0.44–1.08 (n.s.)

RCT comparing TIPS to sclerotherapy, the trials were designed as the initial therapy, not treatment of medical failures. A meta-analysis of these trials found TIPS superior for prevention of recurrent bleeding but at a cost of an increase in hepatic encephalopathy with no difference in survival[27,28]. In a trial comparing TIPS with endoscopic variceal ligation, patients were randomized within 24 hours after control of acute variceal bleeding with a mean follow-up of 16 months[29]. Rebleeding was significantly more frequent in patients treated with variceal ligation (51.9%) compared to TIPS (9.87%) ($p < 0.006$). The development or worsening of encephalopathy was similar for both treatment groups, with no survival differences. These results were confirmed in two additional RCT in which TIPS was superior to variceal ligation for the prevention of recurrent variceal hemorrhage, with no significant differences in encephalopathy or survival[30,31]. Why the incidence of new and/or worsening encephalopathy is significantly greater when TIPS is compared to endoscopic sclerotherapy than when compared to variceal ligation is unclear, but the sample size for the latter trials is small, with only the study by Jalan et al. published.[29]

In an RCT confined to Child–Pugh class B/C cirrhotics, patients were randomized to a combination of propranolol and isosorbide-5-mononitrate versus TIPS for the initial prevention of variceal rebleeding and followed for a mean of 15 months[32]. Rebleeding occurred in 13% of patients treated with TIPS compared to 39% receiving combination drug therapy ($p = 0.007$). However, encephalopathy was significantly more common in patients receiving TIPS (38%) than pharmacologic therapy (14%) ($p = 0.007$), with no difference in survival. The cost of TIPS treatment was double the cost of pharmacologic therapy (21 603 vs 10 692 Euros).

Not surprisingly, TIPS is more effective than medical therapy for the prevention of recurrent variceal hemorrhage, but with more encephalopathy, a higher cost, and no survival benefit. All of these trials were designed as initial therapy for prevention of recurrent bleeding, not for treatment of medical failures; perhaps a more appropriate role for TIPS. RCT to evaluate TIPS as a rescue procedure are needed.

## TIPS VERSUS SURGICAL SHUNTS

For the past 50 years, surgically created total or selective shunts have been effective treatment for the prevention of recurrent variceal bleeding. Recurrent bleeding was reported in 11% of patients treated with a total shunt compared to 17% receiving a distal splenorenal shunt[33]. However, hepatic encephalopathy is more common after a total shunt, especially in patients with non-alcoholic cirrhosis. In patients with alcoholic cirrhosis, reversal of prograde portal venous blood flow occurs over time, with an associated increase in encephalopathy[34]. Rebleeding after a surgical shunt is usually due to shunt thrombosis, and occurs within the first year postoperationally. Unlike TIPS, recurrent bleeding after 1 year is unusual.

In a trial designed for failures of sclerotherapy for prevention of recurrent variceal hemorrhage, Rosemurgy et al. compared a small-diameter prosthetic H-graft portacaval shunt with TIPS for prevention of rebleeding[35]. Patients were predominantly Child–Pugh class B/C with 70% having ascites at the time of randomization. Eleven percent of patients had a major variceal bleed after TIPS compared to none after a surgical shunt. Failure defined as major variceal hemorrhage, need for liver transplantation or death was 57% after TIPS placement compared to 26% for surgical shunts ($p < 0.02$). Using a decision analysis model, Zacks et al. found the DSRS more cost-effective than TIPS for Child–Pugh class A patients with no significant difference in survival[36]. Henderson et al. are currently conducting a multi-center, NIH-sponsored trial comparing TIPS and the distal splenorenal shunt in an attempt to determine the appropriate role for each procedure.

With the development of coated stents for TIPS, the efficacy and complications of TIPS will need reassessment. Comparing a polytetrafluoroethylene-coated stent with standard non-coated stents, Bureau et al. reported significantly less shunt dysfunction (13% vs 44%) and clinical relapse defined as uncontrolled bleeding, recurrent bleeding or refractory ascites (8% vs 29%) with coated stents[37]. There was also a trend toward less encephalopathy and a better 2-year survival that did not reach statistical significance.

## CONCLUSIONS

Both non-selective β-blockers and endoscopic variceal ligation are effective for decreasing the risk of recurrent variceal bleeding, and should be considered first-line therapy. Factors to consider when making a decision are patient compliance and the portal hemodynamic response to pharmacologic therapy. Non-compliant patients should be treated with variceal ligation. The roles of combination pharmacologic therapy or pharmacologic therapy combined with variceal ligation are evolving. For now their use should probably be restricted to very high-risk patients or patients who have failed monotherapy. Both surgically created shunts and TIPS are effective for treatment of medical failures. The advent of coated stents may redefine the role of TIPS, but appropriate RCT will need to be done. Finally, liver transplantation is life-saving for appropriate candidates, based on their MELD score.

## References

1. D'Amico G, Pagliaro L, Bosch J. The treatment of portal hypertension. A meta-analytic review. Hepatology. 1995;22:332–54.
2. Graham D, Smith JL. The course of patients after variceal hemorrhage. Gastroenterology. 1981;80:800–9.
3. D'Amico G, DeFranchis R, Cooperative Study Group. Upper digestive bleeding in cirrhosis. Post-therapeutic outcome and prognostic indicators. Hepatology. 2003;38:599–612.
4. Chalasani N, Kahi C, Francois F et al. Improved patient survival after acute variceal bleeding: a multicenter, cohort study. Am J Gastroenterol. 2003;98:653–9.
5. Grace ND, Groszmann RJ, Garcia-Tsao G et al. Portal hypertension and variceal bleeding. An AASLD single topic symposium. Hepatology. 1998;28:868–80.
6. De Franchis R, ed. Portal Hypertension II. Proceedings of the Second Baveno International Consensus Workshop on Definitions, Methodology and Therapeutic Strategies. Oxford: Blackwell Science, 1996:10–17.
7. De Franchis R, ed. Portal Hypertension III. Proceedings of the Third International Consensus Workshop on Definitions, Methodology and Therapeutic Strategies. Oxford: Blackwell Science, 2001:13–21.
8. Lebrec D, Nouel O, Corbic M, Benhamou JP. Propanolol – a medical treatment for portal hypertension? Lancet. 1980;2:180–2.
9. Lebrec D, Poynard T, Hillon P, Benhamou JP. Propanolol for prevention of recurrent gastrointestinal bleeding in patients with cirrhosis, a controlled study. N Engl J Med. 1981;305:1371–4.
10. D'Amico G, Pagliaro L, Bosch J. Pharmacological treatment of portal hypertension: an evidence-based approach. Semin Liver Dis. 1999;19:475–503.
11. Grace ND, Bhattacharya K. Pharmacologic therapy of portal hypertension and variceal hemorrhage. Clin Liver Dis. 1997;1:59–75.
12. Bernard B, Lebrec D, Mathurin P, Opolon P, Poynard T. Beta-adrenergic antagonists in the prevention of gastrointestinal rebleeding in patients with cirrhosis: a meta-analysis. Hepatology. 1997;25:63–70.
13. DeFranchis R, Primignani M. Endoscopic treatments for portal hypertension. Semin Liver Dis. 1999;19:439–55.
14. Stiegmann GV, Cambret, Sun JH. A new endoscopic elastic band ligating device. Gastrointest Endosc. 1986;32:230–3.
15. Stiegmann GV, Goff, JS, Michaletz-Onody PA et al. Endoscopic sclerotherapy as compared with endoscopic ligation for bleeding esophageal varices. N Engl J Med. 1992;326:1527–32.
16. Ryan BM, Stockbrugger RW, Ryan JM. A pathophysiologic, gastroenterologic and radio-logic approach to the management of gastric varices. Gastroenterology. 2004;126:1175–89.
17. Garcia-Pagan JC, Navasa M, Bosch J, Bru C, Pizcueta P, Rodes J. Enhancement of portal pressure reduction by the association of isosorbide-5-mononitrate to propranolol admin-istration in patients with cirrhosis. Hepatology. 1990;11:230–8.
18. Garcia-Pagan J, Feu F, Bosch J, Rodes J, Propranolol compared with propranolol plus isosorbide-5-mononitrate for portal hypertension in cirrhosis. A randomized controlled trial. Ann Intern Med. 1991;114:869–73.
19. Feu F, Garcia-Pagan JC, Bosch J et al. Relations between portal pressure response to pharmacotherapy and risk of recurrent variceal hemorrhage in patients with cirrhosis. Lancet. 1995;346:1056–9.

20. Gournay J, Masliah C, Martin T, Perrin D, Galmiche JP. Isosorbide mononitrate and propranolol compared with propranolol alone for the prevention of variceal rebleeding. Hepatology. 2000;31:1239–45.
21. Pasta L, D'Amico G, Patti R et al. Isosorbide mononitrate with nadolol compared to nadolol alone for prevention of recurrent bleeding in cirrhosis. A double-blind placebo-controlled randomized trial. Gastroenterology. 2001;120:A375.
22. Villanueva C, Minana J, Ortiz J et al. Endoscopic ligation compared with combined treatment with nadolol and isosorbide mononitrate to prevent recurrent variceal bleeding. N Engl J Med. 2001;345:647–55.
23. Patch D, Sabin A, Goulis J et al. A randomized controlled trial of medical therapy versus endoscopic ligation for the prevention of variceal rebleeding in patients with cirrhosis. Gastroenterology. 2002;123:1013–19.
24. Lo GH, Chen WC, Chen MH et al. Banding ligation versus nadolol and isosorbide mononitrate for the prevention of esophageal variceal rebleeding. Gastroenterology. 2002; 123:728–34.
25. Groszmann RJ, Garcia-Tsao G. Endoscopic variceal banding vs pharmacological therapy for the prevention of recurrent variceal hemorrhage: what makes a difference? Gastroenterology. 2002;123:1388–91.
26. Lo GH, Lai KH, Cheng JS et al. Endoscopic variceal ligation plus nadolol and sucralfate compared with ligation alone for the prevention of variceal rebleeding: a prospective, randomized trial. Hepatology. 2000;32:461–5.
27. Grace ND. TIPS: the search for a proper role. In: Arroyo V, Bosch J, Bruguera M. Rodes J, editors. Therapy in Liver Diseases: The Pathophysiologic Basis of Therapy. Barcelona: Spain Masson SA, 1997:435–40.
28. Burroughs AK, Patch D. Transjugular intraheaptic portosystemic shunt. Semin Liver Dis. 1999;19:457–73.
29. Jalan R, Forrest EH, Stanley AJ et al. A randomized trial comparing transjugular intrahepatic portosystemic stent–shunt with variceal band ligation in the prevention of rebleeding from esophageal varices. Hepatology. 1997;26:1115–22.
30. Pomier-Layrargues G, Dufresne MP, Bui B et al. TIPS versus endoscopic variceal ligation in the prevention of variceal rebleeding in the cirrhotic patient: a comparative randomized clinical trial (interim analysis). Hepatology. 1997;26:137A.
31. Sauer P, Benz C, Theilmann L, Richter G, Stremmel W, Stiehl A. Transjugular intrahepatic portosystemic stent shunt (TIPS) vs endoscopic banding in the prevention of variceal rebleeding: final results of a randomized study. Gastroenterology. 1998;114:A1334.
32. Escorsell A, Banares R, Garcia-Pagan JC et al. TIPS versus drug therapy in preventing variceal rebleeding in advanced cirrhosis: a randomized controlled trial. Hepatology. 2002;35:385–92.
33. Grace ND, Conn HO, Resnick RH et al. Distal splenorenal vs portal–systemic shunts after hemorrhage from varices: a randomized controlled trial. Hepatology. 1988;8:1475–81.
34. Widrich WC, Robbins AH, Johnson WC et al. Long-term follow-up of distal splenorenal shunts: evaluation by arteriography, shuntography, transhepatic portal venography, and cinefluorography. Radiology. 1980;134:341–5.
35. Rosemurgy AS, Goode SE, Zweibel BR, Black TJ, Brady PG. A prospective trial of transjugular intrahepatic portosystemic stent shunts versus small-diameter prosthetic H-graft portacaval shunts in the treatment of bleeding varices. Ann Surg. 1996;224:378–86.
36. Zacks SL, Sandler RS, Biddle AK, Mauro MA, Brown RS. Decision-analysis of transjugular intrahepatic portosystemic shunt versus distal splenorenal shunt for portal hypertension. Hepatology. 1999;29:1399–405.
37. Bureau C, Garcia-Pagan JC, Otal P et al. Improved clinical outcome using polytetrafluoroethylene-coated stents for TIPS: results of a randomized study. Gastroenterology. 2004; 126:469–75.

# 28
# Cost-effectiveness of primary prophylaxis for esophageal variceal bleeding

JAYANT A. TALWALKAR

## INTRODUCTION

A recent examination of control groups in acute variceal hemorrhage trials is noted for an overall 40% risk reduction in mortality over the past three decades[1]; however, the probability of death remains high (25–30%) despite advances in medical management. From a number of high-quality randomized controlled trials the use of beta-adrenergic blocking agents (beta-blockers) as primary prophylaxis is associated with a 50% risk reduction in esophageal variceal bleeding[2]. Among patients ineligible or intolerant of beta-blocker therapy, clinical benefits from endoscopic variceal ligation (EVL) versus observation alone are also recognized[3].

Independent of the primary prophylaxis method used, the clinical effectiveness of these strategies remains unknown based on limited evidence. Even less is known about the extent of resource utilization and subsequent impact on health status associated with primary prophylaxis. Recently, a number of economic analyses[4-7] have been developed to answer these questions and identify gaps in knowledge. This chapter will provide a systematic overview of results from these studies and explore areas of need for future investigations. A single investigation employing decision analysis methods alone is recognized[8], but will not be included in this chapter.

## PRINCIPLES OF COST-EFFECTIVENESS ANALYSIS

Based on the recognition of limited resources, there continues to be a need for identifying clinical strategies associated with fiscally responsible healthcare. Several methods for conducting an economic evaluation between two or more competing strategies have been developed. Common to these designs is the determination of a ratio involving consequences of health (outcomes) and the costs required to execute a particular strategy. The most commonly employed technique is known as cost-effectiveness analysis. A cost-effectiveness (C/E) ratio can be defined by the following equation:

$$C/E = \frac{[\text{Cost}]_{\text{Program B}} - [\text{Cost}]_{\text{Program A}}}{[\text{Health benefit}]_{\text{Program B}} - [\text{Health benefit}]_{\text{Program A}}}$$

When two or more strategies are compared, the measure of choice is called an incremental cost-effectiveness ratio (ICER). The ICER represents the additional cost required to prevent one additional outcome (i.e. variceal bleed) when choosing the more expensive of two competing strategies. It is calculated by ranking strategies from the least to the most expensive and performing calculations as done for a C/E ratio. The recommended metric for ICER is "cost per quality-adjusted life year (QALY)". Quality of life is best determined by health state preferences (or utilities) elicited from patients who are enrolled in the program of interest. The product of health state utility with number of life years gained from an intervention is used to calculate QALY values[9,10].

Disease states characterized by well-defined stages of progression are best suited for the application of mathematical modeling. A technique called the Markov state-transition process (or Markov model) is commonly used to simulate the natural history of chronic disease and its attendant complications[11]. The transition probabilities for moving from one stage to the next are based on evidence from observational and intervention studies published in the literature. When using a Markov model, individuals are not allowed to return to an earlier stage of their disease. The inability to have esophageal varix regression over time is an example of this concept.

## REVIEW OF PUBLISHED COST-EFFECTIVENESS ANALYSES FOR PRIMARY PROPHYLAXIS

To date, a number of cost-effectiveness analyses[4-7] examining various primary prophylaxis strategies have been published. The most frequently studied approaches include: (1) observation alone, (2) universal beta-blocker therapy without performing screening endoscopy, (3) beta-blockers after endoscopy, and (4) variceal band ligation at the time of endoscopy. Other methods including endoscopic sclerotherapy, surgical shunt, and transjugular portosystemic shunt (TIPSS) have been studied in only one investigation[4]. The rationale for including observation as a clinical strategy, despite the ethical questions raised by this approach, has not been well-described in these models.

### Teran et al. (1997)[4]

The first published analysis was from Teran and colleagues. Using a Markov model, a total of four primary prophylaxis strategies were compared. These comprised observation alone, propranolol, endoscopic sclerotherapy, and shunt surgery. Patients were stratified according to known prognostic factors for variceal hemorrhage including varix size and Child–Turcotte–Pugh (CTP) classification. Primary model endpoints were: (1) incidence rate of variceal bleeding, (2) bleed-related mortality rate, (3) overall mortality rate, (4) life expectancy, and (5) quality-adjusted life expectancy.

Among hypothetical cohorts of 40-year-old men with cirrhosis, the most cost-saving method of primary prophylaxis was propranolol. Quality-adjusted life expectancy increased by 1–3 months in all subgroups with propranolol compared to observation alone. The remaining strategies were cost-prohibitive and without gains in quality-adjusted life expectancy. The model's results were stable after varying the probabilities of variceal bleeding rate, bleed-related mortality rate, and all-cause mortality rate.

### Arguedas et al. (2002)[6]

An examination of the entire process for initiating primary prophylaxis in clinical practice was performed by Arguedas and colleagues. This included endoscopic screening, surveillance, and the treatment of primary prophylaxis failures. A Markov model was used to compare four clinical strategies: observation alone, beta-blockers following endoscopic screening, variceal band ligation following endoscopic screening, and universal beta-blocker treatment without screening. Patients with compensated cirrhosis (CTP A) and decompensated cirrhosis (CTP B and C) were examined separately. In accordance with consensus practice guidelines[12–14], patients without esophageal varices at screening endoscopy underwent repeat examination in 2 years. If small varices were identified, surveillance endoscopy was performed in 1 year and annually thereafter until large varices developed. Beta-blockers were instituted when large varices on screening or surveillance endoscopy were found with no further endoscopy performed. The intolerance rate to beta-blockers was assumed to be 15% with affected patients referred for variceal band ligation as primary prophylaxis. Model outcomes included: (1) life expectancy, (2) number of bleeding episodes, and (3) expected costs for each strategy.

For a 50-year-old patient with compensated cirrhosis the ICER for endoscopic screening and beta-blocker therapy versus endoscopic variceal ligation was $4700 (US dollars) per QALY. Universal beta-blocker prophylaxis was considered cost-prohibitive compared to other strategies. Variceal ligation was preferred in this patient population if the risk reduction with beta-blockers was < 30%, intolerance rate to beta-blockers was > 27%, and the cost of beta-blocker treatment exceeded $400 annually.

For a 50-year-old patient with decompensated cirrhosis the ICER for endoscopic screening and beta-blocker therapy versus endoscopic variceal ligation was $4000 per QALY. However, the ICER for universal beta-blocker treatment was more favorable compared to endoscopic screening and beta-blockers ($2000 per QALY) and endoscopic variceal ligation ($2727 per QALY).

### Saab et al. (2003)[5]

A Markov model was also used by Saab and colleagues to compare three strategies for primary prophylaxis. These strategies included universal beta-blocker treatment without endoscopic screening, endoscopic screening followed by beta-blocker therapy, and observation alone. Endoscopic surveillance for patients with no or small esophageal varices at index endoscopy was according to consensus practice guidelines. Again, the intolerance rate to beta-blocker therapy was assumed to be 15%. Model outcomes included: (1) the number of patients who bled, (2) the number of patients who rebled, and (3) the number of patients with bleed-related death.

Among a hypothetical cohort of 1000 patients (CTP class unknown), the dominant strategy in this model was universal prophylaxis with beta-blockers compared to endoscopic screening and observation. If compliance with the strategy of endoscopic screening and beta-blocker therapy is high, then this strategy was the preferred method compared to universal primary prophylaxis.

## Spiegel et al. (2003)[7]

The most recent cost-effectiveness analysis was published by Spiegel and colleagues. In this study a total of six clinical strategies were examined comprising: (1) observation alone, (2) universal beta-blocker therapy without endoscopic screening, (3) endoscopic screening then beta-blocker therapy, (4) endoscopic screening then variceal ligation, (5) screening only high-risk patients based on clinical prediction rules followed by beta-blocker therapy, and (6) screening only high-risk patients with clinical prediction rules followed by variceal ligation. Both intolerance and non-compliance rates with beta-blocker therapy were included in the model. The primary model outcome was cost per initial variceal bleed prevented by each strategy.

Among 50-year-old patients with CTP class A or B cirrhosis, the strategy of observation alone was noted for a cost of $2401 per initial bleed prevented. The ICER for universal beta-blocker therapy versus observation alone was $12 408 per additional bleed prevented. When comparing screening endoscopy followed by beta-blocker therapy versus universal beta-blocker therapy, the ICER was $175 833 per additional bleed prevented. Screening endoscopy followed by variceal ligation cost $178 400 per additional bleed prevented compared to endoscopy and beta-blocker therapy. Both strategies using clinical prediction models were more expensive and less effective than universal beta-blocker therapy. The authors concluded that beta-blocker therapy was the optimal strategy.

As the probability of beta-blocker non-compliance increased to 80%, the ICER for endoscopic screening with variceal ligation dropped to < $50 000 per additional bleed prevented compared to universal beta-blockers. When the cost of screening endoscopy was reduced by 66% (or less than $300), the ICER for endoscopic screening with variceal ligation was $50 000 per additional bleed prevented compared to universal beta-blockers.

## FACTORS TO CONSIDER IN COST-EFFECTIVENESS ANALYSIS OF PRIMARY PROPHYLAXIS

### Variation in methodology used for analysis

Specific recommendations for the appropriate conduct of cost-effectiveness analyses have been reported[10]. The use of incremental cost-effectiveness ratios (ICER) does not appear in all primary prophylaxis models[4], making comparisons between studies difficult. In turn, the use of QALY to measure health benefits was not uniformly applied (see below). The exclusion of liver-related and all-cause mortality as model outcomes may compromise the validity of model results since these events influence the effectiveness of primary prophylaxis[7]. An important observation is the exclusion of decompensated patients (CTP C) in some models[6,7]. Finally, the cost of endoscopic screening should be included in all models as part of the process-of-care for instituting preventive therapy[4].

## Level of evidence used for analysis

The evidence used in published models is derived from randomized controlled trials, meta-analyses, and well-performed observational studies. Applying these data to simulate clinical experience in a consistent fashion, however, has not been observed. In two studies where universal beta-blocker therapy was considered the optimal strategy, the use of different estimates for risk reduction with variceal ligation occurred[15]. This resulted in an inconsistent recommendation for universal beta-blockers in patients with both compensated and decompensated cirrhosis. All studies have extrapolated the short-term data available for primary prophylaxis to 3- and 5-year time horizons. The linearity of these assumptions, however, may not be true in actual practice. In turn, a longer time horizon would be more applicable for patients with compensated cirrhosis who are expected to survive for an additional 5–10 years.

## Adherence to prophylaxis strategy

The majority of existing models do not address the issue of adherence to primary prophylaxis[4–6]. Knowledge regarding patient compliance with long-term treatment (for either beta-blockers or endoscopic variceal ligation) is critical for understanding the actual effectiveness of these strategies. Clinical experience suggests that adverse events from beta-blockers are more common and severe in patients with decompensated cirrhosis. Based on this observation, it becomes difficult to comprehend that universal beta-blocker treatment would be the most effective strategy for this population. The costs for treating adverse events and bleeding episodes in the face of inadequate prophylaxis from drug discontinuation would be quite large. Better information on patient preference and adherence, therefore, is needed before this recommendation can be introduced into routine clinical practice.

## GAPS IN KNOWLEDGE

1. The effectiveness of primary prophylaxis strategies in community-based patients and individuals not participating in clinical trials remains unknown. For example, the effectiveness of long-acting beta-blocker agents, which are being increasingly used to improve adherence, would be of interest.
2. The measurement and validation of patient preferences for primary prophylaxis has not been widely performed. Existing models which recognize

health state preference (utilities) have used opinion-based data[6] or information extrapolated from other clinical situations involving patients with cirrhosis. Small changes in health status can result in large changes in ICER. Health status assessment, therefore, is one of the most pressing issues for determining the true cost-effectiveness of any intervention aimed at patients with cirrhosis and portal hypertension.

3. The ability to individualize therapy based on existing data is not possible. Decision-making with regard to primary prophylaxis, therefore, rests initially on determining which patients are at highest risk for variceal bleeding. Practice guidelines recommend that if large esophageal varices are found during screening endoscopy, the institution of either beta-blockers or EVL should be performed[12-14]. To date, efforts to develop prediction models for reducing the number of unnecessary procedures in low-risk patients are limited by poor sensitivity and remain clinically unhelpful[16]

4. The degree of clinical practice variation for recommending screening and surveillance endoscopy among referral and community-based health-care providers remains unknown.

## References

1. McCormick PA, O'Keefe C. Improving prognosis following a first variceal haemorrhage over four decades. Gut. 2001;49:682–5.
2. D'Amico G, Pagliaro L, Bosch J. Pharmacological treatment of portal hypertension: an evidence-based approach. Semin Liver Dis. 1999;19:475–505.
3. Imperiale TF, Chalasani N. A meta-analysis of endoscopic variceal ligation for primary prophylaxis of esophageal variceal bleeding. Hepatology. 2001;33:802–7.
4. Teran JC, Imperiale TF, Mullen KD, Tavill AS, McCullough AJ. Primary prophylaxis of variceal bleeding in cirrhosis: a cost-effectiveness analysis. Gastroenterology. 1997;112:473–82.
5. Saab S, DeRosa V, Nieto J, Durazo F, Han S, Roth B. Costs and clinical outcomes of primary prophylaxis of variceal bleeding in patients with hepatic cirrhosis: a decision analytic model. Am J Gastroenterol. 2003;98:763–70.
6. Arguedas MR, Heudebert GR, Eloubeidi MA, Abrams GA, Fallon MB. Cost-effectiveness of screening, surveillance, and primary prophylaxis strategies for esophageal varices. Am J Gastroenterol. 2002;97:2441–52.
7. Spiegel BM, Targownik L, Dulai GS, Karsan HA, Gralnek IM. Endoscopic screening for esophageal varices in cirrhosis: is it ever cost effective? Hepatology. 2003;37:366–77.
8. Aoki N, Kajiyama T, Beck JR, Cone RW, Soma K, Fukui T. Decision analysis of prophylactic treatment for patients with high-risk esophageal varices. Gastrointest Endosc. 2000;52:707–14.
9. Drummond M. The role of health economics in clinical evaluation. J Eval Clin Pract. 1995;1:71–5.
10. Weinstein MC, Siegel JE, Gold MR, Kamlet MS, Russell LB. Recommendations of the Panel on Cost-effectiveness in Health and Medicine. J Am Med Assoc. 1996;276:1253–8.
11. Sonnenberg F, Beck JR. Markov models in medical decision making: a practical guide. Med Decis Making. 1993;13:322–38.
12. Grace N. Diagnosis and treatment of gastrointestinal bleeding secondary to portal hypertension. Am J Gastroenterol. 1997;92:1081–91.
13. Grace ND, Groszmann RJ, Garcia-Tsao G et al. Portal hypertension and variceal bleeding: an AASLD single topic symposium. Hepatology. 1998;28:868–80.
14. Jalan R, Hayes PC. UK guidelines on the management of variceal haemorrhage in cirrhotic patients. Gut. 2000;46(Suppl. 3–4):III1–5.

15. Rubenstein JH, Inadomi JM. Empiric beta-blockers for the prophylaxis of variceal hemorrhage: cost effective or clinically applicable? Hepatology. 2003;37:249–52.
16. Ong J. Clinical predictors of large esophageal varices: how accurate are they? Am J
Gastroenterol. 1999;94:3103–5.

# Section VIII
# Problems in treatment

# 29
# The cirrhotic patient with no varices and with small varices

CARLO MERKEL, MASSIMO BOLOGNESI
and ANGELO GATTA

## INTRODUCTION

The history of treatment of portal hypertension is characterized by a progressive tendency to treat patients in earlier stages of the disease. Indeed, in the beginning, treatment of portal hypertension was limited to treatment of acute bleeding and prevention of recurrent variceal bleeding; from the end of the 1980s it was shown that patients with high-risk varices but without previous bleeding are good candidates for a pharmacologic prophylaxis (and in some instances for an endoscopic prophylaxis). Recent research has been devoted to investigating whether prophylaxis of variceal bleeding should be started early, when varices are not yet present (in order to prevent varices formation), or when small varices with low risk of bleeding are seen, in order to decrease the risk of growth of varices and eventually the risk of variceal bleeding[1]. This area of research, sometimes called "pre-primary prophylaxis", is the background on which the clinical decisions on single patients with cirrhosis without varices or with small varices should be made.

## PATIENTS WITHOUT VARICES

Therapeutic options for patients without esophageal varices are limited to non-selective beta-blockers, or endoscopic surveillance without treatment. A rational decision may be based on the pathophysiology and epidemiology of this condition, and on the few data arising from clinical trials.

From a pathophysiological point of view, patients without esophageal varices represent a heterogeneous condition, including patients with initial portal hypertension, which has not yet reached the level necessary for the formation and growth of esophageal varices, and patients with full-blown portal hypertension, in whom a collateral circulation different from esophageal varices has already developed, and who eventually (but not necessarily) may also develop esophageal varices. This heterogeneity has been known

**Table 1.** Incidence of esophageal varices in the natural history of cirrhotic patients, according to the published series

| Author | Risk of developing varices | Observations |
|---|---|---|
| Calés et al. 1990[9] | 18/41 after 15.8 months of follow-up | Mostly alcoholic, one-third with advanced disease |
| Pagliaro et al. 1994[10] | 16% after 2 years of follow-up | Mostly virus-related, with compensated disease |
| Merli et al. 2003[11] | 5% after 1 year of follow-up; 28% after 3 years of follow-up | |

for more than 20 years, since the time when the first investigations of hepatic venous pressure gradient (HVPG) in patients with or without varices consistently showed that some patients without varices showed minor elevations on HVPG, and some showed elevated levels, very similar to those of patients with varices[2-4]. In this area, despite an overall agreement between extension of collateral circulation in gastroesophageal and peritoneal areas, we also observed that there was a minority of cases showing extensive collateral peritoneal circulation, but no esophageal varices[4]. This implies that anatomical factors may be responsible for a preferential development of collateral circulation in different districts, including gastroesophageal circulation. It is not established, however, if the risk of developing esophageal varices is different in these subgroups of patients.

Despite these uncertainties the majority of cirrhotic patients without varices have initial portal hypertension, and the question is whether these patients may benefit from an early treatment with beta-blockers. Beta-blockers act by decreasing cardiac output and splanchnic blood inflow, which are increased due to the hyperdynamic syndrome induced by the initial formation of collateral circulation and the activation of splanchnic vasodilation due to endogenous factors, in particular nitric oxide. In most experimental models (portal vein stenosis in rats, carbon tetrachloride-induced cirrhosis in rats, schistosomiasis in mice) it was shown that beta-blockers prevent the formation of collateral circulation, hamper the increase in portal pressure, and lessen the increase in portal blood inflow[5-7], although the same was not observed in the bile-duct ligated rat[8].

For these reasons it was reasonable to test the hypothesis that beta-blockers may prevent the formation of esophageal varices, and all the clinical complications of portal hypertension. Studies on this subject are very difficult to perform, due to the long time-course of the disease. Epidemiologic data support an incidence of esophageal varices ranging from 16% to 50% after 2 years of follow-up (Table 1), and the incidence of further complications of portal hypertension is much lower.

A single clinical study has been specifically addressed to evaluating the role of beta-blockers in preventing varices formation and the occurrence of the other complications of portal hypertension, and it was recently presented in part at the 2003 AASLD meeting[12]. However, complete data are not yet available. This was a double-blind study of patients with cirrhosis, without esophageal varices, with HVPG higher than 6 mmHg, who were randomized to the non-selective beta-blocker, timolol (108 patients) or placebo (105 patients). The authors did not observe any significant difference in occurrence of esophageal varices, variceal bleeding, occurrence of ascites or encephalopathy, or survival, between the two groups. The only clear-cut difference was that patients with baseline HVPG higher than 10 mmHg had a much higher rate of occurrence of varices, irrespective of the treatment received. It appears that in this condition beta-blockers are ineffective in preventing varices formation. Apart from possible problems related to the size of the treatment effect, which may have been too small to be observed with the current sample size and time of follow-up, a possible interpretation of these data is related to the mechanisms of action of beta-blockers. It is possible that, in patients with initial portal hypertension, pathophysiological mechanisms leading to portal hypertension (hyperdynamic circulation, increase in portal inflow) are weakly operating, and beta-blockers may have lacked the site on which to act.

Whatever the reason for this lack of effect, current data do not support the use of beta-blockers in patients without esophageal varices. Therefore, endoscopic surveillance is advisable.

## PATIENTS WITH SMALL ESOPHAGEAL VARICES

Therapeutic options for patients with small esophageal varices (less than 5 mm in size, or F1 according to Beppu's classification) are limited to non-selective beta-blockers, or endoscopic surveillance without treatment. Here too, a rational decision may be based on pathophysiology and epidemiology of this condition, and on the few data arising from clinical trials.

Usually the term "small esophageal varices" is considered synonymous with "low-risk esophageal varices"; F1 varices, according to the Japanese classification, the first two classes of the NIEC classification, and all varices smaller than 5 mm are all considered "small esophageal varices".

From a pathophysiological point of view, patients with small esophageal varices are not markedly different from patients with large esophageal varices. In many series no significant difference in HVPG was found between patients with small or large varices[2,3,13]; when a significant difference was reported, it was not shown to be very relevant[4,14]. The risk of bleeding in patients with small varices is definitely lower than that in patients with large varices, reaching approximately half of the value of high-risk varices (approximately 7% vs 15% at 2 years)[15–18]. Overall, patients with small esophageal varices show a quantitative more than qualitative difference compared with patients with large esophageal varices.

Beta-blockers also decrease HVPG in patients with small esophageal varices (Figure 1)[19], and it was also shown that they are more effective in decreasing HVPG in patients with less developed collateral circulation[20].

Clinical trials on the effect of beta-blockers in preventing growth of esophageal varices and decreasing risk of bleeding are very few. Prevention of growth of esophageal varices was assessed in two studies, one of which, coming from our study group, is currently reported as an abstract. In a series of patients with small esophageal varices or without varices, Calés

273

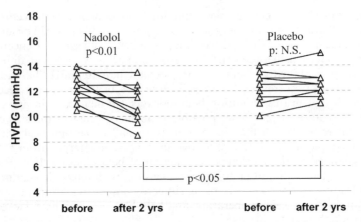

**Figure 1.** Hepatic venous pressure gradient in a group of patients with small esophageal varices treated with nadolol or placebo for 2 years (from ref. 19)

et al.[21] investigated the value of propranolol in preventing the occurrence of large esophageal varices. After 2 years of follow-up they observed a detrimental effect of propranolol, and after 3 years of follow-up propranolol was also less effective than placebo, although this difference was not significant. Some drawbacks, however, limit the value of this report. In particular, an excessive fraction of patients were lost to follow-up during the study, and treatment was given as a fixed dose, without adjustments related to the individual needs.

In October 2003 we presented the final results of a large multicenter study, comparing nadolol vs placebo in the prophylaxis of growth of small esophageal varices[19]. Previously, an interim analysis, suggesting a possible beneficial effect of treatment, was reported in 1998, after a mean follow-up of 18 months[22]. In the complete study, which included 83 patients randomized to nadolol and 78 to placebo, followed for up to 60 months, we observed a significantly lower rate of growth of esophageal varices in patients randomized to nadolol, and a significantly lower probability of variceal bleeding. This effect was evident when patients were analyzed from the beginning of follow-up, but was not observed when analysis was started from the moment at which patients reached a condition of large varices, and were all treated with nadolol. Survival was not affected by the treatment. Side-effects requesting withdrawal of treatment were similar in rate to the previous studies of prophylaxis of variceal bleeding with beta-blockers, and were always reversible after discontinuation of the drug. Therefore, it appears that treatment delayed the occurrence of large varices, and decreased the overall time spent by patients in a condition of high-risk varices.

Our results on the effect of beta-blockers on risk of bleeding in patients with small esophageal varices can be compared with a subgroup analysis of patients with small varices who were included in placebo-controlled trials of varices of any size. In two studies in which data are available[23,24] a tendency to improvement in outcome with beta-blockers was observed,

**Table 2.** Meta-analysis of beta-blockers vs placebo in the prophylaxis of first variceal bleeding in patients with small varices

| Reference | Odds ratio | Lower 95% CI | Higher 95% CI |
|---|---|---|---|
| Andreani et al. 1990[23] | 0.14 | 0.01 | 2.41 |
| Conn et al. 1991[24] | 1.12 | 0.15 | 8.46 |
| Merkel et al. 2003[19] | 0.24 | 0.07 | 0.82 |
| Typical | 0.32 | 0.12 | 0.87 |

although the numbers were too small to draw any statistical conclusions. A preliminary meta-analysis of the clinical results on risk of bleeding from the data reported in the three studies is reported in Table 2. From these figures it seems that a significant improvement in risk of bleeding may be obtained using beta-blockers in patients with small varices; however, the amount of available data is small. Therefore we should wait further studies on this topic before drawing definite conclusions about the treatment of patients with small esophageal varices.

From a pharmacoeconomic point of view, early treatment with beta-blockers may be favorably compared with the conventional strategy of endoscopic surveillance and treatment when varices become large. Indeed, drug treatment with beta-blockers is inexpensive and, when patients are included in a treatment program, there is no reason to continue endoscopic surveillance; in addition, early treatment decreases the overall risk of first variceal bleeding, reducing the global cost of treatment of these patients. A preliminary sensitivity analysis demonstrated that the cost of early treatment is also lower than that of the conventional strategy if the risk of developing large varices, or the difference in risk of bleeding between the two strategies, is decreased by half, or if the interval between surveillance endoscopies is changed from 12 months to 18 or 24. Therefore, if the results of our trial are confirmed in further studies, prophylaxis of variceal bleeding starting from small esophageal varices may also become the best option from a pharmacoeconomic point of view.

Until further clinical trials are available, although early treatment is not definitely proven to be superior to the conventional strategy, I feel that, for all the reasons outlined above, it may be reasonable to start prophylaxis with non-selective beta-blockers when patients have small esophageal varices.

## References

1. Merkel C, Escorsell A, Sieber CC, Lee FY, Groszmann RJ. Pre-primary prophylaxis: can (and should) we prevent the formation and growth of varices? In: de Franchis R, editor. Portal Hypertension III. Oxford: Blackwell, 2001:97–111.
2. Lebrec D, De Fleury P, Rueff B, Nahum H, Benhamou JP. Portal hypertension, size of esophageal varices, and risk of gastrointestinal bleeding in alcoholic cirrhosis. Gastroenterology. 1980;79:1139–44.
3. Garcia-Tsao G, Groszmann RJ, Fisher RL, Conn HO, Atterbury CE, Glickman M. Portal pressure, presence of gastroesophageal varices, and variceal bleeding. Hepatology. 1985;5:419–24.

4. Zuin R, Gatta A, Merkel C et al. Evaluation of peritoneoscopic and oesophagoscopic findings as indexes of portal hypertension in patients with liver cirrhosis. Ital J Gastroenterol. 1982;14:214–19.
5. Sarin SK, Groszmann RJ, Mosca PG et al. Propranolol ameliorates the development of portal–systemic shunting in a chronic murine schistosomiasis model of portal hypertension. J Clin Invest. 1991;87:1032–6.
6. Colombato LA, Albillos A, Genecin P. Prevention of portal–systemic shunting in propranolol-treated and in sodium-restricted cirrhotic rats. Gastroenterology. 1991;100:A730.
7. Lin HC, Soubrane O, Cailmail S, Lebrec D. Early chronic administration of propranolol reduces the severity of portal hypertension and portal–systemic shunts in conscious portal vein stenosed rats. J Hepatol. 1991;13:213–19.
8. Oberti F, Rifflet H, Maiga MY et al. Prevention of portal hypertension by propranolol and spironolactone in rats with bile duct ligation. J Hepatol. 1997;26:167–73.
9. Calès P, Desmorat H, Vinel JP et al. Incidence of large esophageal varices in patients with cirrhosis: application to prophylaxis of first bleeding. Gut. 1990;31:1298–302.
10. Pagliaro L, D'Amico G, Pasta L et al. Portal hypertension in cirrhosis: natural history. In: Bosch J, Groszmann RJ, editors. Portal Hypertension: Pathophysiology and Treatment. Oxford: Blackwell, 1994:72–92.
11. Merli M, Nicolini G, Angeloni S et al. Incidence and natural history of small esophageal varices in cirrhotic patients. J Hepatol. 2003;38:361–3.
12. Groszmann RJ, Garcia-Tsao G, Makuch R et al. Multicenter randomized placebo-controlled trial of non-selective beta-blockers in the prevention of the complications of portal hypertension: final results and identification of a predictive factor. Hepatology. 2003;38 (Suppl. 1):206 (abstract).
13. Le Moine O, Hadengue A, Moreau R et al. Relationship between portal pressure, esophageal varices and variceal bleeding on the basis of the stage and cause of cirrhosis. Scand J Gastroenterol. 1997;32:731–5.
14. Gluud C, Henriksen JH, Nielsen G, Copenhagen Study Group for Liver Disease. Prognostic indicators in alcoholic cirrhotic man. Hepatology. 1988;8:222–7.
15. North Italian Endoscopic Club for the Study and Treatment of Esophageal Varices. Prediction of the first variceal hemorrhage in patients with cirrhosis of the liver and esophageal varices. N Engl J Med. 1988;319:983–9.
16. Rigo GP, Merighi A, Chahin NJ et al. A prospective study of the ability of three endoscopic classifications to predict hemorrhage from esophageal varices. Gastrointest Endosc. 1992;38:425–9.
17. Prada A, Bortoli A, Minoli G, Carnovali M, Colombo E, Sangiovanni A. Prediction of oesophageal variceal bleeding: evaluation of the Beppu and North Italian Endoscopic Club scores by an independent group. Eur J Gastroenterol Hepatol. 1994;6:1009–13.
18. Zoli M, Merkel C, Magalotti D, Marchesini G, Gatta A, Pisi E. Evaluation of a new endoscopic index to predict first bleeding from the upper gastrointestinal tract in patients with cirrhosis. Hepatology. 1996;24:1047–52.
19. Merkel C, Marin R, Angeli P, Zanella P et al. Beta-blockers in the prevention of aggravation of esophageal varices in patients with cirrhosis and small esophageal varices: a placebo-controlled clinical trial. Hepatology. 2003;38(Suppl. 1):217 (abstract).
20. Escorsell A, Ferayorni L, Bosch J et al. The portal pressure response to beta-blockade is greater in cirrhotic patients without varices than in those with varices. Gastroenterology. 1997;112:2012–16.
21. Calès P, Oberti F, Payen JL et al. Lack of effect of propranolol in the prevention of large esophageal varices in patients with cirrhosis: a randomized trial. French-Speaking Club for the Study of Portal Hypertension. Eur J Gastroenterol Hepatol. 1999;11:741–5.
22. Merkel C, Angeli P, Marin R et al. Beta-blockers in the prevention of aggravation of esophageal varices in patients with cirrhosis and small esophageal varices. interim analysis of a controlled clinical trial. Hepatology. 1998;28(Suppl. 1):453A (abstract).
23. Andreani T, Poupon RE, Balkau BJ et al. Preventive therapy of first gastrointestinal bleeding in patients with cirrhosis: results of a controlled trial comparing propranolol, endoscopic sclerotherapy and placebo. Hepatology. 1990;12:1413–19.
24. Conn HO, Grace ND, Bosch J et al. Propranolol in the prevention of the first hemorrhage from esophagogastric varices: a multicenter, randomized clinical trial. Hepatology. 1991;13:902–12.

# 30
# Gastric varices

## S. K. SARIN

The prevalence of gastric varices (GV) in patients with portal hypertension has been reported to vary between 2% and 70%[1-3]. This substantial variability in the prevalence of GV is probably related to the differences in the patient populations, stage of cirrhosis and bleeding status, the techniques used for the diagnosis, and the classifications used for GV. In general, GV are present in about one in five patients with portal hypertension. On the other hand, about 5–10% of patients with gastric varices may not have esophageal varices[4]. It is worthwhile to note that GV are significantly more common in bleeders than in non-bleeders (27% vs. 4%), perhaps indicating that GV develop at a more advanced stage of portal hypertension[5].

GV are more difficult to detect by endoscopy, especially if they are small and isolated. Small varices in the fundus are often mistaken for mucosal folds. Their identity as varices is based on their shape (grape-like clusters) and their bluish tinge. On endoscopic ultrasound[6,7], they can be seen as circular or linear anechoic channels within the gastric wall. The addition of color Doppler may confirm blood flow within varices and document obliteration of GV after endoscopic treatment. MR angiography and multislice CT scanning are likely to further improve our accuracy in diagnosing GV.

## CLASSIFICATION OF GASTRIC VARICES

GV can be satisfactorily classified only by endoscopy. While several classifications have been proposed[3,5,7], the most widely accepted is Sarin's classification which is based on the anatomical location of GV, their relationship with esophageal varices and their origin as primary (GV present at the time of initial presentation) or secondary (GV presenting after the obliteration of esophageal varices) GV (Figure 1)[5]. This classification was evaluated in a prospective manner in a series of 568 patients and was found to be quite useful in defining the natural history and outlining the management of GV. This classification was also prospectively evaluated by Kind et al.[9] in a large study of 657 Italian patients with portal hypertension. They reaffirmed the usefulness of Sarin's classification in determining the natural history and selection of choice of therapy for different types of GV. The same was

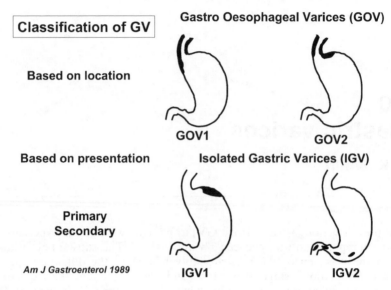

**Figure 1.** Sarin's classification of gastric varices

unanimously accepted at the Baveno III consensus conference on portal hypertension[10]. According to this classification GV are divided into two main types:

*Gastro-oesophageal varices (GOV)*

These varices extend beyond the gastro-oesophageal junction and are always associated with oesophageal varices. They are further subdivided into:

1. Type 1 (GOV1): These appear as continuations of oesophageal varices and extend for 2–5 cm below the gastro-oesophageal junction along the lesser curvature of the stomach. These varices are more or less straight (Figure 2a),
2. Type 2 (GOV2): These varices extend beyond the gastro-oesophageal junction towards the fundus of the stomach (Figure 2b). They appear as long, tortuous and nodular elevations at the cardia.

*Isolated gastric varices (IGV)*

GV in the absence of oesophageal varices are termed "isolated" GV. Depending on their location, they are subdivided into:

1. Type 1 (IGV1): These varices are located in the fundus of the stomach and fall short of the cardia by a few centimeters (Figure 2c).
2. Type 2 (IGV2): These include isolated ectopic varices present anywhere in the stomach (Figure 2d), such as in the antrum, pylorus or body or in the first part of the duodenum.

## Pathogenesis of gastric varices:

To understand the origin of GV, it is necessary to understand the venous drainage of the stomach, lower oesophagus and spleen. The fundus of the

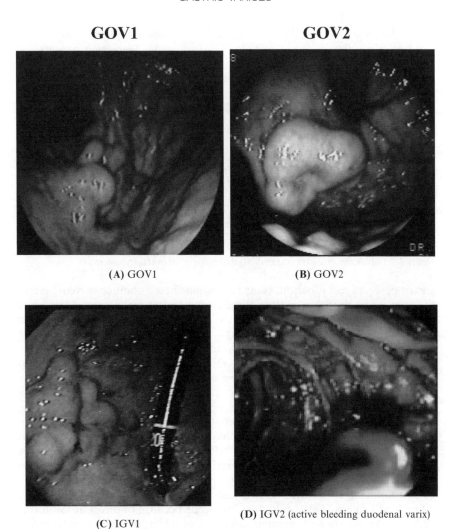

**GOV1**　　　　　　　**GOV2**

(A) GOV1　　　　　　　(B) GOV2

(C) IGV1　　　　(D) IGV2 (active bleeding duodenal varix)

**Figure 2**

stomach has a rich venous plexus in its submucosa. This plexus drains into the splenic vein via the short gastric veins and into the portal vein via the coronary vein. GV can develop in patients with either generalized (e.g. in cirrhosis) or segmental (e.g. in splenic vein thrombosis) portal hypertension. In generalized portal hypertension, the raised portal pressure would be transmitted via the left gastric vein to esophageal varices and via the short and posterior gastric veins to the fundic plexus and cardiac veins. GOV1 or lesser curve varices are formed by the dilation of the left gastric vein at the cardia[11]. Hashizume et al.[12–15] have shown that GOV1 develop because one of the branches of the left gastric vein perforates the gastric wall perpendicularly (Figure 3) and joins the deep submucosal veins about 2 cm below the

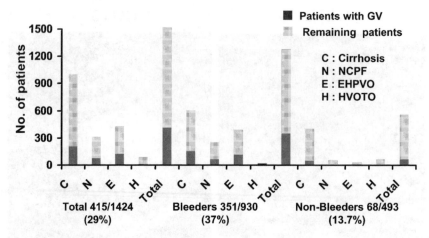

**Figure 3.** Prevalence of gastric varices in different types of portal hypertension

gastro-oesophageal junction. Near the cardia these submucosal veins pierce the muscularis mucosae in the palisade zone and at the proximal border of the palisade zone the veins pierce the muscularis mucosae to run again within the submucosa[13]. Thus, a high pressure zone develops below the palisade zone and explains the appearance of both GOV1 and GOV2.

In segmental portal hypertension, GV develop in the absence of oesophageal varices, mainly due to splenic vein obstruction. The splenic blood flows retrogradely through the short and posterior gastric veins into the submucous space and subsequently varices develop into the fundus and cardiac region from which the blood flows hepatopetally through the coronary vein into the portal vein. The lower oesophageal veins are thus bypassed so that oesophageal varices do not develop[14]. Retrograde flow occurs through the left to the right gastroepiploic vein and also superior mesenteric vein and can explain the development of ectopic varices in the stomach.

Development of isolated GV in the presence of patent splenic vein is difficult to explain. This could possibly occur because of direct anastomosis between the gastric and retroperitoneal veins which open up due to raised portal pressure[15]. However, what determines the route by which major portosystemic collaterals develop when portal pressure increases is not known. The size and length of the potential collateral vein probably determine whether a patient develops oesophageal or gastric varices, and, in the latter case, which type[4].

## Hemodynamics of gastric varices

For oesophageal varices, a higher hepatic vein pressure gradient (HVPG) is generally considered to give a higher risk of first bleed, rebleed and poor outcome. A reduction in the HVPG has been shown to be associated with lower risk of bleeding.

Patients with GV probably have lower hepatic vein pressure gradient than patients with oesophageal varices, though some recent reports dispute

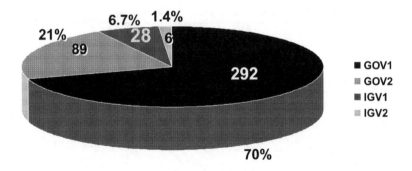

**Total patients : 415**

**Figure 4.** Frequency of different types of gastric varices

this[17,18]. In patients with large GV (those more likely to bleed) are often associated with large gastrorenal shunts which can reduce the portal vein pressure[4,16]. However, these shunts are unable to decompress the pressure and patients do bleed from GV despite an HVPG lower than 12 mmHg.

## PREVALENCE OF DIFFERENT TYPES OF GASTRIC VARICES

The frequency of different types of primary GV is shown in Figures 3 and 4. A nearly similar frequency has been observed by other workers[9]. It is to be noted that, in a proportion of patients, both GOV1 and GOV2 do co-exist[5].

## NATURAL HISTORY OF GASTRIC VARICES

Patients with GV can be asymptomatic and detected incidentally and can present with UGI bleeding or with hepatic encephalopathy. In nearly 3/4 of the patients, GV are detected during treatment of bleeding oesophageal varices or at routine UGI endoscopy in a patient with portal hypertension. Only about 1/4 of the patients present with GV bleeding and a small proportion with hepatic encephalopathy.

### GV bleeding

*Incidence*

There are conflicting reports on how often and how severely GV bleed. The incidence of bleeding from GV has been reported between 3% and 43%[5,9,19,20]. It is generally believed that GV bleed less frequently than oesophageal varices. This however, would depend on the type of GV. We observed in a large prospective study that the incidence of bleeding is higher in IGV1 (78%) and GOV2 (55%) than GOV1 (11%)[9]. Thus, both IGV1 and GOV2 have a higher incidence of bleeding than the oesophageal varices.

**Table 1.** Factors for hemorrhage from fundal varices[20]

| Factor | Risk ratio |
|---|---|
| Size of fundal varices | 2.18 (1.21–3.93)* |
| | 4.75 (1.45–15.5)[†] |
| Child's status | 1.70 (1.11–2.59)[#] |
| | 2.88 (1.21–3.93)[§] |
| Red spot present | 2.06 (1.01–4.19)[‡] |

*Small vs. medium.
[†] Small vs. large.
[#] Class A vs. class B.
[§] Class A vs. class C.
[‡] Absent vs. present.

Kind et al.[9] in a recent study found the frequency of bleeding from GOV2 and IGV1 to be 60.3%. Korula et al.[19] also observed that the number of bleeding episodes in patients with fundal ($4.8 \pm 2.9$) varices was higher than junctional ($2.2 \pm 2.2$) varices.

The bleeding risk factor per year (total number of bleeding episodes/time interval between the first and the last bleed) for oesophageal varices is higher than for GV ($4.3 \pm 0.4$ vs. $2.0 \pm 0.6$, $p < 0.01$)[5]. The mean number of bleeding episodes in patients with gastric and oesophageal varices is however comparable ($2.14 \pm 1.03$ vs. $2.3 \pm 1.8$). Kind et al.[9] observed in a series of 67 patients an overall tendency of bleeding from GV to be lower (43.3%) compared with oesophageal varices (79.8%). Kim et al.[20], in a prospective study of 117 patients with fundal varices, documented cumulative bleeding rates at 1, 3, and 5 years of 16%, 36%, and 44%, respectively. In another recent study, Tomikawa et al. observed bleeding in 87 (29%) of the 300 patients with GV[24].

*Risk factors for bleed*

Kim et al.[20] have identified the size of fundal varices, presence of red spots on fundal varices, and the Child's status of the patient as important risk factors (Table 1). Hashizume et al.[8] have also emphasized the importance of size and red spots on GV. There is however a need to objectively validate these risk factors. Accurate determination of the size of GV is not easy, as quite often these veins form bunches. A simple approach practiced by us is to use the shaft of the retroflexed endoscope as a measuring scale. Varices larger than the scope (approximately 10 mm) are called large GV. This approach was agreed upon unanimously as useful in the Baveno III International conference[10]. However, its predictive value needs to be studied prospectively.

## Influence of oesophageal variceal obliteration on GV

It is now well known that variceal obliteration could alter the natural history of GV. The possible variables are:

(a) Influence on coexisting GV.

(b) Development of new GV following obliteration of oesophageal varices (secondary GV).

(c) Induction of bleeding from GV while performing sclerotherapy or ligation for oesophageal varices.

### (a) Influence on coexisting GV

Logically, only GOV are likely to be influenced by the treatment of oesophageal varices. In nearly 60% of the patients GOV1 and in 25% of patients GOV2 disappear within 6 months of obliteration of oesophageal varices, by either sclerotherapy or variceal ligation. This regression of GOV1 or GOV2 is likely to be due to the flow of the sclerosant towards the stomach or formulation of a thrombus at the GE junction which could propagate caudally[13]. It is recommended that, in patients with GOV1/GOV2, the oesophageal varices should be treated first. If GV persist beyond 6 months, then they should be treated[5].

### (b) Development of secondary GV

GV which develop after obliteration of oesophageal varices are termed secondary GV. The reported frequency of secondary GV varies between 9.7% and 43%[3,5,8,19]. While in some series GOV1 have been reported to develop more frequently than GOV2 (11.2% vs. 4.1%)[6], (9.6% vs. 0.5%)[3], in our experience, GOV2 develop more frequently than GOV1 (11.4% vs. 2.6%) after oesophageal variceal eradication[5]. Using endoscopic ultrasonography, development of secondary GV has been detected in 26–43% of patients[6].

The frequency of bleeding from secondary GV has been reported to be higher than with primary GV. Over a follow-up period of 16.1 and 12.6 months, the bleeding incidence in secondary GOV1 and GOV2 was 37% and 100%, respectively. A high incidence of bleeding from secondary GOV2 and IGV1 has also been reported by Kind et al.[9] These observations raise an important issue: should secondary GV be treated prophylactically? There is a need to evaluate both pharmacotherapy and endoscopic therapy in this group of patients.

### (c) Induction of bleeding from GV

It has been suggested that sclerotherapy blocks the shunting veins which are present in the palisade zone. This leads to increased blood flow in the gastric veins and a rise in portal pressure, possibly leading to dilation and rupture of these veins[21]. However, bleeding from GV due to oesophageal variceal sclerotherapy is quite rare[22–24]. Neverthless, an isolated study has reported bleeding in 10% of patients[25].

## Hepatic encephalopathy

Cirrhotics with GV develop encephalopathy more often than patients with only oesophageal varices (25 vs. 3%)[4]. This is due to the entry of nitrogenous substances from the gut directly into the systemic circulation through the shunts which form the GV The stage of underlying liver disease determines

283

the development of encephalopathy to a large extent. This, however, is not true for patients with non-cirrhotic portal hypertension who, despite having a higher reported incidence of GV[5], do not have an increased incidence of hepatic encephalopathy[26].

## Correlation with portal hypertensive gastropathy

There are limited data on this aspect. Cales et al., in an anecdotal experience, observed no influence of GV on the development of PHG[27]. On the other hand, in our prospective study of 107 patients, 36 had coexisting GV and the rest had only oesophageal varices before sclerotherapy. PHG developed in 42% of the former and 11% of the latter patients after sclerotherapy ($p < 0.01$)[28]. This suggests that the chances of development of PHG are increased nearly fourfold when GV are present compared to when oesophageal varices alone are there. The higher frequency of association of PHG with GV could be explained by redistribution and an increase in gastric blood flow after obliteration of oesophageal varices. However, Eleftheriadis et al.[29], using the endoscopic laser-Doppler technique, found an increase in the gastric microcirculation after sclerotherapy only in the pyloric area, and not in the fundic area, where gastropathy is more common.

## MANAGEMENT OF GASTRIC VARICEAL BLEED

Current protocols for bleeding GV have been adopted from the treatment of bleeding oesophageal varices. Hemostatic methods that use standard therapy for oesophageal varices have not been found effective for gastric varices. Most reports of endoscopic treatment of bleeding gastric varices are small series, case reports, or retrospective reviews. Only a few studies have prospectively compared the effectiveness and safety of different treatment modalities. Hence, despite nearly 25 years of active interest, the management of GV remains largely empirical.

### Primary prophylaxis of bleeding from GV

Should non-bleeding GV that accompany bleeding oesophageal varices or non-bleeding IGV be prophylactically treated? This can only be answered if more data on the natural history of GV bleeding and survival become available in relation to the location, size, presence of red signs and Child's status of the patient. Thus, prophylactic treatment of GV is not warranted in general at the present time. However, as mentioned above, since patients in whom GOV1 persist after obliteration of oesophageal varices, bleed significantly more often, they form a group which requires prophylactic treatment. In these patients prophylactic β-blockers or endoscopic intervention could be tried, though their value is empirical (GE).

It is known that fundal (GOV2 and IGV1) varices are at a higher risk of bleeding than junctional varices (GOV1)[5,9]. Similarly, large fundal varices and those with red signs are even more likely to bleed[20]. Therefore, large fundal varices should constitute the subset which could be treated prophylactically. Kim et al.[20] in their prospective study have documented a bleed rate

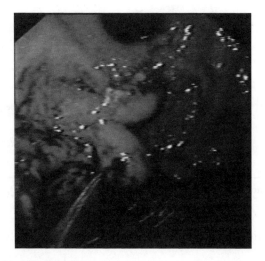

**Figure 5.**  Active bleeding from GV

of 53% from fundal varices $> 2$ cm in size in a median follow-up of 15.2 months. According to the available data, rebleed rate after glue injection or transjugular intrahepatic portosystemic shunt (TIPS) is $< 30\%$ over a similar follow-up period. Therefore, it seems logical to undertake clinical studies to assess the utility of treating large fundal varices prophylactically.

## MANAGEMENT OF ACUTE GASTRIC VARICES BLEEDING

The treatment goals are the same as for oesophageal varices: to control acute bleeding and to prevent rebleeding.

### Indications of treatment

i)   Active bleed from GV (Figure 5);
ii)  Stigmata of recent bleed on GV adherent clot or a nipple;
iii) History of previous bleed and presence of GV as the only source of bleed.

These patients need to be treated according to the type of GV and the expertise available. Sometimes, however, it is not possible to determine whether a patient with oesophagogastric varices is bleeding from oesophageal or gastric varices. In such a situation, opinions differ on which varix should be injected first, oesophageal or gastric! We recommend to inject the GOV2 with glue and then ligate the oesophageal varices at the same session.

## SECONDARY PROPHYLAXIS

The end-point of treatment in patients who have bled from GV should be obliteration of varices as rebleeding rate is significantly higher in those in

**Table 2.** Endoscopic sclerotherapy for gastric varices in active gastric variceal bleeding[10]

| Reference | Agent | n | Success (%) | Rebleed (%) | Complications |
|---|---|---|---|---|---|
| Trudeau 1986[33] | STD | 9 | 100 | 90 | Ulcer 89% |
| Gimson 1991[35] | EO/Glue | 41 | 40 | 16 | Ulcer 29% Perforation |
| Oho 1995[36] | EO (5%) | 24 | 67 | 25 | — |
| Chang 1996[37] | STD (1.5%) | 25 | 80 | 70 | Ulcer 30% |
| Chang 1996[37] | GW (50%) | 26 | 92 | 30 | Ulcer 30% |
| Chiu 1997[38] | STD (1.5%) | 27 | 66.7 | — | — |
| Sarin 1997[39] | AA (95%) | 18 | 67 | 34 | Ulcer 100% |
| Ogawa 1999[40] | EO (5%) | 21 | 81 | 100 | — |
| Sarin 2002[42] | AA (95%) | 8 | 62 | 25 | — |

AA, absolute alcohol; EO, ethanolamine oleate; GW, glucose water; STD, sodium tetradecyl sulfate.

whom eradication is achieved than in those in whom varices do not disappear[30].

## Interventional strategies

The various treatment modalities employed for the management of GV bleeding include the following:

### Balloon tamponade

Two types of balloons are available for the control of active bleeding from GV, namely the Sengstaken–Blakemore tube and the Linton–Nachlas tube. In the former the gastric balloon is small (volume 200 ml) while in the latter the gastric balloon is large (capacity 600 ml), The Linton tube is preferred for controlling acute GV bleeding with a success rate of up to 50%[31].

### Pharmacological agents

Since the primary pathology in patients with GV is raised pressure and splanchnic vasodilation, it is reasonable to presume that vasoactive drugs could be as effective in GV bleed as in oesophageal variceal bleeding. There are however limited published data on the role of vasoactive drugs in the control of acute bleeding from GV.

Propranolol and nitrates, the main drugs in oesophageal variceal bleeding, have not been studied for GV. In a small open label study, β-blockers and nitrates were not found to be useful in reducing rebleeding or improving survival[32].

### Gastric variceal sclerotherapy

Gastric variceal sclerotherapy (GVS) can be performed intravariceally or by a combination of intravariceal and paravariceal injections. Much larger volumes of sclerosant are required for GVS than oesophageal variceal sclero-therapy. This could be associated with more side-effects. Initial control of active bleeding has been reported with GVS in 40–100% of cases (Table 2)[33–40]. Two studies have shown equal efficacy of emergency GVS for

**Table 3.** Endoscopic sclerotherapy for gastric varices for prevention of rebleeding[10]

| Reference | Agent | n | Obliteration (%) | Rebleeding (%) | Recurrence (%) | Follow-up (months) |
|---|---|---|---|---|---|---|
| Gimson 1991[35] | EO/Glue | 31 | 32.3 | 16 | — | — |
| Chang 1996[37] | STD (1.5%) | 25 | 32 | 70 | 25 | 52±37 |
| Chang 1996[37] | GW (50%) | 26 | 81 | 30 | 4.8 | 57±32 |
| Sarin 1997[39] | AA (95%) | 60 | 72 | 23 | 0 | 24±23 |

AA, absolute alcohol; EO, ethanolamine oleate; GW, glucose water; STD, sodium tetradecyl sulfate.

GOV1 and GOV2[37–39], while studies by Korula et al. and Gimson et al. show higher success rate for GOV1 as compared to GOV2[19,35]. Chiu et al. did emergency GVS in 27 patients with isolated GV with a success rate of 67% and rebleed rate of 18% at 48 hours[38]. GVS is least effective in achieving hemostasis in IGV1.

Using repeated GVS, variceal eradication can be achieved in 17–81%, with a bleed rate of 16–70% (Table 3)[35,37,39,41]. Variceal obliteration is achieved in a higher proportion of patients with GOV1 (94%) than in patients with GOV2 (70%) and IGV1 (41%). Rebleeding is seen in 5.5%, 19% and 53% patients respectively, in the three types of GV, respectively[39]. The recurrence rate of gastric varices has been variably reported from 0% to 25%.[35,37,39,41]

The major problem with GVS is a high rebleed rate. This rebleeding could be due to rapid blood flow in GV, making formation of a thrombus difficult. Also the early appearance of ulceration in incompletely obliterated varices is another major factor for recurrent bleed which usually occurs after the first or second GVS session. Moreover, unlike oesophageal variceal ulcers, which are generally mucosal, ulcers following GVS are deep and submucosal. Approximately 50% of the post-GVS bleeds are from ulcers[33,37,41]. Chang et al. have shown a higher rebleeding rate (70% vs. 30%) with sodium tetradecyl sulfate (STD) as compared to 50% glucose water and delayed ulcer healing (13±5 days vs. 6±2 days)[37]. Once rebleeding occurs, it is difficult to control with repeat GV, the success rate being only 9–44%[33,37–39].

If an agent produces less mucosal ulceration and achieves complete and rapid obliteration of GV, it will significantly reduce the early rebleed rate following GVS. Poly-N-acetyl glucosamine, a polysaccharide polymer originating from marine microalgae, has been demonstrated to produce rapid and effective hemostasis by stimulating erythrocyte aggregation and variceal eradication by inducing an inflammatory reaction in a rabbit model[47]. Clinical studies are awaited with this agent.

### Gastric variceal obliteration

Variceal obliteration refers to obliteration of varix with a solidifying agent, such as glue or thrombin. Two tissue adhesive agents, n-butyl-2-cyanoacrylate (Histoacryl) and isobutyl-2-cyanoacrylate (Bucrylate) have been used[42–50], although the latter agent has been withdrawn from the

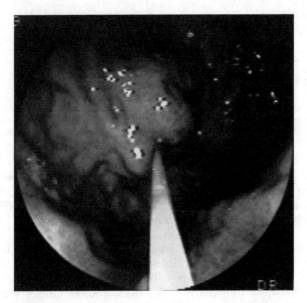

**Figure 6.** Injection of cyanoacrylate glue in a GOV2

European market because of concerns about carcinogenicity. Native cyano-acrylate is a liquid with consistency similar to water and therefore lends itself to intravariceal injection. When added to a physiologic medium such as blood, the cyanoacrylate rapidly polymerizes, forming a hard substance. Thus, after injection into a varix (Figure 6), the cyanoacrylate plugs the lumen and results in rapid hemostasis. Several weeks after the injection (2 weeks to 3 months), the mucosa overlying the injected area sloughs off and a glue cast is extruded into the stomach (Figure 7). Since ulceration over the varix appears quite late as compared to GVS, it does not hinder repeat glue injections and also reduces the risk of ulcer bleeding. Tissue adhesives, therefore, come close to the requirements of an ideal sclerosing agent for GV.

Cyanoacrylate injection has been shown to achieve hemostasis in more than 90% of patients with acute GV bleeding, with an early rebleeding rate of 0–28%[9,36,40,42–50]. Glue injection in 1–2 sessions can achieve variceal obliteration in 87–100% of patients (Table 4).[44–48] The term obliteration more accurately describes the desired immediate endpoint for glue injection of GV than eradication since a varix occluded with cyanoacrylate may remain endoscopically visible for many weeks. The methods used to assess the success of variceal obliteration include palpating the varix with a blunt instrument (soft versus hard), radiographic visualization of varices filled with lipiodol and cyanoacrylate mixture, and endoscopic ultrasound[50] (absence of hypoechoic vascular channels in fundus and cardia (Figure 8).

Though the glue is injected like a sclerosant, its unique adhesive properties necessitate some modifications in the technique. It is important to ensure the intravariceal position of the needle. To prevent damage to the scope due to the adhesive, lipiodol, an oily contrast agent, or silicone oil could be

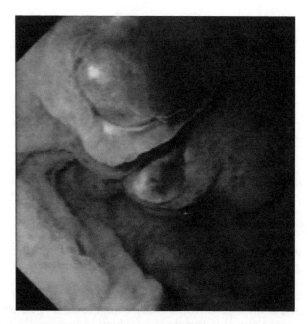

**Figure 7.** Cast extrusion 3 weeks after glue injection in a gastric varix

**Table 4.** Histoacryl injection for treatment of gastric varices

| References | n | Hemostasis (%) | Rebleeding (%) | Mortality (%) | Follow-up (months) |
|---|---|---|---|---|---|
| Lee 2000[50] | 47 | 95.7 | 12.8[a]/44.7[b] | 17 | 24 |
| Kind 2000[9] | 174 | 97.1 | 15.5 | 19.5 | 36 |
| Battaglia 2000[58] | 32 | 96.8 | 34.4 | 18.7 | 45.4 |
| Huang 2000[49] | 90 | 93.3 | 23.3 | 2.2 | 13 |
| Sarin 2002[42] | 11 | 100 | 27 | 9 | — |

[a] $\leq 48$ h; [b] $> 48$ h.

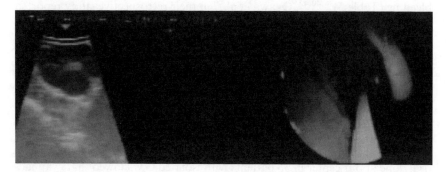

**Figure 8.** Glue injection of gastric varix under endoscopic ultrasound guidance

**Table 5.** Gastric variceal sclerotherapy versus glue injection for active gastric variceal bleeding[10,36,40,58]

| Reference | Agent | n | Hemostasis (%) | Rebleeding (%) | Ulcer (%) | Mortality (%) |
|-----------|-------|---|----------------|----------------|-----------|---------------|
| Oho 1995[36] | EO | 24 | 67 | 12.5 | 25 | 67 |
|  | HC | 29 | 93 | 10 | 30 | 38 |
| Ogawa 1999[40] | EO | 21 | 81 | 35 | — | 23.8 |
|  | HC | 17 | 100 | 0 | — | 0 |
| Sarin 2002[42] | AA | 9 | 44 | 33 | — | 33 |
|  | HC | 11 | 100 | 27 | — | 9 |

AA, absolute alcohol; EO, ethanolamine oleate; HC, histoacryl.

smeared at the tip of the scope and in the working channel. Lipiodol is mixed with cyanoacrylate (in a ratio of 0.5 to 0.8 ml, respectively) to prevent premature solidification within or at the tip of the catheter during injection and to help in radiological evaluation. Unnecessary suction should be avoided during the procedure.

The total amount of histoacryl injection per aliquot should not exceed 2 ml to decrease the risk of thrombotic complications[51]. Cerebral stroke, presumably due to anomalous right to left shunt in two cases[52], fatal pulmonary embolization in one patient[53], bacteremia in a patient with portal vein embolization[54], splenic infarction[55] and formation of retrogastric abscess[56] have been reported after injection of cyanoacrylate in patients with bleeding GV.

These complications caution us about the indiscriminate use of glue in all patients with variceal bleeding. However, for patients with GV the benefits of glue injection outweigh the potential risks. The concern about the potential carcinogenicity of cyanoacrylate observed in rats[57] is probably ill-founded.

*Comparison of gastric variceal sclerotherapy and oturation*

Three studies have compared sclerotherapy using ethanolamine oleate (5%) or absolute alcohol and cyanoacrylate injection in acute gastric variceal bleeding (Table 5)[36,40,42]. Ogawa et al.[40] in their retrospective study reported a significantly higher hemostasis rate with cyanoacrylate compared with ethanolamine oleate (100% vs. 81%). While 6 of 17 (35%) patients rebled at 2 weeks in the ethanolamine oleate group, none rebled in the histoacryl group. While 5 of 21 (23.8%) patients died in the ethanolamine group, none died of bleed in the cyanoacrylate glue group. Oho et al.[36] in their prospective, nonrandomized study of 53 patients with acute GV bleed, reported histoacryl to be significantly more efficacious in achieving hemostasis than ethanolamine oleate (93% vs. 67%). Three patients in each group rebled at 1 month. Three patients in the cyanoacrylate group rebled 6 months after treatment from the site of polymer elimination. A randomized controlled trial done at our center in 35 patients with isolated GV showed that cyanoacrylate is more effective in achieving initial hemostasis and in achieving faster variceal obliteration. The need for emergency surgical rescue was also much less in the glue injected group[42]. The results of these three comparative studies indicate that cyanoacrylate is more effective than sclerosants like ethanolamine oleate or absolute alcohol.

## Thrombin

Human and bovine thrombin have been safely used in oesophageal as well as gastric variceal sclerotherapy, without any report of distant thrombosis. Williams et al.[59], using bovine thrombin, reconstituted to 1000 u/ml intravariceally, achieved initial hemostasis and obliteration in all 11 cases with 2 injection sessions. Rebleeding was observed in only one patient over a median follow-up of 9 months. Similar results have been reported in another study[60].The most important advantage of this approach is the absence of any mucosal damage and post-sclerotherapy ulceration that is characteristic of sclerosants and tissue adhesives. The widespread evaluation of this technique is limited by cost and lack of availability of the product, which is yet to be approved by the FDA.

## Endoscopic variceal ligation

Endoscopic variceal band ligation (EVL) is an effective and safe method for the management of bleeding oesophageal varices. The development of multiband ligating devices has made EVL technically easier even with the endoscope retroflexed in the stomach.

Gastric variceal ligation (GVL) has been evaluated for the treatment of bleeding GV in a prospective uncontrolled study by Shiha et al. They were able to achieve hemostasis in 89%, with rebleeding in 18.5% of cases[61]. Obliteration of GV could be achieved in all patients with a median of 3 sessions. Ulcers were seen at the ligation site in all the patients one week later. In the only RCT, GVL was found to be less effective than glue injection in controlling acute GV bleed (45% vs. 87%) with a higher rebleed rate (54% vs. 31%) though with comparable efficacy for variceal eradication (45% vs. 51%).

More randomized studies are needed before variceal band ligation can be recommended as a safe and effective modality for the treatment of GV.

## Endoscopic snare ligation

The major concern with GVL is incomplete inclusion of large GV during ligation and subsequent bleeding[62,63]. Many workers have therefore used a snare for ligation of GV which are more than 1 cm in size.

Yoshida et al.[64] used a detachable snare with an inner diameter of 4 cm to tighten around the varix base, grasping the periphery of varix with a forceps through the second channel of the double channel scope. High success rates (83–100%) in the control of acute GV bleed and variceal eradication with low recurrence rates have been reported by them and other workers (Table 6)[65–68]. While no significant ulcer-related complications were seen, gastric perforation was reported in two patients in one study[65].

A combination of variceal ligations and sclerotherapy has been evaluated. After putting and partially tightening a detachable snare around the varix,

**Table 6.** Gastric variceal ligation in the management of gastric variceal bleeding

| Reference | Therapy | n | Active bleed (%) | Success (%) | Rebleeding (%) | Obliteration (%) |
|-----------|---------|---|------------------|-------------|----------------|-------------------|
| Yoshida 1994[64] | GVL-S | 10 | 10 | 100 | 10 | 100 |
| Harada 1997[66] | GVL-S | 5 | 100 | 100 | 20 | — |
| Cipolletta 1998[67] | GVL-S | 7 | 100 | 100 | 0 | — |
| Yoshida 1999[68] | GVL-S and EIS | 35 | 23 | 100 | 3 | 97 |
| Shiha 1999[61] | GVL | 27 | 7 | 89 | 18.5 | 100 |

GVL, gastric variceal ligation; GVL-S, gastric variceal snare ligation.

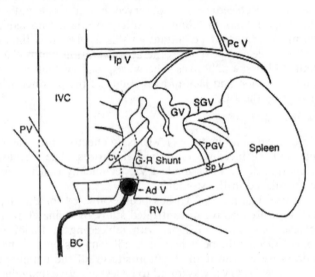

**Figure 9.** Balloon occluded retrograde transvenous obliteration (BRTO)

a sclerosant is injected into the GV followed by tightening of the snare around the varices. Anecdotal data suggest high success rates[69,71].

### Balloon-occluded retrograde transvenous obliteration of gastric varices (BRTO)

Gastrorenal shunt is often present between GV and left renal vein in patients with fundal varices[4]. A balloon catheter is introduced in the gastrorenal shunt via the left renal vein, and the shunt is occluded by inflating the balloon and then a sclerosant (usually a mixture of ethanolamine oleate and a noniodinated contrast medium) is injected into the gastric varices and left to remain for a few hours till injection of the contrast medium shows that clots have formed in the varices (Figure 9). BRTO has been reported to achieve a high success rate (100%) of GV obliteration and a low recurrence rate[72-74]. BRTO is only feasible in patients who have a gastrorenal shunt. It has been largely used in primary prophylaxis of GV bleeding[34,75-80]. In one study, 100% hemostasis was reported in patients with active GV bleeding with no rebleeding up to 2 years[78]. The same technique has been used

**Table 7.** Transjugular intrahepatic portosystemic shunt (TIPS) in gastric varices

| Reference | Patient characteristics | Number of patients | Active bleed (%) | Hemostasis (%) | Rebleed (%) | Follow-up (months) |
|---|---|---|---|---|---|---|
| Stanley 1997[16] | Unresponsive to endoscopic therapy in 18 | 32 | 34.4 | NA | 15.6 | 14.2 |
| Chau 1998[17] | Unresponsive to vasoconstrictors | 28 | 100 | 96.4 | 29 | 7 |
| Barange 1999[83] | Unresponsive to vasoconstrictors, sclerotherapy, tamponade | 32 | 62.5 | 90 | 31 | 12 |
| Rees 2000[18] | Naïve patients | 12 | NA | NA | 16 | 17 |

to treat chronic portosystemic encephalopathy[69,70,77]. Therefore, it could serve as a feasible alternative to TIPS for patients with large gastrorenal shunts or hepatic encephalopathy where TIPS is contraindicated. The major problem with BRTO however is aggravation of oesophageal varices in up to 50% of the patients because of a rise in portal pressure subsequent to occlusion of gastrorenal shunt[72–74]. The other reported complications include hemoglobinuria, abdominal pain, pleural effusion, abdominal pain and shock.

Recently balloon-occluded endoscopic injection sclerotherapy has been reported from Japan. The preliminary results in 20 patients are encouraging[81].

## Transjugular intrahepatic portosystemic shunt (TIPS)

TIPS is considered to be the current standard therapy for bleeding oesophagogastric varices unresponsive to endoscopic and pharmacologic treatment, especially for GV[51,82]. Placement of TIPS abruptly reduces the outflow hepatic resistance, lowers portal pressure, and diverts portal flow from gastro-oesophageal collaterals through the stent. TIPS has been shown to achieve control of bleeding in more than 90% of patients with actively bleeding GV[17,83]. Once the acute bleed is controlled the reported one-year survival is up to 58–79%[83–86]. The rebleeding rate is ~15–30% within one year often due to stenosis or obstruction of the stent (Table 7)[84,85]. TIPS dysfunction occurs in ~50–60% of patients at 6 months, requiring close monitoring and repeated interventions to keep it patent. With the introduction of covered stents, this problem is likely to significantly decrease[86]. The majority of the studies have shown TIPS to be equally effective in treatment of GV and oesophageal varices, but one study has shown a significantly higher rebleed in GV as compared to oesophageal varices (53% vs. 11%)[87]. However, other workers have reported higher survival rates at 5 years after TIPS in patients with GV compared with oesophageal varices (50% vs. 25%)[88]. Since most patients with fundal varices have well-developed gastrorenal shunts[4], there is a risk of causing intractable hepatic encephalopathy by TIPS. Furthermore, in such patients the HVPG is often low. The efficacy of TIPS in such patients has been questioned[88]. The most common causes of death are advanced liver disease, sepsis, and multiorgan failure.

*Surgery*

Several studies have reported good results with surgical intervention in GV[89,90]. The recommended operations include portosystemic shunt, distal splenorenal shunt, and oesophageal transection. The role of surgery in the treatment of GV has howerver changed with the emergence of new treatment modalities, such as glue injection, TIPS and BRTO.

The application of surgical techniques in the management of GV can be divided into: (i) segmental portal hypertension without any liver disease; and (ii) generalized portal hypertension.

*Segmental portal hypertension*    Splenectomy effectively cures most patients with left-sided, segmental portal hypertension without liver disease. Madsen et al.[91] reviewed the literature and described the course of 72 patients up to 24 years after splenectomy for segmental portal hypertension. Only two patients rebled after splenectomy. Mortality after splenectomy has been reported to be around 7%[92]. It needs to be emphasized here that endoscopic intervention is not quite effective in these patients. The success rate of both GVS and glue injection has been reported to be around 30%. In the Italian study, failure to control bleeding resulted in reduced (16.6%) long term survival[9].

*Generalized portal hypertension*    There is abundant information available on the surgical management of gastro-oesophageal varices. Little, however, is mentioned specifically about the management of GV. There are no clear guidelines available on the selection of patients for a given surgical procedure. For patients with generalized portal hypertension and isolated GV, a definitive treatment is advisable. Hosking and Johnson[3] advocate variceal ligation with gastric devascularization for the control of active bleeding from such varices. However, if lesser-curve varices are associated, a shunt procedure may be better, according to them. Alternatively, for patients with acute gastric variceal bleeding, an emergency shunt can be equally effective. According to Wood et al.[93], the shunt of choice is a large-bore H-graft mesocaval or mesorenal shunt. This shunt effectively controls the acute bleeding, is relatively simple to perform, does not influence the subsequent transplant, and can be ligated after the transplant is completed. For an elective procedure, a distal splenorenal shunt is preferred by many surgeons because it maintains hepatic portal perfusion and does not require dissection of the porta hepatis[94,95]. We at our center have used devascularization in patients with active bleed from GV and portosystemic shunt in elective setting. No recurrence or rebleed was observed in the shunt group (31 patients) while 2 of 10 patients who underwent devascularization developed oesophageal varices[96]. Tomikawa et al.[24] have used gastric devascularization and splenectomy in 42 patients with isolated GV and showed eradication of GV in 100% of patients and no recurrence was reported in a follow-up of 46 months. Shunt surgery has been recommended as an alternative to TIPS for prevention of GV rebleeding or as second-line treatment of refractory acute GV bleeding[97].

*Orthotopic liver transplantation (OLT)*    The survival rates in transplanted patients project OLT as a useful alternative to other modalities of treating GV. The differences become more prominent when the survival rates of Child's class C patients who received liver transplant (79% at 1 year and 71% at 5 years) are compared with those of Child's C patients who were treated with shunts (30–70% 1-year and 15–35% 5-year)[93]. These results of OLT bring a ray of hope for the large number of patients with cirrhosis and portal hypertension, including those with GV. At present, however, for a significant proportion of patients, transplant remains an expensive and difficult option.

## LONG-TERM FOLLOW-UP OF GASTRIC VARICES

While a number of trials have reported the long-term outcome of endoscopic management of oesophageal varices, there is scanty long-term follow-up data after gastric variceal obliteration[39].

The available data indicate that the recurrence rates after obliteration with sclerotherapy are much lower in patients with GV compared to oesophageal varices.

## APPROACH TO A PATIENT WITH GASTRIC VARICES

### Active bleeding

A rational approach to control acute bleeding from GV is shown in Figure 10 It needs to be pointed out that the definitions of success and failure of control of bleeding have been specifically developed only for oesophageal varices (Baveno) and not for GV[10].

When it is not clear whether the active bleeding is from oesophageal or GV, we prefer to inject the GV and ligate the oesophageal varices.

### Elective therapy

Secondary prophylaxis for GV bleeding is essential and is outlined in Figure 11. In conclusion, patients with active GV bleed or those who have bled in the past from GV are candidates for endoscopic intervention. The agent of choice for injection of GV is cyanoacrylate glue since it achieves more rapid and effective hemostasis with high obliteration rates. Gastric variceal sclerotherapy using absolute alcohol or ethanolamine oleate is an effective alternative treatment. With both techniques, more so with sclerotherapy, attention needs to be paid to decreasing the frequency of ulcers developing following injection, which cause recurrent bleed. The data on the efficacy and safety of gastric variceal ligation are preliminary and the technique could be recommended if proven in large randomized prospective clinical trials. TIPS and surgery remain good options for patients with uncontrolled GV bleeding or with IGV1 where the endoscopic therapies

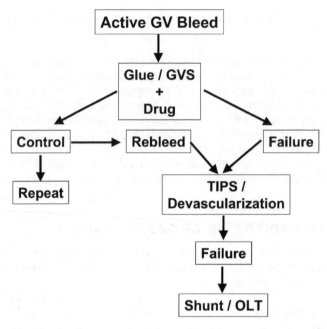

**Figure 10.** Algorithm for the management of acute bleed from gastric varices

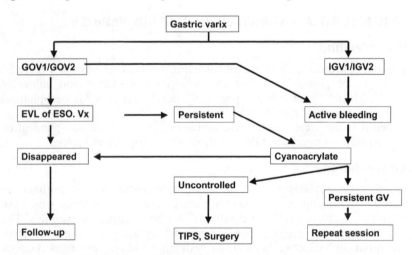

**Figure 11.** Algorithm for the elective management of gastric varices

have limited efficacy. Further advances in the management and outcome of GV bleeding can come only when the natural history, risk factors for bleeding and the mechanism of GV rupture are better defined. Prophylactic management of GV is receiving more and more attention. The use of BRTO and, in specific situations, glue injection, may decrease the risk of first bleed from GV.

# References

1. Feldman M, Feldman M Jr. Gastric varices. Gastroenterology. 1956;30:318–21.
2. Sarin SK, Kumar A. Gastric varices: profile, classification, and management. Am J Gastroenterol. 1989;84:1244–9.
3. Hosking SW, Johnson A. Gastric varices: a proposed classification leading to management. Br J Surg. 1988;75:195–6.
4. Watanabe K, Kimura K, Matsutani S, Masao O, Okuda K. Portal hemodynamics in patients with gastric varices: a study of 230 patients with oesophageal and gastric varices using portal vein catheterization. Gastroenterology. 1988;95:434–40
5. Sarin SK, Lahoti D, Saxena SP, Murthi NS, Makwane UK. Prevalence, classification and natural history of gastric varices: a long-term follow-up study in 568 portal hypertension patients. Hepatology. 1992;16:1343–9.
6. Lo GH, Lai KH, Cheng JS, Huang RL, Wang SJ, Chiang HT. Prevalence of paraesophageal varices and gastric varices in patients achieving variceal obliteration by banding ligation and by injection sclerotherapy. Gastrointest Endosc. 1999;49:428–36.
7. Iwase H, Suga S, Morise K, Kuroiwa A, Yamaguchi T, Horiuchi Y. Color Doppler endoscopic ultrasonography for the evaluation of gastric varices and endoscopic obliteration with cyanoacrylate glue. Gastrointest Endosc. 1995;41:150–4.
8. Hashizume M, Kitano S, Yamaga H, Koyanagi N, Sugimachi K. Endoscopic classification of gastric varices. Gastrointest Endosc. 1990;36:276–80.
9. Kind R, Guglielmi A, Rodella I et al. Bucrylate treatment of bleeding gastric varices: 12 years' experience. Endoscopy. 2000;32:512–19.
10. Sarin SK, Primignani M, Agarwal SR. Gastric varices. In: de Franchis R, ed. Portal hypertension. Proceedings of the third Baveno international consensus workshop on definitions, methodology and therapeutic strategies. Blackwell Science, London: 2001;76–96.
11. Takashi M, Igarashi M, Hino S et al. Esophageal varices: correlation of left gastric venography and endoscopy in patients with portal hypertension. Radiology. 1985;154:327–31.
12. Hashizume M, Kitano S, Sugimachi K, Sueishi K. Three-dimensional view of the vascular structure of the lower esophagus in clinical portal hypertension. Hepatology. 1988;8:1482–7.
13. Vianna A, Hayes PC, Moscoso G et al. Normal venous circulation of the gastroesophageal junction: a route to understanding varices. Gastroenterology. 1987;93:876–89.
14. Marshall JP, Smith PD, Hoyumpa AM Jr. Gastric varices, problems in diagnosis. Dig Dis Sci. 1977;22:947–55.
15. Fleming RJ, Seaman WB. Roentgenographic demonstration of unusual extraesophageal varices. Am J Roentgenol Radium Ther Nucl Med. 1968;103:281–90.
16. Stanley AJ, Jalan R, Ireland HM, Redhead DN, Bouchier IA, Hayes PC. A comparison between gastric and oesophageal variceal haemorrhage treated with transjugular intrahepatic portosystemic stent shunt (TIPSS). Aliment Pharmacol Ther. 1997;11:171–6.
17. Chau TN, Patch D, Chan YW, Nagral A, Dick R, Burroughs AK. Salvage transjugular intrahepatic portosystemic shunts: gastric fundal compared with esophageal variceal bleeding. Gastroenterology. 1998;114:981–7.
18. Rees CJ, Nylander DL, Thompson NP, Rose JD, Record CO, Hudson M. Do gastric and esophageal varices bleed at different portal pressures and is TIPS an effective treatment? Liver. 2000;20:253–6.
19. Korula J, Chin K, Ko Y, Yamada S. Demonstration of two distinct subsets of gastric varices observed during a 7 year study of endoscopic sclerotherapy. Dig Dis Sci. 1991;36:303–9.
20. Kim T, Shijo H, Kokawa H et al. Risk factors for hemorrhage from gastric fundal varices. Hepatology. 1997;25:307–12.
21. Korula J, Ralls P. The effect of chronic endoscopic variceal sclerotherapy on portal pressure in cirrhosis. Gastroenterology. 1991;101:800–6.
22. Zanasi G, Rossi A, Grosso C et al. The effect of endoscopic sclerotherapy of esophageal varices on the development of gastric varices. Endoscopy. 1996;28:234–8.
23. Sarin SK, Nanda R, Sachdev G. Follow-up of patients after variceal eradication: a comparison of patients with cirrhosis, non-cirrhotic portal fibrosis and extrahepatic portal vein obstruction. Ann Surg. 1986;204:78–82.
24. Tomikawa M, Hashizume M, Saku M, Tanoue K, Ohta M, Sugimachi K. Effectiveness of gastric devascularization and splenectomy for patients with gastric varices. J Am Coll Surg 2000 (under publication).

25. Schubert TT, Schnell GA, Walden JM. Bleeding from varices in the gastric fundus complicating sclerotherapy. Gastrointest Endosc. 1989;35:268–9.
26. Sarin SK, Nundy S. Subclinical encephalopathy after portosystemic shunts in patients with non-cirrhotic portal fibrosis. Liver. 1985;5:142–6.
27. Cales P, Zabotto B, Meskens C et al. Gastric endoscopic features in cirrhosis. Observer variability, interassociations and relationship to hepatic dysfunction. Gastroenterology. 1990;98:156–62.
28. Sarin SK, Sreniwas DV, Lahoti D, Saraya A. Factors influencing development of congestive gastropathy in patients with portal hypertension. Gastroenterology. 1992;102:994–9.
29. Eleftheriadis F, Kotzampassi K, Aletras H. The influence of sclerotherapy on gastric mucosal blood flow distribution. Am Surg. 1990;56:593.
30. Miyazaki S, Yoshida T, Harada T, Shigemitsu T, Takeo Y, Okita K. Injection sclerotherapy for gastric varices using N-butyl-2-cyanoacrylate and ethanolamine oleate. Hepato-Gastroenterology. 1998;45:1155–8.
31. Teres J, Cecilia A, Bordas JM et al. Oesophageal tamponade for bleeding varices. Controlled trial between the Sengstaken–Blakemore tube and the Linton–Nachlas tube. Gastroenterology. 1978;75:566–9.
32. Wu CY, Yeh HZ, Chen GH. Pharmacological efficacy in gastric variceal rebleeding and survival: including multivariate analysis. J Clin Gastroenterol. 2002;35:127–32.
33. Trudeau W, Prindiville T. Endoscopic injection sclerosis in bleeding gastric varices. Gastrointest Endosc. 1986;32:264–8.
34. Bretagne JF, Dudicourt JC, Morisot D et al. Is endoscopic variceal sclerotherapy effective for the treatment of gastric varices? Dig Dis Sci. 1986;31:A505S .
35. Gimson AES, Westaby D, Williams R. Endoscopic sclerotherapy in the management of gastric variceal haemorrhage. J Hepatol. 1991;13:274–8.
36. Oho K, Iwao T, Sumino M, Toyonaga A, Tanikawa K. Ethanolamine oleate versus butyl cyanoacrylate for bleeding gastric varices: a nonrandomized study. Endoscopy. 1995;27:349–54.
37. Chang KY, Wu CS, Chen PC. Prospective randomized trial of hypertonic glucose water and sodium tetradecyl sulfate for gastric variceal bleeding in patients with advanced liver cirrhosis. Endoscopy. 1996;28:481–6.
38. Chiu KW, Changchien CS, Chuah SK et al. Endoscopic injection sclerotherapy with 1.5% sotradecol for bleeding cardiac varices. J Clin Gastroenterol. 1997;24:161–4.
39. Sarin SK, Long-term follow-up of gastric variceal sclerotherapy: an eleven year experience. Gastrointest Endosc. 1997;46:8–14.
40. Ogawa K, Ishikawa S, Naritaka Y et al. Clinical evaluation of endoscopic injection sclerotherapy using n-butyl-2-cyanoacrylate for gastric variceal bleeding. J Gastroenterol Hepatol. 1999;14:245–50.
41. Yassin MY, Eita MS, Hussein AMT. Endoscopic sclerotherapy for bleeding gastric varices. Gut. 1985;26:A1105.
42. Sarin SK, Jain AK, Jain M, Gupta R. A randomized controlled trial of cyanoacrylate vs. alcohol injection in patients with isolated fundic varices. Am J Gastroenterol. 2002; 97:1010–15.
43. Ramond MJ, Valla D, Gotlib JP et al. Endoscopic obliteration of oesophagogastric varices with bucrylate. I. Clinical Study in 49 patients. Gastroenterol Clin Biol. 1986;10:8–9.
44. Sohendra N, Grimm H, Nam V, Berger B. N-Butyl-2-cyanoacrylate: A supplement to endoscopic sclerotherapy. Endoscopy. 1987;19:221–4.
45. Ramond MJ, Valla D, Mosnier JF et al. Successful endoscopic obturation of gastric varices with butyl cyanoacrylate. Hepatology. 1989;10:488–93.
46. Rauws EAJ, Jansen PLM, Tytgat GNJ. Endoscopic sclerotherapy of gastric varices with bucrylate: treatment of acute bleeding and long- term follow-up. Gastrointest Endosc. 1991;37:242.
47. Grimm H, Maydeo A, Noar M, Sohendra N. Bleeding esophagogastric varices: is endoscopic treatment with cyanoacrylate the final answer? Gastrointest Endosc. 1991;37:275.
48. D'Imperio N, Piemontese A, Baroncini D et al. Evaluation of undiluted N-butyl-2-cyanoacrylate in the endoscopic treatment of upper gastrointestinal tract varices. Endoscopy. 1996;28:239–43.
49. Huang YH, Yeh HZ, Chen GH et al. Endoscopic treatment of bleeding gastric varices by N-butyl-2-cyanoacrylate (Histoacryl) injection: long-term efficacy and safety. Gastrointest Endosc. 2000;52:160–7.

50. Lee YT, Chan FK, Ng EK et al. EUS-guided injection of cyanoacrylate for bleeding gastric varices. Gastrointest Endosc. 2000;52:168–74.
51. Binmoller KF, Sohendra N. Nonsurgical treatment of variceal bleeding: new modalities. Am J Gastroenterol. 1995;90:1923–31.
52. See A, Florent C, Lamy P et al. Cerebral infarction following endoscopic obliteration of esophageal varices using isobutyl-2-cyanoacrylate: Report of two cases. Gastroenterol Clin Biol. 1986;10:604–7.
53. Moustafa I, Omar MM, Nooh A. Endoscopic control of gastric variceal bleeding with butyl cyanoacrylate. Endoscopy. 1993;25:A11.
54. Thakeb F, Salama Z, Salama H, Raouf TA, Kader SA, Hamid HA. The value of combined use of N-butyl-2-cyanoacrylate and ethanolamine oleate in the endoscopic treatment of upper gastrointestinal tract varices. Endoscopy. 1995;27:358–64.
55. Chang PN, Sheu BS, Chen CY, Chang TT, Lin XZ. Splenic infarction after histoacryl injection for bleeding gastric varices. Gastrointest Endosc. 1998;48:426–7.
56. Verter P, Blais J, Gruau M, Haffaf Y. Retrogastric abscess secondary to gastric varices obturation with cyanoacrylate. Gastroenterol Clin Biol. 1998;22:248–9.
57. Recter A. Induction of sarcomas by the tissue binding substance histoacryl in the rat. Z Exp Chir Transplant Kumstticherorgane. 1987;20:55–60.
58. Battaglia G, Morbin T, Paterello E, Ancona E, Merkel C, Corona M. Visceral fistulae as a complication of sclerotherapy for esophageal and gastric varices using isobutyl-2-cyanocrylate. Gastrointest Endosc. 2000;52:267–70.
59. Williams SG, Peters RA, Westaby D. Thrombin – an effective treatment for gastric variceal hemorrhage. Gut. 1994;35:1287–9.
60. Przemioslo RT, McNair A, Williams R. Thrombin is effective in arresting bleeding from gastric variceal hemorrhage. Dig Dis Sci. 1999;44:778–81.
61. Shiha G, El-Sayed SS. Gastric variceal ligation: a new technique. Gastrointest Endosc. 1999;49:437–41.
62. Takeuchi M, Nakai Y, Syu A, Okamoto E, Fujimoto J. Endoscopic ligation of gastric varices. Lancet. 1996;348:1038.
63. Vitte RL, Eugene C, Fingerhut A, Felsenheld C, Merrer J. Fatal outcome following endoscopic fundal variceal ligation. Gastrointest Endosc. 1996;43:82.
64. Yoshida T, Hayashi N, Suzumi S et al. Endoscopic ligation of gastric varices using a detachable snare. Endoscopy. 1994;26:502–5.
65. Takeuchi M, Nakai Y, Syu A, Okamoto E, Fujimoto J. Endoscopic ligation of gastric varices. Lancet. 1996;348:1038.
66. Harada T, Yoshida T, Shghnitsu T, Takeo Y, Tada H, Okita K. Therapeutic results of endoscopic variceal ligation for acute bleeding esophageal and gastric varices. J Gastroenterol Hepatol. 1997;12:331–5.
67. Cipolletta L, Bianco MA, Rotondano G, Piscopo R, Prisco A, Garofano ML. Emergency endoscopic ligation of actively bleeding gastric varices with a detachable snare. Gastrointest Endosc. 1998;47:400–3.
68. Yoshida T, Harada T, Shigemitsu T, Takeo Y, Miyazaki S, Okita K. Endoscopic management of gastric varices using a detachable snare and simultaneous endoscopic sclerotherapy and O-ring ligation. J Gastroenterol Hepatol. 1999;14:730–5.
69. Kanagawa H, Mima S, Kouyama H et al. Treatment of gastric fundal varices by balloon-occluded retrograde transvenous obliteration. J Gastroenterol Hepatol. 1996;11:51–8.
70. Hirota S, Matsumoto S, Tomita M, Sako M, Kono M. Retrograde transvenous obliteration of gastric varices. Radiology. 1999;211:349–56.
71. Matsumoto A, Hamamoto N, Nomura T et al. Balloon-occluded retrograde transvenous obliteration of high risk gastric fundal varices. Am J Gastroenterol. 1999;94:643–9.
72. Kanagawa H, Mima S, Kouyama H et al. Treatment of gastric fundal varices by balloon-occluded retrograde transvenous obliteration. J Gastroenterol Hepatol. 1996;11:51–8.
73. Hirota S, Matsumoto S, Tomita M, Sako M, Kono M. Retrograde transvenous obliteration of gastric varices. Radiology. 1999;211:349–56.
74. Matsumoto A, Hamamoto N, Nomura T et al. Balloon-occluded retrograde transvenous obliteration of high risk gastric fundal varices. Am J Gastroenterol. 1999;94:643–9.
75. Chikamore F, Kuniyoshi N, Shibuya S, Tkase Y. Eight years of experience with transjugular retrograde obliteration for gastrorenal shunts. Surgery. 2001;129:414–20.

76. Fukuda T, Hirota S, Sugimura K. Long-term results of balloon occluded retrograde transvenous obliteration for the treatment of gastric varices and hepatic encephalopathy. J Vasc Interv Radiol. 2001;12:327–36.
77. Kato T, Uematsu T, Nishigaki Y, Sugihara J, Tomita E, Moriwaki H. Therapeutic effect of balloon-occluded retrograde transvenous obliteration on portal–systemic encephalopathy in patients with liver cirrhosis. Intern Med. 2001;40:688–91.
78. Tanikawa K. Randomized prospective trial for bleeding fundal varices: endoscopic sclerotherapy versus transvenous obliteration. Gastroenterology. 1997;112:A1351.
79. Kiyosue H, Matsumoto S, Onishi R et al. [Balloon-occluded retrograde transvenous obliteration (B-RTO) for gastric varices: therapeutic results and problems]. Nippon Igaku Hoshasen Gakkai Zasshi. 1999;59:12–19.
80. Kin H, Kubota Y, Tsuji K et al. MR imaging in the evaluation of the therapeutic effect of B-RTO for gastric varices. Hepatogastroenterology. 1998;45:677–83.
81. Shiba M, Higuchi K, Nakamura K et al. Efficacy and safety of balloon-occluded endoscopic injection for sclerotherapy as a prophylactic treatment for high-risk gastric varices: a prospective, randomized, comparative clinical trial. Gastrointest Endosc. 2002;56:522–8.
82. Sanyal AJ, Freedman AM, Luketic VA et al. Transjugular intrahepatic portosystemic shunt for patients with active variceal hemorrhage unresponsive to sclerotherapy. Gastroenterology. 1996;111:138–46.
83. Barange K, Peron JM, Imani K et al. Transjugular intrahepatic portosystemic shunt in the treatment of refractory bleeding from ruptured gastric varices. Hepatology. 1999;30:1139–43.
84. Song HG, Lee HC, Park YH et al. (Therapeutic efficacy of transjugular intrahepatic portosystemic shunt on bleeding gastric varices). Taehan Kan Hakhoe Chi. 2002;8:448–57.
85. Lind CD, Malisch TW, Chong WK et al. Incidence of shunt occlusion or stenosisment. Gastroenterology. 1994;106:1277–83.
86. Ryan BM, Stockbrugger RW, Ryan JM. A pathophysiological, gastroenterologic and radiologic approach to the management of gastric varices. Gastroenterology. 2004;126:1175–89.
87. Spahr L, Dufresene MP, Bui BT et al. Efficacy of TIPS in the prevention of rebleeding from esophageal and fundal varices: a comparative study (abstr.). Hepatology. 1995;22:296A.
88. Tripathi D, Therapondos G, Jackson E, Redhead DN, Hayes PC. The role of the transjugular intrahepatic portosystemic stent shunt (TIPSS) in the management of bleeding gastric varices: clinical and haemodynamic correlations. Gut. 2002;51:270–4.
89. Greig ID, Garden OJ, Anderson JR, Carter DC. Management of gastric variceal hemorrhage. Br J Surg. 1990;77:297–9.
90. Merican I, Burroughs AK. Gastric varices. Eur J Gastroenterol Hepatol. 1992;4:511–20.
91. Madsen MS, Petersen TH, Sommer H. Segmental portal hypertension. Ann Surg. 1986;204:72–7.
92. Toder OC. Splenic vein thrombosis with bleeding gastroesophageal varices. Report of 2 splenectomized cases and review of the literature. Acta Chir Scand. 1984;150:265–8.
93. Wood RP, Shaw BW Jr, Rikkers LF. Liver transplantation for variceal hemorrhage. Surg Clin N Am. 1990;70:449–61.
94. Warren WD, Henderson JM, Millikan WJ et al. Distal splenorenal shunt versus endoscopic sclerotherapy for long-term management of variceal bleeding. Preliminary report of a prospective, randomized trial. Ann Surg. 1986;203:454–62.
95. Thomas PG, D'Cruz AJ. Distal splenorenal shunting for bleeding gastric varices. Br J Surg. 1994;81:241–4.
96. Choudhary A, Dhar P, Aggarwal A, Sarin SK. Long-term outcome of surgical treatment for gastric varices (abstract). Hepatology. 2000;32:519A.
97. Jalan R, Hayes PC. UK guidelines on the management of variceal haemorrhage in cirrhotic patients. British Society of Gastroenterology. Gut. 2000;46(Suppl. 3–4):III1–15.

# 31
# The patient who cannot receive beta-blockers

THOMAS D. BOYER

## INTRODUCTION

During the past 15–20 years management of patients with varices and portal hypertensive gastropathy has been made much easier by the finding that non-selective beta-blockers reduce portal pressure[1]. Subsequent controlled trials have shown that non-selective beta-blockers are effective in the primary and secondary prevention of variceal bleeding, and they are the standard form of treatment for these complications of portal hypertension[2–5]. In addition, bleeding from portal hypertensive gastropathy is reduced following treatment with beta-blockers[6]. Unfortunately, many patients are intolerant of beta-blockers and thus must be treated with alternative therapies. In this chapter the alternatives to beta-blocker therapy for the treatment of the above conditions are discussed. Controlled trials examining different therapies in this subgroup of patients would allow for determination of the best approach. However, we lack these controlled trials and the conclusions in this chapter are based on data extracted from trials in which beta-blockers were compared to other therapies. I have assumed that the patient intolerant of beta-blockers will respond to alternative therapies in the same manner as patients who can tolerate beta-blockers.

## CONTRAINDICATIONS AND SIDE-EFFECTS OF BETA-BLOCKERS

Listed in Table 1 are the most common contraindications to the use of beta-blockers in patients with cirrhosis. Problems such as congestive heart failure, severe asthma, and heart rates less than 50 beats/min are absolute contraindications to the use of beta-blockers. Hypotension, however, is a relative contraindication as patients with cirrhosis frequently have a hyperdynamic circulation and therefore are hypotensive. Systolic values of $< 85$ mmHg have been used by some investigators to exclude patients from receiving beta-blockers[7], but it is unknown whether cirrhotics with lower pressures

**Table 1.** Contraindications to use of beta-blockers

Heart block grade II
Severe chronic obstructive pulmonary disease or asthma
Severe insulin-dependent diabetes
Aortic stenosis
Congestive heart failure
Hypotension
Sinus bradycardia < 50/min
Symptomatic peripheral vascular disease

**Table 2.** Complications of beta-blocker therapy

Asthenia
Impotence
Bradycardia
Hypotension
Asthma
Shortness of breath
Congestive heart failure

would be intolerant of beta-blocker therapy. The number of cirrhotic patients with contraindications to the use of beta-blockers varies from study to study. In one recent report fully 27% of patients eligible for the study had contraindications to the use of beta-blockers[7]. Hence, many patients with cirrhosis and complications of portal hypertension will not be candidates for treatment with beta-blockers.

In addition to having a contraindication to the use of beta-blockers, many will also develop side-effects while on therapy, leading to discontinuation of the medication. Some of the more common side-effects are listed in Table 2. The most common side-effect appears to be asthenia or generalized weakness. In primary prophylaxis studies the frequency of side-effects ranges from 24% to 46%, and therapy is discontinued due to intolerance in 4–30% of patients[7-12]. When beta-blockers are used to prevent rebleeding the frequency of side-effects is 10–21% and therapy is withdrawn secondary to side-effects in 0–8% of patients[13-16]. This variability in the number withdrawn from therapy due to side-effects in these different studies suggests that there is a significant subjective component to the decision to withdraw therapy. However, it is clear that many patients who are in need of beta-blocker therapy cannot receive beta-blockers and thus require an alternative form of therapy.

## PRIMARY PREVENTION

One of the major uses of beta-blockers is in the primary prevention of variceal bleeding. Multiple controlled trials have been performed in which beta-blockers are compared to placebo and other forms of therapy in the prevention of bleeding from varices[2,3]. Beta-blocker therapy is clearly better than placebo and is cost-effective[17,18]. If the patient cannot take beta-blockers then is there an alternative form of pharmacologic therapy? One alterna-

**Table 3.** Agents that may be effective in preventing variceal bleeding

| |
|---|
| Clonidine |
| Diuretics |
| Verapamil pentoxifylline |
| Metoclopramide |
| Endothelin receptor antagonists |
| NO-URSO |

tive is isosorbide-5-mononitrate (ISMN), which lowers portal pressure in cirrhotics. Unfortunately, ISMN does not appear to be very effective for primary prophylaxis. In one trial in which ISMN was compared to propranolol, the percentage of patients free of bleeding at 24 months was 82% with ISMN and 86% with propranolol[19]. However, in a second study ISMN was significantly less effective (61% free of bleeding at 24 months) than was treatment with nadolol (87% free of bleeding at 24 months)[11]. The efficacy of ISMN in primary prevention of bleeding in patients who cannot receive beta-blockers has been examined in a placebo-controlled trial. Garcia-Pagan and colleagues randomized 67 patients who had contraindications to the use of beta-blockers to either ISMN or placebo[20]. The 2-year risk of bleeding was 29% in the ISMN group and 14% in the placebo group (difference n.s.). Based on the results of these three studies it appears that ISMN is an ineffective form of therapy for the primary prophylaxis of patients with varices. A number of other drugs have been suggested as possible therapies for the prevention of bleeding from varices (Table 3); however, none has been proven to be effective as a single agent in controlled trials, and their use cannot be recommended.

Variceal band ligation (VBL) is another form of therapy that is used in the primary prevention of variceal bleeding. Although endoscopic sclerosis of varices has also been used in primary prevention of bleeding, its use is not recommended because of concerns as to efficacy and better outcomes using VBL[2,3,21]. In a meta-analysis VBL appears to be at least equal to, if not better than, beta-blocker therapy in the primary prevention of variceal bleeding[22]. In a more recent study[12] VBL was compared to monotherapy with propranolol or ISMN. The 2-year actuarial risk of bleeding was greatest with ISMN (28%), less with propranolol (19%) and least with VBL (6%). Treatment with ISMN was significantly less effective than VBL in the prevention of bleeding in this report. In addition, the side-effect profile of VBL was significantly better than either form of pharmacologic therapy. VBL therefore appears to be an excellent form of therapy for patients with varices who have never bled, and who are intolerant of beta-blockers.

## SECONDARY PREVENTION

Once patients have bled from varices more than 70% of patients will suffer an episode of rebleeding within 2 years; thus treatment is essential[23]. A number of different treatments, including beta-blockers, are used in the prevention of rebleeding, and it is beyond the scope of this chapter to review all of those studies[2,3,23]. The best pharmacologic therapy is thought to be the combination of a beta-blocker plus ISMN[24]. At least three published studies have compared combination pharmacologic therapy to VBL[24]. The rebleeding rate in those receiving a beta-blocker plus ISMN ranged from 33% to 57%, whereas with VBL the rebleeding rates ranged from 38% to 53%. Thus, VBL was as good as combination pharmacologic therapy in the prevention of rebleeding. Alternatives such as sclerotherapy or transjugular intrahepatic portosystemic shunts (TIPS) are not recommended because of a lack of efficacy relative to VBL, i.e. sclerotherapy, or because of increased costs and risk of encephalopathy, i.e. TIPS[21,25].

## PORTAL HYPERTENSIVE GASTROPATHY (PHG)

The other complication of portal hypertension for which beta-blockers are prescribed is PHG. PHG is a common finding in patients with cirrhosis, with a reported incidence of 65–90%. Most patients have mild gastropathy whereas 10–25% have severe gastropathy. Bleeding is uncommon, with 2.5% suffering acute bleeding and 10% having chronic blood loss[26,27]. A small number of studies suggest that beta-blockers reduce the bleeding in patients with portal hypertensive gastropathy. Alternatives to beta-blockers include portacaval shunts, TIPS and liver transplantation. For the acutely bleeding patient somatostatin and octreotide appear effective but, other than beta-blockers, there is no medical therapy for the patient with chronic bleeding[26].

## TREATMENT OF PATIENTS WHO ARE INTOLERANT OF BETA-BLOCKERS

Before discussing alternatives to beta-blocker therapy it is important to decide which patients should be treated if beta-blockers cannot be used (Table 4). Beta-blockers have been used to prevent the development of new varices and to stop the growth of small varices. Although use of beta-blockers for these two indications is controversial, some have suggested that all cirrhotic patients should be treated with beta-blockers[18]. Recent work, however, suggests that patients with no or small varices have a low likelihood of bleeding. Merli and colleagues reported on 206 cirrhotics, 113 without varices and 93 with small varices, who were followed for a mean of 37 months[28]. After 2 years of follow-up, 17% of patients developed new varices, but in only 2.6% were high-risk varices seen, and only 2% of the patients bled. In contrast, after 2 years 25% of patients with small varices progressed to large varices, but still the risk of bleeding was only 12%. Thus, if patients with cirrhosis have no or small varices at the index endoscopy they have a low risk of bleeding during the next 2 years and the use of alternative forms of treatment is not warranted.

In contrast, patients with large varices are at the greatest risk of bleeding, and if intolerant of beta-blockers should receive another form of therapy. As there are no pharmacologic agents that have proven effective in primary prevention, VBL is the treatment of choice. If bleeding occurs following

**Table 4.** Treatment of patient intolerant of beta-blockers

| Indication | Recommendation |
| --- | --- |
| Primary prevention | |
| No or small varices | Observe |
| High risk varices | VBL |
| | Failure = |
| | shunt/TIPS |
| Secondary prevention | VBL |
| | Failure = |
| | shunt/TIPS |
| Gastropathy | |
| Present no bleeding | Observe |
| Moderate bleeding | Observe |
| Severe bleeding | TIPS/OLTx |

OLTx, orthotopic liver transplant; TIPS, transjugular intrahepatic portosystemic shunt; VBL, variceal band ligation.

VBL then either a TIPS or surgical shunt should be performed, depending on the patient's liver function. A similar approach should be taken with secondary prevention of bleeding. VBL is an effective form of therapy for this group of patients and should be used in those who are intolerant of beta-blockers. Bleeding not responding to VBL should lead to a surgical shunt or a TIPS.

Portal hypertensive gastropathy has a relatively benign prognosis with the risk of bleeding either acutely or chronically being less than 15% over an 18-month period[27]. Thus, portal hypertensive gastropathy irrespective of its appearance should not be treated in the absence of bleeding. When bleeding develops the only two options in the beta-blocker-intolerant patient are a transplant or a TIPS. If the bleeding is mild to moderate then observation would be the most appropriate course. If the bleeding is more significant then a liver transplant, if possible, is the treatment of choice as these patients are more likely to have advanced liver disease. TIPS can be used as a bridge to transplant.

## CONCLUSIONS

At least 25% of cirrhotics who are candidates for use of beta-blockers to treat the complications of portal hypertension cannot receive beta-blockers because of intolerance to these drugs. This large group of patients has not been the subject of controlled trials with one exception[20]; therefore the management of these patients is based on extrapolations from other studies. Currently the only options for these patients are limited to VBL, TIPS/shunts or liver transplantation. We clearly need other forms of pharmacologic therapy to better manage patients who cannot receive beta-blockers. As we develop new therapies for the treatment of the complications of portal hypertension, patients intolerant of beta-blockers are an ideal group to study. From the results of these future studies we will be able to better manage this interesting and large group of patients.

## References

1. Lebrec D, Nouel O, Corbic M, Benhamou P-P. Propranolol – a medical treatment for portal hypertension? Lancet. 1980;2:180–2.
2. D'Amico G, Pagliaro L, Bosch J. Pharmacological treatment of portal hypertension: an evidence-based approach. Semin Liver Dis. 1999;19:475–505.
3. Luketic VA, Sanyal AJ. Esophageal varices. I. Clinical presentation, medical therapy and endoscopic therapy. Gastroenterol Clinics N Am. 2000;29:337–85.
4. Garcia-Pagan, JC, Grace N. Primary prophylaxis. In: de Franchis R, editor. Portal Hypertension III. Oxford: Blackwell Science, 2001:127–33.
5. Lebrec D, Stiegmann GV. Prevention of recurrent variceal hemorrhage (Secondary Prophylaxis). In: de Franchis R, editor. Portal Hypertension III. Oxford: Blackwell Science, 2001:170–9.
6. Burak KW, Lee SS, Beck PL. Portal hypertensive gastropathy and gastric antral vascular ectasia (GAVE) syndrome. Gut. 2001;49:866–72.
7. Garcia-Pagan JC, Morillas R, Banares R et al. Propranolol plus placebo versus propranolol plus isosorbide-5-mononitrate in the prevention of a first variceal bleed: a double-blind RCT. Hepatology. 2003;37:1260–6.
8. Angelico M, Carli L, Piat C et al. Isosorbide-5-mononitrate versus propranolol in the prevention of first bleeding in cirrhosis. Gastroenterology. 1993;104:1460–5.
9. Merkel C, Marin R, Sacerdoti D et al. Long-term results of a clinical trial of nadolol with or without isosorbide mononitrate for primary prophylaxis of variceal bleeding in cirrhosis. Hepatology. 2000;31:324–9.
10. Sarin SK, Lamba GS, Kumar M, Misra A, Murthy NS. Comparison of endoscopic ligation and propranolol for the primary prevention of variceal bleeding. N Engl J Med. 1999; 340:988–93.
11. Borroni G, Salerno F, Cazzaniga M et al. Nadolol is superior to isosorbide mononitrate for the prevention of the first variceal bleeding in cirrhotic patients with ascites. J Hepatol. 2002;37:315–21.
12. Lui HF, Stanley AJ, Forrest EH et al. Primary prophylaxis of variceal hemorrhage: a randomized controlled trial comparing band ligation, propranolol, and isosorbide mononitrate. Gastroenterology. 2002;123:735–44.
13. Lebrec D, Poynard T, Hillon P, Benhamou JP. Propranolol for prevention of recurrent gastrointestinal bleeding in patients with cirrhosis. N Engl J Med. 1981;305:1371–4.
14. Gournay J, Maslian C, Martin T, Perrin D, Galmiche J-P. Isosorbide mononitrate and propranolol compared with propranolol alone for the prevention of variceal rebleeding. Hepatology. 2000;31:1239–45.
15. Teres J, Bosch J, Bordas JM et al. Propranolol versus sclerotherapy in preventing variceal rebleeding: a randomized controlled trial. Gastroenterology. 1993;105:1508–14.
16. Westaby D, Polson RJ, Gimson AES, Hayes PC, Hayllar K, Williams R. A controlled trial of oral propranolol compared with injection sclerotherapy for the long-term management of variceal bleeding. Hepatology. 1990;11:353–9.
17. Arguedas, MR, Heudebert, GR, Eloubeidi, MA, Abrams, GA, Fallon, MB. Cost-effectiveness of screening, surveillance, and primary prophylaxis strategies for esophageal varices. Am J Gastroenterol. 2002;97:2442–52.
18. Spiegel BM, Targownik L, Dulai GS, Karsan HA, Gralnek IM. Endoscopic screening for esophageal varices in cirrhosis: Is it ever cost effective? Hepatology. 2003;37:366–77.
19. Angelico M, Carli L, Piat C, Gentile S, Rinaldi V, Bologna E, Capocaccia L. Isosorbide-5-mononitrate versus propranolol in the prevention of first bleeding in cirrhosis. Gastroenterology. 1993;104:1460–5.
20. Garcia-Pagan JC, Villanueva C, Vila MC et al. Isosorbide mononitrate in the prevention of first variceal bleed in patients who cannot receive β-blockers. Gastroenterology. 2001; 121:908–14.
21. Laine L, Cook D. Endoscopic ligation compared with sclerotherapy for treatment of esophageal variceal bleeding. Ann Intern Med. 1995;123:280–7.

22. Imperiale T, Chalasani N. A meta-analysis of endoscopic variceal ligation for primary prophylaxis of esophageal variceal bleeding Hepatology. 2001;33:802–7.
23. Sharara AI, Rockey DC. Gastroesophageal variceal hemorrhage. N Engl J Med. 2001; 34:669–81.
24. Groszmann RJ, Garcia-Tsao G. Endoscopic variceal banding vs. pharmacologic therapy for the prevention of recurrent variceal hemorrhage: what makes the difference? Gastroenterology. 2002;123:1388–91.
25. Boyer TD. Transjugular intrahepatic portosystemic shunt: current status. Gastroenterology. 2003;124:1700–10.
26. Burak KW, Lee SS, Beck PL. Portal hypertensive gastropathy and gastric antral vascular ectasia (GAVE) syndrome. Gut. 2001;49:866–72.
27. Primignani M, Carpinelli L, Preatoni P et al. Natural history of portal hypertensive gastropathy in patients with liver cirrhosis. Gastroenterology. 2000;119:181–7.
28. Merli M, Nicolini G, Angeloni S et al. Incidence and natural history of small esophageal varices in cirrhotic patients. J Hepatol. 2003;38:266–72.

# 32
# Hepatic venous pressure gradient: the facts

**JULIO D. VOROBIOFF, JUAN G. ABRALDES and ROBERTO J. GROSZMANN**

*Fact:* An assertion, statement, or information containing or purporting to contain something having objective reality

*Webster's Third New International Dictionary*

## INTRODUCTION

Many of the clinical complications of cirrhosis are the direct consequences of the elevation of portal venous pressure (PVP). Portal hypertension is defined as a PVP of greater than the normal 5–10 mmHg. The degree of portal hypertension has been shown to correlate with the severity of liver disease, both functionally[1] and histologically[2,3]. However, direct portal venous measurement is invasive and cannot be routinely performed. As a surrogate, hepatic venous pressure gradient (HVPG) has been widely accepted as a measurement for PVP. The ease and safety of HVPG measurement has made it a valuable tool not only in the research arena, but also more and more in clinical practice.

## PVP MEASUREMENT

PVP was first measured in 1896 by Hallion and Francois-Frank, who inserted a cannula into the mesenteric vein of a dog and read the result from a water manometer[4]. The first determination of PVP in humans was performed in 1937 by Thompson et al.[5], who recorded PVP by means of a water manometer in a branch of the portal system during abdominal surgery. Normally, portal pressure ranges from 7 to 12 mmHg.

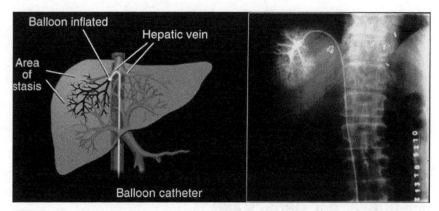

**Figure 1.** Measurement of HVPG with the balloon occlusion method. The catheter in the wedged position (balloon inflated) measures the sinusoidal pressure of a large area of the liver. (Modified from Groszmann et al. *Gastroenterology*, 1979, with permission)

Indirect measurement of PVP was first described in 1951 by Myers and Taylor[6]. By advancing a small catheter into a hepatic venule until it could go no further, they were able to demonstrate that this wedged hepatic venous pressure (WHVP) was closely correlated with the directly measured PVP. The difference between the WHVP and the free hepatic venous pressure (FHVP) constitutes the HVPG, that represents the gradient between portal vein and intra-abdominal vena cava pressure. Both the WHVP and FHVP are affected equally by intra-abdominal pressure; their gradient, HVPG, is not. Therefore, the measurement of HVPG incorporates its own zero reference point and is not affected by increases in intra-abdominal pressure. Thus an important source of error, such as an external zero reference point, is eliminated by the use of the HVPG[7]. Normally the HVPG ranges from 1 to 5 mmHg; pressure values above this limit define the presence of portal hypertension.

Currently, the most widely used technique in evaluating HVPG is a modification of Myer's method[8]. A fluid-filled balloon catheter is introduced into the jugular or the femoral vein and advanced under fluoroscopic guidance into a hepatic vein. FHVP is the pressure measured with the balloon deflated and the catheter floating freely within the vein. The balloon is then inflated until that branch of hepatic vein is completely occluded. In this situation the static column of blood formed by the occluding balloon results in a pressure reading that is slightly lower than the actual portal pressure (sinusoidal pressure) (Figure 1). The advantage of the balloon catheter is that serial measurements of FHVP and WHVP can be obtained with ease using the same catheter, inflated and deflated as needed. In addition, the catheter can be safely left in place for hours; hence the effects of pharmacologic agents on portal hemodynamics can be studied over time. Furthermore, unlike the conventional catheter where the WHVP is measured in a small hepatic venule, the balloon catheter allows measurement in the hepatic veins at lobar and sublobar levels; therefore, the pressure obtained averages the pressure of several segments of the liver and is more likely to represent the true PVP[7]. The rate of successful hepatic vein catheterization is greater than 95%, and the procedure has been shown to be extremely safe[9]. Moreover, if necessary, it can be performed under conscious sedation without effects on hepatic pressures[10].

## CLINICAL APPLICATIONS OF PORTAL HEMODYNAMICS ASSESSMENT

HVPG measurement has found many applications in clinical practice, as well as in the research field. HVPG is a valuable tool in diagnosing the etiologies of liver disease, in determining the prognosis and in evaluating the efficacy of various treatments of portal hypertension. It has also been advocated as a predictor of the outcome of hepatic resection for hepatocellular carcinoma.

### HVPG as a diagnostic tool

A normal liver is a low-resistance system and the sinusoidal network dissipates some of the pressure of the occluded catheter. In this situation the static column of blood formed by the occluding balloon results in a pressure reading that is slightly lower than actual portal pressure (sinusoidal pressure). Portal hypertension develops when there is an increase in resistance to portal venous flow. The sites of increased resistance can be prehepatic, intrahepatic or posthepatic. Portal hypertension from intra-hepatic causes can be conceptually subdivided into presinusoidal, sinusoidal and postsinusoidal portal hypertension[11]; nevertheless, it is worth noting that a disease process can involve more than one anatomic site.

Keeping this classification in mind, patterns of PVP, WHVP and FHVP can be used to delineate the types of portal hypertension, as well as its possible etiologies (Figure 2). For instance, in patients who have a clinical syndrome of portal hypertension, but have normal WHVP, a presinusoidal (whether intrahepatic or extrahepatic) cause of portal hypertension should be suspected. In these cases the catheter is not in continuity with the area of increased resistance; therefore the recorded pressure will be that of the normal sinusoids (with normal intersinusoidal anastomosis) and not of the area of increased pressure. HVPG will thus underestimate the PVP gradient (PVPG = PVP − FHVP). In primary biliary cirrhosis, and in chronic active hepatitis, a predominantly presinusoidal portal hypertension picture is observed initially because the early lesion is located mainly in the portal area[12]. In the advanced stages the fibrosis involves most areas of the lobule; and the pattern of portal hypertension eventually becomes mixed sinusoidal. In alcoholic cirrhosis, and in most cases of hepatitis B- and C-induced cirrhosis, connections between sinusoids are decreased because of narrowing of the sinusoidal vascular bed (collagen deposition in the space of Disse, compression by regenerative nodules, microthrombosis, etc.). In these cases HVPG is virtually equal to PVPG because there is little dissipation of pressure in the occluded sinusoids[12-17]. Finally, a posthepatic cause such as

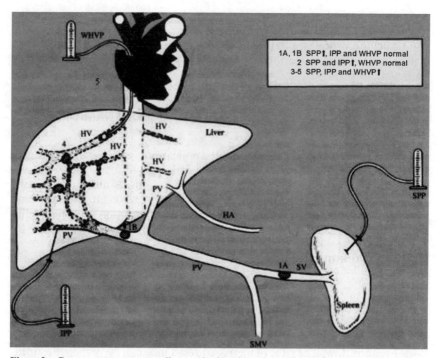

**Figure 2.** Pressure patterns according to the location of the obstruction to portal vein flow. When the obstruction is located at the splenic vein (1A) or extrahepatic portal vein (1B) only splenic pulp pressure (SPP) is increased, with normal intrahepatic portal pressure (IPP) and wedged hepatic venous pressure (WHVP). When the obstruction is located at the intrahepatic portal vein (2), both SPP and IPP are increased, with normal WHVP. When all SPP, IPP and WHVP are found increased, obstruction can be located at the liver sinusoids (3), at the hepatic veins (4) or can be of cardiac origin (5). Differential diagnosis between these three cases is generally straightforward, by measuring right atrial pressure (which would be increased in cardiac conditions and normal in sinusoidal and hepatic vein obstruction), and by the injection of a contrast agent in the hepatic veins, which readily discloses hepatic vein obstruction. SV: splenic vein. SMV: superior mesenteric vein. PV: portal vein. HV: hepatic vein. S: liver sinusoids. HA: hepatic artery. (Modified from Groszmann RJ and Atterbury C. *Semin Liver Dis.* 1982, with permission)

right heart failure will give rise to elevation in both WHVP and FHVP while HVPG remains normal.

## HVPG as a clinical prognostic parameter

HVPG has also been used to assess prognosis of cirrhotic patients, and has been shown to correlate with severity of liver disease and Child–Pugh classification[1-3], a tool used to predict survival in patients with end-stage liver disease[18].

## HVPG as a predictor of survival

The relationship between HVPG and survival has been assessed in several studies. Many of these trials showed that HVPG measurement is valuable in predicting survival in cirrhotic patients[19-30]. Two of these studies[22,25] found that, by adding the HVPG to the Child–Pugh score, survival prediction improved significantly better than analysis considering Child–Pugh classification alone.

However, another study failed to demonstrate a relationship between HVPG and survival. In this study the prognostic significance of HVPG was compared to that of the aminopyrine breath test, and it was found that, while the higher-level aminopyrine correlated significantly with survival, the HVPG did not. Urbain et al.[31] did not specify a history of previous variceal hemorrhage and, if so, when such hemorrhage occurred in the test subjects. Since HVPG has been shown to decrease spontaneously shortly after the acute bleeding episodes[32], such lack of information makes interpretation of the studies difficult.

In the studies by Groszmann et al.[24] and Vorobioff et al.[26], a decrease in HVPG to $\leq 12$ mmHg or $\geq 15\%$ respectively, was associated with significantly longer survival.

In a more recent multicenter trial Groszmann et al.[33] performed sequential measurements of HVPG in 213 cirrhotic patients without esophageal varices, followed during a median time of 4.2 years. An HVPG $> 10$ mmHg at baseline and at year 1 after inclusion in the study was highly predictive of death.

In 73 cirrhotic patients pharmacologically treated for the prevention of variceal rebleeding and having two separate HVPG measurements, Abraldes et al.[30] reported that the 8-year cumulative probability of survival was significantly higher in responders (i.e. patients whose HVPG decreased $\geq 20\%$ or to $\leq 12$ mmHg) than in non-responders (95% vs 52%, respectively; $p < 0.003$).

Regarding the timing of HVPG measurement in patients who develop variceal hemorrhage, some authors have suggested that HVPG obtained close to the bleeding episode may have a higher predictive value with regard to survival. Vinel et al.[21] measured HVPG within 48 h of the bleeding episode, and showed that patients who survived after the first month had significantly lower HVPG than patients who expired ($19.1 \pm 7.9$ mmHg vs $23.9 \pm 8.0$ mmHg; respectively; $p < 0.025$). Patch et al.[28] observed that a single HVPG measurement, performed within the first 2 weeks from bleeding, was an independent predictor of survival. In the same study a HVPG $\geq 16$ mmHg appeared to identify patients with a greatly increased risk of dying. Finally Moitinho et al.[29] measured the HVPG in 65 cirrhotic patients within 48 h after admission for acute variceal bleeding. The only variable associated with outcome was the HVPG, which was higher in patients with poor evolution ($23.7 \pm 6.1$ vs $19.2 \pm 3.3$ mmHg; $p < 0.0004$). An initial HVPG $\geq 20$ mmHg was associated with a worse actuarial probability of survival (1-year mortality, 64% vs 20%, $p < 0.002$).

## HVPG as a predictor of variceal hemorrhage

While it is widely accepted that HVPG is a good prognostic indicator of survival, it is less clear whether HVPG is a good predictor of variceal hemorrhage. Several studies have been published on this subject with conflicting results. The early studies were retrospective and included HVPG measurements at varying time points after the index bleeding episodes[34–37]. Since HVPG has been shown to change spontaneously after an acute hemorrhage[32], it is important to establish a standardized time frame in portal hemodynamic evaluation. Nevertheless, an HVPG of 12 mmHg was shown by several authors to be a minimal threshold below which variceal rupture is unlikely[34–36].

Among prospective studies involving patients who never bled, or had no recent bleeding, there are conflicting results with regard to the relationship between risks of variceal bleeding and HVPG. In four studies, using Cox regression analysis, HVPG was shown to be an independent predictor of variceal bleeding[22,25,38,39]. On the other hand, Lebrec et al.[40] failed to show a significant correlation.

In the above-cited trial by Groszmann et al.[33], a HVPG $> 10$ mmHg at baseline and at year 1 after inclusion in the study was also predictive of the development of varices and variceal hemorrhage.

In studies examining the relationship between HVPG and recurrent variceal hemorrhage after a recent bleeding episode, again the results are conflicting. Adamson et al.[41] first suggested that the height of HVPG influenced whether the acute hemorrhage would or would not resolve with non-operative treatment. This correlation was later confirmed by Ready et al.[42], who further suggested that HVPG $\geq 16$ mmHg was associated with 50% of uncontrolled bleeding. Nevertheless, two other studies by Westaby et al.[43] and Patch et al.[28] failed to find a significant correlation between HVPG and the risk of recurrent hemorrhage. Two recent studies have added valuable information in this area. In one of them Moitinho et al.[29], by performing early measurement of HVPG, observed that patients with an initial HVPG $\geq 20$ mmHg had a poor evolution, in terms of failure to control bleeding (23% vs 0%; $p < 0.004$) and early rebleeding (50% vs 12%; $p < 0.003$) when compared with patients whose HVPG was $< 20$ mmHg. In the other study, Villanueva et al.[44] continuously monitored portal pressure in 40 patients with acute variceal bleeding, receiving somatostatin or placebo. HVPG decreased significantly only in patients without further bleeding. One of 27 patients with HVPG $< 20$ mmHg at baseline or decreased $> 10\%$ rebled vs 9 of 13 who had neither of these two criteria ($p < 0.0001$); therefore, monitoring HVPG may stratify further bleeding risk and discriminate treatment response.

Changes in HVPG from baseline, during serial measurements, may represent a more accurate predictor of bleeding than a single measurement. In 1996 Vorobioff et al.[26] reported that the risk of first variceal bleeding was significantly reduced in alcoholic cirrhotic patients whose HVPG showed a spontaneous decrease of at least 15%, in a median time of 10 months.

## HVPG as a predictor of other clinical events

In 1958 Leevy et al.[45] performed serial measurements of WHVP in 50 alcoholic cirrhotic patients, at baseline and within 3–6 months after medical management. A decrease in WHVP, accompanied by an improvement in clinical and biochemical findings, was observed in 12 of these patients. On the other hand, WHVP increased in patients whose clinical condition was impaired. Serial measurements of HVPG were also performed by Reynolds et al.[46] in 18 alcoholic cirrhotic patients showing evidence of clinical improvement during follow-up. Nine of these patients showed a significant fall in the HVPG while only minor changes were observed in the other nine. Interestingly, mean baseline value in the nine patients decreasing their HVPG (16.3 mmHg) was substantially lower than that observed in the other nine patients (20.2 mmHg). Beyond recent and more sophisticated diagnostic and therapeutic advances, Leevy and Reynolds then added a new prognostic parameter to alcoholic liver disease, whether at its cirrhotic stage or within the context of acute alcoholic hepatitis, as many of their patients certainly had.

More recently, similar observations were reported by Groszmann et al.[24] (almost 80% of alcoholic cirrhotic patients) and Vorobioff et al.[26] (100% alcoholics). In both of these studies the HVPG seemed to be related to the improvement or worsening of liver disease. An improvement in the Child–Pugh score accompanied decreases in HVPG of $> 10\%$ and $\geq 15\%$; respectively. In the the study by Vorobioff et al.[26] changes in HVPG and variations in the Pugh score were significantly correlated. The mean HVPG variation between abstainers and non-abstainers also differed significantly ($-15.9\% \pm 3.5\%$ vs $18.4\% \pm 5.7\%$, respectively; $p < 0.01$). Finally, patients decreasing their HVPG to values below the bleeding threshold ($\leq 12$ mmHg)[24] or $\geq 15\%$[26] showed significantly larger reductions in variceal size.

In 73 cirrhotic patients having two separate HPVG measurements for the evaluation of pharmacologic therapy, during an 8-year follow-up study, Abraldes et al.[30] observed that non-responders (those decreasing their HVPG $\leq 20\%$ or not reaching $\geq 12$ mmHg) had a significantly higher risk of developing ascites ($p < 0.025$), spontaneous bacterial peritonitis ($p < 0.003$), hepatorenal syndrome ($p < 0.026$) and hepatic encephalopathy ($p < 0.024$) (Figure 3); therefore, in cirrhotic patients receiving pharmacologic treatment, a decrease in HVPG $\geq 20\%$ or to $\leq 12$ mmHg is associated with a marked reduction in the long-term risk of developing complications of portal hypertension.

Among the 213 well-compensated cirrhotic patients studied by Groszmann et al.[33] an HVPG $> 10$ mmHg at baseline and at year 1 after inclusion in the study was highly predictive of the development of ascites and encephalopathy ($p < 0.0001$). Thus an HVPG $> 10$ mmHg is a powerful prognostic predictor of the development of complications of portal hypertension. According to this study the presence of "clinically significant portal hypertension", manometrically defined, given that no patient had esophageal varices at entry into the study, seems by itself to be a prognostic indicator in cirrhotic patients. Of note, during the Baveno III conference, experts in the field reached a consensus defining "clinically significant portal hypertension" as an increase in HVPG to a threshold above approximately 10 mmHg[47].

## HVPG as an assessment of efficacy of therapy

The two most devastating consequences of portal hypertension are ascites and esophageal varices, both of which can lead to lethal complications

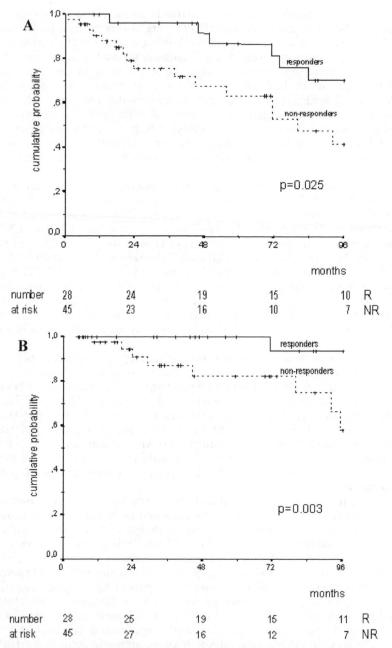

**Figure 3.** In patients under pharmacologic treatment for portal hypertension for the prevention of variceal rebleeding, a good hemodynamic response (a decrease in HVPG of more than 20% from baseline or to less than 12 mmHg) is associated with a significantly lower risk of ascites (panel **A**) and spontaneous bacterial peritonitis (panel **B**) (From Abraldes et al.[30], with permission)

including spontaneous bacterial peritonitis, hepatorenal syndrome and variceal hemorrhage. The main objective of therapeutic trials for portal hypertension should therefore aim at preventing these complications. Studies have shown that there appear to be threshold HVPG necessary for the formation of ascites and gastroesophageal varices which are 8 mmHg[48,49] and 10–12 mmHg[50], respectively. Furthermore, there also appears to be a threshold HVPG for variceal rupture, since it has been shown that variceal hemorrhage is unlikely if HVPG is less than 12 mmHg[24]. It was suggested that, during pharmacologic treatment, a decrease in the HVPG to $\leq 12$ mmHg is the single most useful prognostic indicator, and that a reduction in portal pressure to that level should be the aim of the pharmacologic therapy of portal hypertension[24].

Feu et al.[51] have subsequently reported that even a 20% reduction in HVPG from baseline can result in a significant protection against recurrent variceal hemorrhage even though the post-treatment HVPG is still higher than 12 mmHg. In this study the cumulative probability of rebleeding at 1, 2 and 3 years was 4%, 9% and 9% in patients who achieved a decrease in HVPG of $\geq 20\%$. In other patients, however, the probability of recurrent hemorrhage was 28%, 39% and 66% at 1, 2 and 3 years respectively. In a subsequent study McCormick et al.[52] failed to observe such a correlation.

Villanueva et al.[53] compared endoscopic and pharmacologic treatment for the prevention of variceal rebleeding. By serial measurements of HVPG they observed that the probability of remaining free of rebleeding and the probability of survival were both shown to be significantly greater in patients in whom the HVPG, measured 1–3 months after initiating therapy, was reduced $> 20\%$ or to $\leq 12$ mmHg. Interestingly, this applied to both therapies (endoscopic variceal banding and combination drug therapy), indicating that the important factor is the reduction in HVPG, whether this is achieved pharmacologically or spontaneously by an improvement in liver disease. This study confirms the earlier findings of Groszmann et al.[24].

A good hemodynamic response, as assessed by HVPG monitoring 1–3 months after starting treatment, was observed in 30 of 49 cirrhotic patients treated for the prophylaxis of first variceal bleeding and followed for up to 5 years. Among these, none of the 12 in whom HVPG decreased to $\leq 12$ mmHg bled. The probability of bleeding was higher in poor responders (41%) than in good responders (7%) ($p < 0.0008$). Merkel et al.[54] conclude that the assessment of hemodynamic response to drugs in terms of HVPG is the best predictor of efficacy in the pharmacologic treatment.

The results of adapting medical therapy to the monitoring of hemodynamic response in 34 cirrhotic patients for the prevention of first variceal bleeding or rebleeding were recently published. After being followed for a mean of 28 months and whether being treated with propranolol alone or with propranolol + I-5MN, none of the eight patients in whom HVPG decreased $< 12$ mmHg and only two of 12 whose HVPG decreased $\geq 20\%$ bled. Meanwhile, nine of 14 non-responders bled during the observation period. Bureau et al.[55] reinforce previous assertions regarding clinical–hemodynamic correlations and also demonstrate the benefit of sequential HVPG measurements for adapting treatment according to the patient's response.

On the other hand Patch et al.[56] performed serial HVPG measurements, the second measurement being performed 3 months after the baseline study, in 26 patients on pharmacologic therapy for the prevention of recurrent variceal hemorrhage. The authors were unable to show a downward trend in HVPG in survivors and in patients not rebleeding. However, none of the five patients decreasing their HVPG to $\leq 12$ mmHg rebled. These findings are consistent with a previous study from the same group of investigators[52].

Given that most rebleeding events occur during the first month after the index bleed, and in an attempt to minimize differences among studies, the second HVPG measurement should be performed no later than 2 or 3 weeks after stabilization of the patient. In order to maximize the portal pressure-reducing effect in these high-risk patients, dosing of pharmacologic therapy should be achieved within 2–3 weeks after the index bleed[57].

Beyond its usefulness for monitoring pharmacologic treatment of portal hypertension, serial HVPG measurements could be of additional benefit in the assessment of the progression of chronic liver diseases[58].

## HVPG as a tool for preoperative assessment in cirrhotic patients

It is generally accepted that cirrhotic patients carry a much higher operative risk than non-cirrhotic patients, and elective surgery should be avoided. For intra-abdominal surgery the mortality rates were found to range from 5% to 67% and the morbidity rate 7% to 39%. Traditionally, operative risks are stratified using the Child–Pugh classification score[59]. More recently it has been shown that the HVPG is associated with surgical outcome after hepatic resection for early hepatocellular carcinoma (HCC)[60].

Bruix et al. first reported in 1996 that, by multivariate analysis, an elevated HVPG was the only parameter significantly associated with unresolved decompensation at 3 months after hepatic resection for HCC[60]. Subsequently, using an intention-to-treat model, the same group of investigators demonstrated that clinically significant portal hypertension, as well as serum bilirubin, were independent predictors of survival after hepatic resection[61]. In this study the patients were selected to undergo hepatic resection (as opposed to liver transplantation) if a single tumor of less than 5 cm was present and if the patient's Child–Pugh score was less than 6 (Child class A). Among these patients the 5-year survival probability was drastically better in patients whose bilirubin was less than 1 mg/dl and HVPG less than 10 mmHg (74% vs 25%). The survival rate after resection for a "good" candidate is comparable to the survival outcome of patients undergoing liver transplantation for early HCC[62–64].

## SUMMARY

"Despite its unquestionable value in the differential diagnosis of portal hypertension and as predictor of long-term outcome in patients with chronic liver diseases, the popularity of this technique has never gone beyond the realm of research"[65]. This sentence, written by one of us 8 years ago, was a pessimistic and an almost resigned view of what, by then, were HVPG measurement frontiers. Have we accomplished enough information and more objective experience in order to expand these frontiers?

The advent of the balloon catheter technique allows us to perform safe, convenient and accurate measurements of HVPG. Moreover, practice guidelines are now available in order to give HVPG measurement more reliability[7]. Evaluation of portal hemodynamics not only provides information in diagnosing the etiologies of portal hypertension, it is also essential in evaluating the efficacy of various treatments for this devastating syndrome. Furthermore, HVPG has also been shown to correlate with survival in patients with end-stage liver disease. HVPG can be considered a reliable predictor of variceal hemorrhage, even by being monitored during the bleeding episode or serially measured during prophylactic and/or preventive pharmacologic therapy. Moreover, other frequent and serious clinical events in portal hypertensive cirrhotic patients can be reasonably predicted according to HVPG changes. Recently, HVPG has assumed an importance in preoperative assessment in cirrhosis, even though this prognostic value was derived from a specific situation, hepatic resection in early HCC. In summary, HVPG measurement, and its clinical applicability, have reached a point of experience and maturity, developed from a significant number of clinical trials and allied to deep self-criticisms, even by some of their more enthusiastic supporters[7,66,67].

So, without doubt, HVPG is a valuable tool in the clinical management of cirrhotic patients; therefore should we be more optimistic and expect a wider application and applicability of HVPG measurements? It appears so, as there is mounting evidence that HVPG may be a better prognostic marker than other currently available parameters. These data make both the technique and its results reliable enough for no longer considering it as something to be performed exclusively on research grounds. The available information indeed contains something having objective reality; and those are facts.

## Acknowledgements

This work was funded by the Veterans Administration Merit Review; Dr Juan G Abraldes received funding from the Fundacion Ramon Areces and Asociacion Española para el Estudio del Higado.

## References

1. Braillon A, Calès P, Valla D, Gaudy D, Geoffroy P, Lebrec D. Influenece of the degree of liver failure on systemic and splanchnic hemodynamics and on response to propranolol in patients with cirrhosis. Gut. 1986:27:1204–9.
2. Krogsgaard K, Gluud C, Henriksen JH, Christoffersen P. Correlation between liver morphology and portal pressure in alcoholic liver disease. Hepatology. 1984:4:699–703.
3. Picchiotti R, Mingazzini PL, Scucchi L et al. Correlations between sinusoidal pressure and liver morphology in cirrhosis. J Hepatol. 1994:20:364–9.
4. Hallion L, Francois-Frank CA. Recherches experimentales executees a l'aide d'um novel appareil volumetrique sur l'innervation vaso-motrice de l'intestin. Arch Physiol Norm Pathol. 1896:8:493–508.
5. Thompson WP, Caughey JL, Whipple AO et al. Splenic vein pressure and congestive splenomegaly (Banty's syndrome). J Clin Invest. 1937:16:571.
6. Myers JD, Taylor WJ. An estimation of PVP by occlusive catheterization of a hepatic venule. J Clin Invest.1951:30:662–3.

7. Groszmann RJ, Wongcharatrawee S. The hepatic venous pressure gradient: anything worth doing should be done right. Hepatology. 2004:39:280–2.
8. Groszmann RJ, Glickman MC, Blei AT, Storer E, Conn HO. Wedged and free hepatic venous pressure measured with a balloon catheter. Gastroenterology. 1979:76:253–8.
9. Bosch J, Mastai R, Kravetz D, Navasa M. Rodes J. Hemodynamic evaluation of patients with portal hypertension. Semin Liver Dis. 1986:6:309–17.
10. Seinlauf AF, García-Tsao G, Gupta T, Dickey K, Zakko MF, Groszmann RJ. Low-dose midazolam sedation: an option for patients undergoing serial hepatic venous pressure measurements. Hepatology. 1999:29:1070–3.
11. Groszmann RJ, de Franchis R. Portal hypertension. In: Schiff ER, Sorrell MF, Maddrey W, editors. Schiff's Diseases of the Liver. Philadelphia: Lippincott-Raven, 1999:387–442.
12. Boyer TD, Triger DR, Horisawa M, Redeker AG, Reynolds TB. Direct transhepatic measurement of portal vein pressure using a thin needle: comparison with wedged hepatic venous pressure. Gastroenterology. 1977:72:584–9.
13. Groszmann RJ, Atterbury CE. Clinical applications of the measurement of portal venous pressure. J Clin Gastroenterol. 1980:2:379–86.
14. Pomier-Layrargues G, Kusielewicz D, Willems B et al. Presinusoidal portal hypertension in non-alcoholic cirrhosis. Hepatology. 1985:5:415–18.
15. Perello A, Escorsell A, Bru C et al. Wedged hepatic venous pressure adequately reflects portal pressure in hepatitis C virus-related cirrhosis. Hepatology. 1999:30:1393–7.
16. Deplano A, Migaleddu V, Pischedda A et al. Portohepatic gradient and portal hemodynamics in patients with cirrhosis due to hepatitis C virus infection. Dig Dis Sci. 1999:44:155–62.
17. Loureiro-Silva MR, Cadelina GW, Groszmann RJ. Deficit in nitric oxide production in cirrhotic rat livers is located in the sinusoidal and postsinusoidal areas. Am J Physiol Gastrointest Liver Physiol. 2003:284:G567–74.
18. Infante-Rivard C, Esnaola S, Villeneuve JP. Clinical and statistical validity of conventional prognostic factors in predicting short-term survival among cirrhotics. Hepatology. 1987:7:660–4.
19. Arroyo V, Bosch J, Gaya-Beltran J et al. Plasma renin activity and urinary sodium excretion as prognostic indicators in nonazotemic cirrhosis with ascites. Ann Intern Med. 1981:94:198–201.
20. Vinel JP, Cassigneul J, Louis A, Levade M, Pascal JP. Clinical and prognostic significance of portohepatic gradient in patients with cirhosis. Surg Gynecol Obstet. 1982:155:347–52.
21. Vinel JP, Cassigneul J, Levade M, Voigt JJ, Pascal JP. Assessment of short-term prognosis after variceal bleeding in patients with alcoholic cirrhosis by early measurement of portohepatic gradient. Hepatology. 1986:6:116–17.
22. Gluud C, Henriksen JH, Nielsen G. Prognostic indicators in alcoholic cirrhotic men. Hepatology. 1988:8:222–7.
23. Tage-Jensen U, Henriksen JH, Christensen E, Widding A, Ring-Larsen H, Christensen NJ. Plasma catecholamine level and portal venous pressure as guides to prognosis in patients with cirrhosis. J Hepatol. 1988:6:350–8.
24. Groszmann RJ, Bosch J, Grace N et al. Hemodynamic events in a prospective randomized trial of propranolol versus placebo in the prevention of a first variceal hemorrhage. Gastroenterology. 1990:99:1401–7.
25. Merkel C, Bolognesi M, Bellon S et al. Prognostic usefulness of hepatic vein catheterization in patients with cirrhosis and esophageal varices. Gastroenterology. 1992:102:973–9.
26. Vorobioff J, Groszmann RJ, Picabea E et al. Prognostic value of hepatic venous pressure measurement in alcoholic cirrhosis: A ten year prospective study. Gastroenterology. 1996:111:701–9.
27. Villanueva C, Aracil C, Lopez-Balaguer JM, Balanzo J. Nadolol plus isosorbide mononitrate compared with sclerotherapy for the prevention of variceal rebleeding. N Engl J Med. 1996:334:1624–9.
28. Patch D, Armonis A, Sabin C et al. Single portal pressure measurement predicts survival in cirrhotic patients with recent bleeding. Gut. 1999:44:264–9.
29. Moitinho E, Escorsell A, Bandi JC et al. Prognostic value of early measurements of portal pressure in acute variceal bleeding. Gastroenterology. 1999:117:626–31.
30. Abraldes JG, Tarantino I, Turnes J Garcia-Pagan JC, Rodes J, Bosch J. Hemodynamic response to pharmacological treatment of portal hypertension and long-term prognosis of cirrhosis. Hepatology. 2003:37:902–8.

31. Urbain D, Muls V, Makhoul E, Jeghers O, Thys O, Ham HR. Prognostic significance of hepatic venous pressure gradient in medically treated alcoholic cirrhosis: comparison to aminopyrine breath test. Am J Gastroenterol. 1993:88:856–9.
32. Pomier-Layrargues G, Villeneuve JP, Willems B, Huet PM, Marleau D. Systemic and hepatic hemodynamics after variceal hemorrhage: effects of propranolol and placebo. Gastroenterology. 1987:93:1218–24.
33. Groszmann, RJ, Garcia-Tsao G, Makuch R et al. Multicenter randomized placebo-controlled trial of non-selective beta-blockers in the prevention of the complications of portal hypertension: final results and identification of a predictive factor. Hepatology. 2003:38 (Suppl. 1):206A (abstract).
34. García-Tsao G, Groszmann RJ, Fisher RL, Conn HO, Atterbury CE. Portal pressure, presence of gastroesophageal varices and variceal bleeding. Hepatology. 1985:5:419–24.
35. Rigau J, Bosch J, Bordas JM et al. Endoscopic measurement of variceal pressure in cirrhosis: correlation with portal pressure and variceal hemorrhage. Gastroenterology. 1989:96: 873–80.
36. Viallet A, Marleau D, Huet M et al. Hemodynamic evaluation of patients with intrahepatic portal hypertension. Relationship between bleeding varices and the portohepatic gradient. Gastroenterology. 1975:69:1297–300.
37. Christensen U, Sorensen TI, Jensen LI, Aagaard J, Burcharth F. The free portal pressure in awake patients with and without cirrhosis of the liver. Liver. 1983:3:147–50.
38. Viola C, Bosch J, Mastai R et al. Prognostic value of measurements of portal pressure in patients with cirrhosis. J Hepatol. 1987:5(Suppl. 1):S71 (abstract).
39. Vlavianos P, Gimson AES, Hayllar K et al. Prognostic significance of systemic and portal hemodynamic parameters in patients with cirrosis and previous variceal bleeding. Gut. 1990:31:A592 (abstract).
40. Lebrec D, De Fleury P, Rueff B, Nahum H, Benhamou JP. Portal hypertension, size of esophageal varices, and risk of gastrointestinal bleeding in alcoholic cirrhosis. Gastroenterology. 1980:79:1139–44.
41. Adamson RJ, Butt K, Dennis CR et al. Prognostic significance of portal pressure in patients with bleeding esophageal varices. Surg Gynecol Obstet. 1977:145:353–6.
42. Ready JB, Robertson AD, Goff JS, Rector WG Jr. Assessment of the risk of bleeding from esophageal varices by continuous monitoring of portal pressure. Gastroenterology. 1991:100:1403–10.
43. Westaby D, Polson RJ, Gimson AE, Hayes PC, Hayllar K, Williams R. A controlled trial of oral propranolol compared with injection sclerotherapy for the long-term management of variceal bleeding. Hepatology. 1990:11:353–9.
44. Villanueva C, Ortiz J, Miñana J et al. Somatostatin treatment and risk stratification by continuous portal pressure monitoring during acute variceal bleeding. Gastroenterology. 2001:121:110–17.
45. Leevy CM, Zinke M, Baber J, Chey WY. Observations on the influence of medical therapy on portal hypertension in hepatic cirrhosis. Ann Intern Med. 1958:49:837–51.
46. Reynolds TB, Geller HM, Kuzma OT, Redeker AG. Spontaneous decrease in portal pressure with clinical improvement in cirrhosis. N Engl J Med. 1960;263:734–9.
47. D'Amico G, García-Tsao G, Calès P et al. Diagnosis of portal hypertension. How and when? In: de Franchis R, editor. Portal Hypertension. III. Proceedings of the Third Baveno International Consensus Workshop on Definitions, Methodology and Therapeutic Strategies. Oxford: Blackwell Science, 2001:36–63.
48. Morali GA, Sniderman KW, Deitel KM et al. Is sinusoidal portal hypertension a necessary factor for the development of hepatic ascites? J Hepatol. 1992:16:249–50.
49. Rector WG Jr. Portal hypertension: a permissive factor only in the development of ascites and variceal bleeding. Liver. 1986:6:221–6.
50. Bosch J, Mastai R, Kravetz D, Navasa M, Rodes J. Hemodynamic evaluation of the patient with portal hypertension. Semin Liver Dis. 1986:6:309–17.
51. Feu F, García-Pagán JC, Bosch J et al. Relation between portal pressure response to pharmacotherapy and risk of recurrent variceal hemorrhage in patients with cirrhosis. Lancet. 1995:346:1056–9.
52. McCormick PA, Patch D, Greenslade L, Chin J, McIntyre N, Burroughs AK. Clinical vs hemodynamic response to drugs in portal hypertension. J Hepatol. 1998:28:1015–19.

53. Villanueva C, Minana J, Ortiz J et al. Endoscopic ligation compared with combined treatment with nadolol and isosorbide mononitrate to prevent recurrent variceal bleeding. N Engl J Med. 2001:345:647–55.
54. Merkel C, Bolognesi M, Sacerdoti D et al. The hemodynamic response to medical treatment of portal hypertension as a predictor of clinical effectiveness in the primary prophylaxis of variceal bleeding in cirrhosis. Hepatology. 2000:32:930–4.
55. Bureau C, Péron JM, Alric L et al. "A la carte" treatment of portal hypertension: adapting medical therapy to hemodynamic response for the prevention of bleeding. Hepatology. 2002:36:1361–6.
56. Patch D, Sabin CA, Goulis J et al. A randomized, controlled trial of medical therapy versus endoscopic ligation for the prevention of variceal rebleeding in patients with cirrhosis. Gastroenterology. 2002:123:1013–19.
57. Groszmann RJ, García-Tsao G. Endoscopic variceal banding vs pharmacological therapy for the prevention of recurrent variceal hemorrhage: what makes the difference? Gastroenterology. 2002:123:1388–91.
58. Burroughs AK, Groszmann RJ, Bosch J et al. Assessment of therapeutic benefit of antiviral therapy in chronic hepatitis C: is hepatic venous pressure a better end point? Gut. 2002:50:425–7.
59. Friedman LS, Maddrey WC. Surgery in the patient with liver disease. Med Clin N Am. 1987:71:453–76.
60. Bruix J, Castells A, Bosch J et al. Surgical resection of hepatocellular carcinoma in cirrhotic patients. Prognostic value of preoperative portal pressure. Gastroenterology. 1996: 111:1018–22.
61. Llovet JM, Fuster J, Bruix J. Intention-to-treat analysis of surgical treatment for early hepatocellular carcinoma: resection versus transplantation. Hepatology. 1999:30:1434–40.
62. Lovet JM, Bruix J, Fuster J et al. Liver transplantation for small hepatocellular carcinoma: the tumor–node–metastasis classification does not have prognosis power. Hepatology. 1998:27:1572–7.
63. Mazzaferro V, Regalia E, Doci R et al. Liver transplantation for the treatment of small hepatocellular carcinomas in patients with cirrhosis. N Engl J Med. 1996:334:693–9.
64. Bismuth H, Chiche L, Adam R, Castaing D, Diamond T, Dennison A. Liver resection versus transplantation for hepatocellular carcinoma in cirrhotic patients. Ann Surg. 1993: 218:145–51.
65. Groszmann RJ. The hepatic venous pressure gradient: has the time arrived for its application in clinical practice? Hepatology. 1996:24:739–41.
66. Thalheimer U, Mela M, Patch D, Burroughs AK. Monitoring target reduction in hepatic venous pressure gradient during pharmacological therapy of portal hypertension: a close look at the evidence. Gut. 2004:53:143–8.
67. Huet PM, Pomier-Layrargues G. The hepatic venous pressure gradient: "remixed and revisited". Hepatology. 2004:39:295–8.

# 33
# Hemodynamic monitoring: implications for randomized controlled trials and clinical practice

ULRICH THALHEIMER, DIMITRIOS SAMONAKIS,
CHRISTOS TRIANTOS, DAVID PATCH
and ANDREW K. BURROUGHS

## INTRODUCTION

Portal hypertension develops during the natural history of cirrhosis, and is responsible for its complications: the development of gastroesophageal varices and bleeding, ascites, hepatorenal syndrome and hepatic encephalopathy. The advent of these complications worsens prognosis as they are a major cause of death and their presence signals the need for liver transplantation in appropriate candidates. For many years the degree of portal hypertension has been recognized as an independent factor for survival in patients with cirrhosis[1]. Conversely, improvement of liver function in abstinent subjects with cirrhosis has been associated with a reduction in portal pressure[2]. Recently, reduction in portal pressure has been shown to result in a reduction of the complications of cirrhosis together with improved survival, although it is unclear if this was linked to an improvement in liver function[3,4]. Measurement of the hepatic venous pressure gradient (HVPG) is a widely used indirect method of assessing the portal pressure gradient, with wedge hepatic venous pressure reflecting values of portal pressure in cirrhosis with a predominantly sinusoidal site of resistance[5-7].

Clinically significant portal hypertension is defined[8] by a portal pressure gradient above about 12 mmHg, as the development of ascites and variceal bleeding usually occur above this threshold. Monitoring of HVPG has been increasingly used to assess target reductions of portal pressure during secondary and primary pharmacologic prophylaxis of variceal bleeding. A decrease of HVPG of $\geq 20\%$ from baseline[9-11] or to $\leq 12$ mmHg[9-12] is considered a favorable hemodynamic response to treatment, as it correlates with a significant reduction in bleeding. In addition, studies[13–15] have shown that cirrhotics who bleed have an HVPG of $\geq 12$ mmHg.

## PREVENTION OF VARICEAL BLEEDING

There have been five major studies[9–11,16,17] and one smaller series published as correspondence[18] in which the HVPG has been measured at baseline and at a subsequent time point (Table 1). Three of these studies are randomized controlled trials comparing pharmacologic prophylaxis with sclerotherapy[10] or endoscopic banding ligation for the prevention of variceal rebleeding[11,17]; two evaluate the prognostic value of HVPG monitoring in the setting of medical therapy for secondary prevention of variceal hemorrhage[9,16]. Three of these studies[9–11] are the ones usually quoted as evidence to justify a routine practice of HVPG monitoring during pharmacologic prevention of recurrent variceal bleeding. Two further studies[19,20] considered the importance of hemodynamic response to drug therapy for the prevention of variceal bleeding, but their study populations combine both patients with and without a history of prior variceal bleeding, making their interpretation very difficult due to the different response rates to pharmacologic prevention and bleeding risks[20,21] in primary and secondary prophylaxis which are not separated one from another in the results. The main data of the five studies are summarized in Tables 1–3 with additional data from our own study[17].

At first glance all five studies appear similar, but there are some marked differences between these investigations, making the hemodynamic data difficult to interpret. As a result, questions arise regarding their value as evidence to justify the clinical performance of HVPG monitoring[22].

The studies vary with regard to treatment used (only beta-blockers in one or combination therapy with nitrates in the remaining four), percentage of patients with alcoholic liver disease (from 50% to 70%), time of follow-up (from 8 to 28 months), percentage of patients in Child class C (from 6% to 47%) and especially in the interval of time after which the second HVPG measurement was performed (Table 2): indeed, this time interval varied as widely as a mean of 57 days[17] to 5.3 months[16] (Table 2). Furthermore, there are several specific issues which complicate the interpretation of the hemodynamic data.

First, the hemodynamic response in these studies is defined as either an HVPG decrease of $\geq 20\%$ from baseline or a decrease to $\leq 12$ mmHg. However, there is overlap so that some patients who achieved a $\geq 20\%$ decrease from baseline also had a final HVPG of $\leq 12$ mmHg; patients with such an overlap had a lower baseline HVPG. Indeed, in the only studies that report the data, 32%[9] to 57%[10] of hemodynamic responders achieved both criteria and 62% of patients with a $\geq 20\%$ decrease also decreased their HVPG to $\leq 12$ mmHg[10]. Thus it is unclear whether the $\geq 20\%$ decrease is *per se* a valid therapeutic target, if an absolute reduction to $\leq 12$ mmHg is not achieved. Unfortunately one cannot derive these data from the published papers.

Second, the determination of the prognostic value of HVPG monitoring is flawed by the fact that, in a percentage ranging from 17%[9] to 65%[17], the

**Table 1.** The key studies of repeated HVPG measurement in the prevention of variceal rebleeding: total populations and hemodynamic responders (absolute numbers of patients in parentheses)

| | Author | | | | |
|---|---|---|---|---|---|
| | Feu[9] | Villanueva[10] | McCormick[16] | Villanueva[11] | Patch[17] |
| Total number of patients | 83 | 43[a] | 63 | 72[b] | 51[c] |
| % of patients with baseline HVPG measured | 83% (69) | 100% (43) | 89% (56) | 100% (72) | 78% (40) |
| % of patients with remeasurement of HVPG | 83% (69) | 72% (31) | 71% (45)[d] | 68% (49) | 35% (18) |
| Hemodynamic responders | 36% (25) | 45% (14) | 64% (28) | 51% (25) | 50% (9) |
| % of patients with repeat HVPG $\leq 12$ mmHg | 12% (8) | 29% (9) | 48% (21) | 14% (7) | 9% (2) |
| Mortality in patients with baseline HVPG measurement | 13% (9) | 9% (4) | n/a | 32% (23) | 33% (17) |

[a] Initial cohort 121 patients, 86 of whom were included (43 for each treatment arm).

[b] Initial cohort 233 patients, 144 of whom were included (72 for each treatment arm).

[c] Initial cohort 205 patients, 102 of whom were included (51 for each treatment arm).

[d] Only 44 patients included in the study (1 patient excluded because of low initial and repeat HVPG (7 mmHg))

**Table 2.** The key studies of repeated HVPG measurement in the prevention of variceal rebleeding: baseline characteristics, time to remeasurement and length of follow-up

| | Author | | | | |
|---|---|---|---|---|---|
| | Feu[9] | Villanueva[10] | McCormick[16] | Villanueva[11] | Patch[17] |
| Time of, or mean interval to, remeasurement (months) | 3 | 3–4 | 5.3 | 1–3 | 2 |
| Child class C | 6% (4) | 16% (7) | 6% (4) | 19% (14) | 47% (24) |
| Alcoholic etiology | 59% (41) | 51% (25) | 70% (31) | 50% (43) | 63% (32) |
| Follow-up in months (range) | 28[b] (1–69) | 18[b] (4–36) | 22 responders[b] 26 nonresponders[b] (0.1–60) | 20[a] (1–65) | 8[a] (0.25–46) |
| Patients with nitrates | 0 | 100% (43) | 68% (30) | 100% (72) | 41% (22) |
| Baseline HVPG | 18.3±3.6 | 17.7±3.4 | 17.5±0.6 responders 18±1.0 nonresponders | 19.9±3.5 | 18.3±4.9 |

[a]Median; [b]mean.

326

**Table 3.** Patients rebleeding in the key study populations of repeated HVPG measurement in the pharmacological prevention of variceal rebleeding (absolute numbers in parentheses)

| | Author | | | | |
|---|---|---|---|---|---|
| | Feu[9] | Villanueva[10] | McCormick[16] | Villanueva[11] | Patch[17] |
| Total number of patients | 83 | 43[a] | 63 | 72[b] | 51[c] |
| HVPG not measured | 17% (14) | 0% | 11% (7) | 0% | 22% (11) |
| HVPG not remeasured | 17% (14) | 28% (12) | 17% (11)[d] | 33% (23) | 65% (33) |
| Rebleeding in non-remeasured | 64% (9/14) | 17% (2/12) | 28% (5/18)[e] | 17% (4/23) | 33% (11/33) |
| Rebleeding (patient groups) | | | | | |
| Total | 36% (25/69) | 26% (11/43) | 37% (16/44) | 33% (24/72) | 37% (19/51) |
| Hemodynamic responders | 8% (2/25) | 7% (1/14) | 43% (12/28) | 16% (4/25) | 11% (1/9) |
| Hemodynamic non-responders | 52% (23/44) | 47% (8/17) | 25% (4/16) | 67% (16/24) | 22% (2/9) |
| Repeat HVPG ≥ 12 mmHg | 0% (0/8) | 0% (0/9) | 30% (7/23) | ? (?/7) | 50% (1/2) |
| Rebleeding before remeasurement | 7% (5/69) | Some[f] | 16% (7/44) | Some[f] | 22% (5/23) |

[a] Initial cohort 121 patients, 86 of whom were included (43 for each treatment arm).
[b] Initial cohort 233 patients, 144 of whom were included (72 for each treatment arm).
[c] Initial cohort 205 patients, 102 of whom were included (51 for each treatment arm).
[d] Only 44 patients included in the study (one patient excluded because of low initial and repeat HVPG (7 mmHg)).
[e] Rebleeding rate in both non-measured and non-remeasured patients (rebleeding occurred in two of seven patients who did not have their baseline HVPG measured and in three of 11 patients who did not have a repeat HVPG measurement).
[f] Number not stated (in the second study (ref. 4) it can be derived that this number must be between 1 and 4).

responder/non-responder status could not be assessed as the HVPG was not measured and/or remeasured (Table 3). One would expect this group to be composed of both potential responders and non-responders, and hence to have a rebleeding rate intermediate to both groups. However, the rebleeding rate in these patients varies widely, from 17%[10,11] to 64%[9] (Table 3). Thus, the rebleeding rate when HVPG was not measured or remeasured was similar to the responder group in Villanueva et al.'s second study (17% vs 16%)[11], and is higher than in the non-responder group in the original study by Feu et al. (64% vs 52%)[9]. This omission represents an important source of bias, and one explanation for the heterogeneity of the results among the different studies.

One reason why remeasurement of HVPG could not take place was that some patients rebled before the scheduled repeated measurement. This percentage varied from 7%[8] to 22%[17]. In the cohort studied by Feu et al.[9], remeasurement was at 3 months, so the rebleeding rate was low during this interval, suggesting a selection of patients with better risk in terms of rebleeding. Conversely, the highest percentage of rebleeding before remeasurement, probably due to the high percentage of Child class C patients, occurred in the study in which HVPG was remeasured soonest (median of 49 days)[17]. These patients are those at greatest risk of rebleeding; if they are excluded from HVPG monitoring, then the value of this approach is greatly reduced and less applicable. The influence of timing of remeasurement has now been accepted as being clinically relevant. Whereas the initial interval used to recommend remeasurement of HVPG was 3 months[9] (with only 7% rebleeding in this interval), the same group now suggests 2 weeks[23]. However, this recommendation has not been tested prospectively. Furthermore, the interval to remeasurement is not only an issue with regard to the proportion of patients rebleeding before a second HVPG measurement, but also with regard to the spontaneous reduction of HVPG[2,12].

## CHRONIC LIVER DISEASE DUE TO HEPATITIS C VIRUS AND ASSESSMENT OF FIBROSIS

Studies of antiviral therapy for chronic hepatitis C have shown that a sustained biochemical or virologic response is associated with a significant decrease in inflammation and more importantly in fibrosis[24-27]. However, histologic response to treatment can be partly independent of biochemical and sustained virologic responses, so that continuing treatment for long periods in biochemical non-responders can improve both grading and staging of liver histology. This could be related to the antifibrogenic and anti-inflammatory effect of interferon[25-35].

However, there are several important limitations and sources of bias which prevent an accurate and reliable evaluation of the histologic benefit of antiviral therapy for chronic hepatitis C. There are inconsistencies in the definition of pathologic features, processing of specimens, sampling errors, and intra/interobserver variability, so that changes in liver histology are not precise quantitative estimates[36]. There is no firm evidence that fibrosis is regularly distributed throughout the liver[35,37-39], thus the usual right-sided biopsy may not be representative of "true" fibrosis.

Although changes in histologic fibrosis can be considered the closest to "the true endpoints" of liver-related morbidity and mortality, obtaining reliable information from biopsies may be difficult and therefore it will be of fundamental importance to look for additional parameters that can be measured more quantitatively and accurately[40].

Measurement of portal pressure may represent this important parameter. Portal hypertension is the most common and lethal complication of chronic and progressive liver disease. Portal pressure has been shown by several studies to be an independent prognostic variable in cirrhotic patients[1]. Once a patient develops portal hypertension this becomes the pacemaker marking the progression of liver disease.

Thus changes in HVPG can be considered as an adjunctive endpoint for the therapeutic evaluation of antiviral therapy for chronic hepatitis C[40]. Picchiotti et al.[41] found that there is an association between the severity of the piecemeal necrosis and sinusoidal pressure, and Nagula et al.[42] found that, in patients with cirrhotic liver biopsies, a significant relationship exists between HVPG and a combination of small nodularity and increasing thickness of fibrous septae. Van Leeuwen et al. found that WHVP increased with histologic progression of chronic hepatitis, and that portal hypertension was present before histologically detectable cirrhosis developed (the increase in HVPG reflecting an increase in intrahepatic vascular resistance)[43].

Thus serial HVPG measurements may be the best way to evaluate response to therapy in chronic hepatitis C, particularly in later stages (III and IV) when fibrous deposition is significant. Two studies have reported results of HVPG measurements in patients with chronic hepatitis C before and after treatment with interferon, finding a greater percentage change in the interferon-treated group compared with the placebo group[44,45].

Current unpublished data in our unit show that HVPG correlates well with the progression of fibrosis but not with the grade of inflammation, after liver transplantation for HCV cirrhosis, possibly providing a reliable prognostic parameter and adding another index of histologic progression for recurrent HCV infection.

The same issues can be valid for the assessment of fibrosis in general, for which HVPG would be an indirect marker of progression or improvement. Given that fibrosis markers are as yet not sufficiently predictive[46], the addition of HVPG should be assessed prospectively in trials of antifibrotic therapy. This would also enable liver biopsy to be performed at the same time by the transjugular route. Its advantage is that multiple cores of liver tissue can be taken at the same time to minimize sampling issues[39].

## PORTAL PRESSURE AND PROGNOSIS

In clinical practice the prognosis of cirrhosis is usually assessed by the Child–Pugh classification or its modifications. This classification is based on clinical and biochemical criteria and has a sensitivity and a specificity of approximately 80%[47]. In recent years greater accuracy of assessment of prognosis has become important with the increasing use of liver transplantation. Many studies have evaluated quantitative liver function tests but these have not conclusively been shown to be better than Child–Pugh's classification in comparative studies[48]; and neither has the more recent MELD classification[49]. HVPG measurement has not received the same attention, although Armonis et al. have reviewed several studies of HVPG measurement for the assessment of prognosis in cirrhotic patients (Table 4)[1]. The vast majority of the patients included in these studies were alcoholics, and all studies except one concluded that the prediction of survival in cirrhosis based on conventional evaluation was significantly improved by information obtained from hepatic vein catheterization[1].

Since then only one study has failed to show that HVPG measurement was helpful in the prognostic assessment, this in a group of patients with alcoholic cirrhosis[50], but many patients were already in an advanced phase of cirrhosis (48% with Child grade C) and a considerable proportion of them (46%) also had alcoholic hepatitis. No data are available on how many of these patients were abstinent or became abstinent, as abstinence from alcohol has been shown to decrease portal pressure[2].

It has been suggested that portal pressure monitoring with serial measurements may offer better prognostic information than a single measurement. Groszmann et al.[12] showed that patients who had a spontaneous or pharmacologic reduction of HVPG to less than 12 mmHg had a significantly better survival than those who had not. Another study[2] confirmed this finding in 30 patients with alcoholic cirrhosis, as it was shown that the cumulative probability of survival was higher in patients whose HVPG values decreased spontaneously during the follow-up by more than 15% of the baseline values.

A recent study found that, in 73 cirrhotic patients receiving pharmacologic treatment for prevention of variceal bleeding, a decrease in HVPG $\geq 20\%$ or to $\leq 12$ mmHg was associated with a marked reduction in the long-term risk of developing complications of portal hypertension (such as variceal bleeding, ascites, spontaneous bacterial peritonitis, hepatorenal syndrome and hepatic encephalopathy) and with improved survival[3]. Importantly, the degree of liver dysfunction was also associated with the advent of these complications, but it is not clear whether the patients with a hemodynamic response also had an improvement in liver function, thus explaining the improved outcome. Another recent study also showed that hemodynamic response to treatment of portal hypertension, besides being usually sustained after a long-term follow-up, decreases the probability of developing complications of cirrhosis and the need for liver transplantation, and significantly improves survival[4]; however, in this study there was a greater improvement in the Child–Pugh score in the responder group. Thus the question arises whether HVPG may be an independent prognostic factor or whether it is linked to liver function. Another issue arising from this last study is whether propranolol treatment should be advocated for all cirrhotic patients irrespective of a history of bleeding, if it does reduce morbidity and mortality in patients with a hemodynamic response, irrespective of an improvement in liver function. If this were true, propranolol could become the "aspirin" of hepatologic therapeutics.

**Table 4.** Summary of studies evaluating the usefulness of portal pressure measurements in the prediction of survival (modified from ref. 1)

| Reference | No. of patients | No. of patients with alcoholic cirrhosis (%) | No. of patients with variceal bleeding (%) | Follow-up (months) | Statistical method | p-Value |
|---|---|---|---|---|---|---|
| Arroyo 1981 | 31 | n.s. | 0 | $10^d$ | Student's $t$ test | <0.05 |
| Vinel 1982 | 89 | 89 (100%) | n.s. | <36 | Student's $t$ test | <0.05 |
| Vinel 1986 | 72 | 72 (100%) | 72 (100%)[a] | $1^d$ | Student's $t$ test | <0.025 |
| Viola 1987 | 290 | 194 (67%) | 148 (51%) | n.s. | Cox' regression | <0.05 |
| Gluud 1988 | 53 | 53 (100%) | 13 (24%) | $31^b$ | Cox's regression | <0.005 |
| Tage-Jensen 1988 | 81 | 81 (100%) | 24 (30%) | 42–96 | Cox' regression | <0.005 |
| Groszmann 1990 | 84 | 64 (76%) | 0 | $16.3 \pm 12^c$ | Linear regression | <0.05 |
| Barrett 1990 | 101 | 78 (77%) | 0 | $32.4 \pm 20.4^c$ | Cox's regression | <0.001 |
| Merkel 1992 | 129 | 92 (71%) | 14 (11%) | $45^a$ | Multiple regression | <0.001 |
| Urbain 1993 | 99 | 99 (100%) | n.s. | >48, <72 | Log-rank test | >0.05 |
| Vorobioff 1996 | 30 | 30 (100%) | 0 | $42 \pm 25^c$ | Cox's regression | <0.05 |
| Deltenre 2002 | 87 | 87 (100%) | 36 (41%) | $35 \pm 29$ | Cox's regression | >0.05 |

n.s., Not stated.
[a] Patients with acute variceal bleeding.
[b] Median.
[c] Mean ± SD.
[d] Total.

## CONCLUSIONS

There is no doubt that pharmacologic therapy of portal hypertension using non-selective beta-blockers is effective in reducing bleeding rates in both primary and secondary prophylaxis, and is at least equivalent to banding ligation for secondary prevention of variceal bleeding[11,17]. Whilst an absolute reduction of HVPG to 12 mmHg confers near-complete protection against bleeding, this is a rare event, and only constitutes a median of 14% of the cohorts in the five studies in which HVPG was measured (Table 1). When considering the target of $\geq 20\%$ reduction there are currently too many difficulties in interpreting its clinical validity from published work, to recommend routine measurement of HVPG for this purpose.

Instituting monitoring of target HVPG reductions instead of the empirical use of propranolol (which is the second cheapest generic drug worldwide after aspirin) would increase the cost of medical therapy for portal hypertension. Its use needs to be substantiated by solid evidence, demonstrating both better therapeutic efficacy and clinical applicability. Monitoring of HVPG used as a splanchnic sphygmomanometer[1] needs to be assessed in a new prospective study in secondary prophylaxis remeasuring HVPG at 2 weeks from bleeding, and randomizing to a change of therapy or no modification, if target reductions of HVPG have not been achieved. In addition changes in liver function need to be assessed during follow-up in order to explore the interaction of liver function with HVPG.

Chronic hepatitis C is a major health-care problem, and response to antiviral therapy has previously been defined biochemically and by virologic response. However, changes in the HVPG could be considered as an adjunctive endpoint for the therapeutic evaluation of antiviral therapy in chronic hepatitis C. It is a validated technique which is safe, well tolerated, well established, and reproducible. Serial HVPG measurements may be the best way to evaluate response to therapy in chronic hepatitis C[40]. In the future it is likely that a panel of fibrosis markers will be used, and portal pressure measurement will be the important link prognostically between histology and serum markers of fibrosis. In order to test this, therapeutic trials should evaluate HVPG combined with transjugular liver biopsy before and after treatment. In patients with normal HVPG, maintaining a normal pressure should be a sign of good prognosis, and in those in whom it becomes normal it should also be a good prognostic sign. In virologic non-responders it is not known whether a liver biopsy after treatment is appropriate to evaluate therapeutic benefit following antiviral therapy, and in cirrhotics it is not clear what should be measured to assess long-term response. In these two groups, HVPG measurement could be particularly useful[40].

Information obtained from hepatic vein catheterization has significant prognostic value in predicting survival. Most of the published studies, especially those that used Cox's regression analysis, have found that the prediction of survival based on a conventional Child–Pugh score is improved significantly by adding the information regarding the level of portal pressure, as it is a statistically independent prognostic variable[1]. As pharmacologic reduction of portal pressure may decrease the risk of the complications of portal

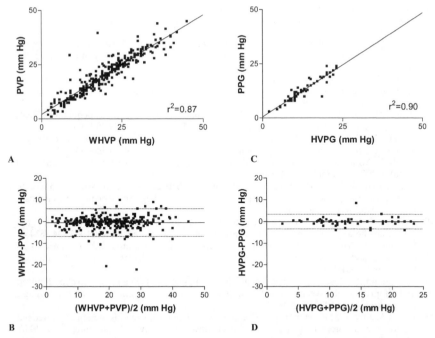

**Figure 1.** Correlation between portal vein pressure and wedged hepatic vein pressure and HVPG and portal pressure gradient in the 11 published studies ($n = 320$ patients). Panels **A** and **B**, correlation; panels **C** and **D**, agreement between measurements according to Altman and Bland[51]

hypertension, and improve survival[3], independent of a concomitant improvement of liver function, measurement of portal pressure becomes clinically very relevant.

In conclusion, HVPG measurement must be considered as the current method of choice in assessing portal pressure in cirrhotic patients (Figure 1). While its role in the management of pharmacologic prevention of variceal rebleeding has to be better defined, it is a valid and useful tool for assessing prognosis in chronic liver disease. Potentially it could be an adjunctive tool to assess histologic and clinical improvement due to antiviral therapy for chronic HCV disease, as well as for the assessment of antifibrotic therapy. Measurement of portal pressure should be more widely used in the clinical practice of hepatology.

## References

1. Armonis A, Patch D, Burroughs AK. Hepatic venous pressure measurement: an old test as a new prognostic marker in cirrhosis? Hepatology. 1997;25:245–8.
2. Vorobioff J, Groszmann RJ, Pibacea E et al. Prognostic value of hepatic venous pressure gradient measurements in alcoholic cirrhosis: a 10-year prospective study. Gastroenterology. 1996;111:701–9.

3. Abraldes JG, Tarantino I, Turnes J et al. Hemodynamic response to pharmacological treatment of portal hypertension and long-term prognosis of cirrhosis. Hepatology. 2003; 37:902–8.
4. Villanueva C, López-Balaguer JM, Aracil C et al. Maintenance of hemodynamic response to treatment for portal hypertension and influence on complications of cirrhosis. J Hepatol. 2004 (In press).
5. Boyer TD, Triger DR, Horisawa M et al. Direct transhepatic measurement of portal vein pressure using a thin needle. Comparison with wedged hepatic vein pressure. Gastroenterology. 1977;72:584–9.
6. Perelló A, Escorsell A, Bru C et al. Wedged hepatic venous pressure adequately reflects portal pressure in hepatitis C virus-related cirrhosis. Hepatology. 1999;30:1393–7.
7. Lin HC, Tsai YT, Lee FY et al. Comparison between portal vein pressure and wedged hepatic vein pressure in hepatitis B-related cirrhosis. J Hepatol. 1989;9:326–30.
8. Bosch J, Abraldes JG, Groszmann R. Current management of portal hypertension. J Hepatol. 2003;38(Suppl. 1):S54–68.
9. Feu F, Garcia-Pagan JC, Bosch J et al. Relation between portal pressure response to pharmacotherapy and risk of recurrent variceal haemorrhage in patients with cirrhosis. Lancet. 1995;346:1056–9.
10. Villanueva C, Balanzo J, Novella MT et al. Nadolol plus isosorbide mononitrate compared with sclerotherapy for the prevention of variceal rebleeding. N Engl J Med. 1996;334:1624–9.
11. Villanueva C, Minana J, Ortiz J et al. Endoscopic ligation compared with combined treatment with nadolol and isosorbide mononitrate to prevent recurrent variceal bleeding. N Engl J Med. 2001;345:647–55.
12. Groszmann RJ, Bosch J, Grace ND et al. Hemodynamic events in a prospective randomized trial of propranolol versus placebo in the prevention of a first variceal hemorrhage. Gastroenterology. 1990;99:1401–7.
13. Viallet A, Joly JG, Marleau D et al. Comparison of free portal venous pressure and wedged hepatic venous pressure in patients with cirrhosis of the liver. Gastroenterology. 1970; 59:372–5.
14. Lebrec D, De Fleury P, Rueff B et al. Portal hypertension, size of esophageal varices, and risk of gastrointestinal bleeding in alcoholic cirrhosis. Gastroenterology. 1980;79:1139–44.
15. Garcia-Tsao G, Groszmann RJ, Fisher RL et al. Portal pressure, presence of gastroesophageal varices and variceal bleeding. Hepatology. 1985;5:419–24.
16. McCormick PA, Patch D, Greenslade L et al. Clinical vs hemodynamic response to drugs in portal hypertension. J Hepatol. 1998;28:1015–19.
17. Patch D, Sabin CA, Goulis J et al. A randomized, controlled trial of medical therapy versus endoscopic ligation for the prevention of variceal rebleeding in patients with cirrhosis. Gastroenterology. 2002;123:1013–19.
18. Sacerdoti D, Merkel C, Gatta A. Importance of the 1-month-effect of nadolol on portal pressure in predicting failure of prevention of rebleeding in cirrhosis [Letter]. J Hepatol. 1991;12:124–5.
19. Escorsell A, Bordas JM, Castañeda B et al. Predictive value of the variceal pressure response to continued pharmacological therapy in patients with cirrhosis and portal hypertension. Hepatology. 2000;31:1061–7.
20. Bureau C, Péron JM, Alric L et al. "A la carte" treatment of portal hypertension: adapting medical therapy to hemodynamic response for the prevention of bleeding. Hepatology. 2002;36:1361–6.
21. De BK, Sen S, Biswas PK et al. Propranolol in primary and secondary prophylaxis of variceal bleeding among cirrhotics in India: a hemodynamic evaluation. Am J Gastroenterol. 2000;95:2023–8.
22. Thalheimer U, Mela M, Patch D et al. Targeting portal pressure measurements: a critical reappraisal. Hepatology. 2004;39:286–90.
23. Bosch J, García-Pagán JC. Prevention of variceal rebleeding. Lancet. 2003;361:952–4.
24. Marcellin P. Interferon alfa for chronic hepatitis C: how do we define cure? Hepatology. 1998;115:501–3.
25. Poynard T, Leroy V, Cohard M et al. Meta-analysis of interferon randomized trials in the treatment of viral hepatitis C: effects of dose and duration. Hepatology. 1996;24:778–89.
26. Grossman HJ, White D, Grossman VL et al. Effect of interferon gamma on intrahepatic haemodynamics of the cirrhotic rat liver. J Gastroenterol Hepatol. 1998;13:1058–60.

27. Sobesky R, Mathurin P, Charlotte F et al. Modeling the impact of interferon alfa treatment on liver fibrosis progression in chronic hepatitis C: a dynamic view. Gastroenterology. 1999;116:378–86.
28. Shiffman M, Hoffmann CM, Thomson EB et al. Relationship between biochemical, virological, and histological response during interferon treatment of chronic hepatitis C. Hepatology. 1997;26:780–5.
29. Baron S, Tyring S, Fleischmann RW et al. The interferons. Mechanisms of action and clinical applications. J Am Med Assoc. 1991;266:1375–83.
30. Camps J, Castilla A, Ruiz J et al. Randomized trial of lymphoblastoid α-interferon in chronic hepatitis C. Effects on inflammation, fibrinogenesis and viremia. J Hepatol. 1993;17:390–6.
31. Capra F, Casaril M, Gabrielli GB et al. α-Interferon in the treatment of chronic viral hepatitis: effects on fibrogenesis serum markers. J Hepatol. 1993;18:112–18.
32. Castilla A, Prieto J, Fausto N. Transforming growth factors beta 1 and alpha in chronic liver disease. Effects on interferon alpha therapy. N Engl J Med. 1991;324:933–40.
33. Hiramatsu N, Hayashi N, Kashara A et al. Improvement of liver fibrosis in chronic hepatitis C patients treated with natural interferon alfa. J Hepatol. 1995;22:135–42.
34. Manabe N, Chevallier M, Chossegros P et al. Interferon-α-2beta therapy reduces liver fibrosis in chronic non-a, non-b hepatitis: a quantitative histological evaluation. Hepatology. 1993;18:1344–9.
35. Hubscher S. Histological grading and staging in chronic hepatitis: clinical applications and problems. J Hepatol. 1998;29:1015–22.
36. Camma C, Giunta M, Linea C et al. The effect of interferon on the liver in chronic hepatitis C: a quantitative evaluation of histology by meta-analysis. J Hepatol. 1997;26:1187–99.
37. Feldman G. Critical analysis of methods used to morphologically quantify hepatic fibrosis. J Hepatol. 1995;22(Suppl. 2):49–54.
38. Bedossa P, Dargère D, Paradis V. Sampling variability of liver fibrosis in chronic hepatitis C. Hepatology. 2003;38:1449–57.
39. Scheuer PJ. Liver biopsy size matters in chronic hepatitis: bigger is better. Hepatology. 2003;38:1356–8.
40. Burroughs AK, Groszmann R, Bosch J et al. Assessment of therapeutic benefit of antiviral therapy in chronic hepatitis C: is hepatic venous pressure gradient a better end point? Gut. 2002;50:425–7.
41. Pichiotti R, Mingazzini PL, Scucchi L et al. Correlations between sinusoidal pressure and liver morphology in cirrhosis. J Hepatol. 1994:20:364–9.
42. Nagula S, Dhanpat J, Groszmann R et al. Histologic–hemodynamic correlations in hepatitis C and other chronic liver diseases – is there a histologically mild and severe cirrhosis? Hepatology. 2003;38(Suppl.):553A.
43. Van Leeuwen DJ, Howe DJ, Scheuer PJ et al. Wedged hepatic venous pressure recording and venography for the assessment of pre-cirrhotic and cirrhotic liver disease. Scand J Gastroenterol. 1989;24:65–73.
44. Garcia-Tsao G, Rodriguez-Perez F, Blei AT et al. Treatment with interferon reduces portal pressure in patients with chronic hepatitis C. A randomized placebo trial. Gastroenterology. 1996;10:A1193.
45. Valla DC, Chevallier M, Marcellin P et al. Treatment of hepatitis C-related cirrhosis: a randomized controlled trial of interferon alfa-2b versus no treatment. Hepatology. 1999;29:1870–5.
46. Rosenberg WMC. Rating fibrosis progression in chronic liver diseases. J Hepatol. 2003;38:357–60.
47. Infante C, Esnaola S, Villeneuve JP et al. Clinical and statistical validity of conventional prognostic factors in predicting short term survival among cirrhotics. Hepatology. 1987;7:660–4.
48. Reichen J. MEGX test in hepatology: the long-sought ultimate quantitative liver function test? J Hepatol. 1993;19:4–7.
49. Hayashi PH, Forman L, Steinberg T et al. Model for End-Stage Liver Disease score does not predict patient or graft survival in living donor liver transplant recipients. Liver Transplant. 2003;9:737–40.

50. Deltenre P, Rufat P, Hillaire S et al. Lack of prognostic usefulness of hepatic venous pressures and hemodynamic values in a select group of patients with severe alcoholic cirrhosis. Am J Gastroenterol. 2002;97:1187–90.
51. Bland JM, Altman DG. Statistical methods for assessing agreement between two methods of clinical measurement. Lancet. 1986;1:307–10.

# 34
# What to do with non-responders

CÀNDID VILLANUEVA, CARLES ARACIL
and JOAQUIM BALANZÓ

## INTRODUCTION

Hemodynamic monitoring provides an accurate stratification of bleeding risk and may enable tailoring of therapy[1]. This may be particularly useful in the prevention of rebleeding, when the risk is much higher than in primary prevention[2].

## CLINICAL IMPLICATIONS OF HEMODYNAMIC MONITORING

A reduction in the hepatic venous pressure gradient (HVPG) below 12 mmHg, or by more than 20% from the baseline value, is currently used to define an adequate response[3,4]. A decrease of HVPG to values below the threshold level of 12 mmHg confers near-complete protection against the risk of bleeding[3–5]; however, such a decrease occurs in only a minority of cases. In patients without previous bleeding a spontaneous HVPG decrease below this threshold occurs in 16–18% of cases[3,6], and has been related to an improvement in liver function induced by alcohol abstinence or other factors[3,6]. Such a spontaneous HVPG decrease has been noted in only 2–6% of patients with a previous bleeding[7,8]. Treatment with β-blockers provides an HVPG reduction below 12 mmHg in 12% of patients treated to prevent rebleeding[4], and in 20–30% of those in primary prophylaxis[3,9]. Even when this target is not reached, a substantial decrease in HVPG of at least 20% from the baseline value also provides a significant reduction in the risk of variceal hemorrhage to below 10%[4].

The risk of variceal bleeding in responders is comparable to that in patients treated with surgical shunts or with transjugular intrahepatic porto-systemic shunt (TIPS) (Figure 1)[1]. Hemodynamic response is also associated with a significant reduction in the probability of developing other complications related to portal hypertension, such as ascites and related conditions[8,10,11]. Furthermore, responders have a significant improvement in liver function, as well as a lower risk of developing encephalopathy[10,11], and

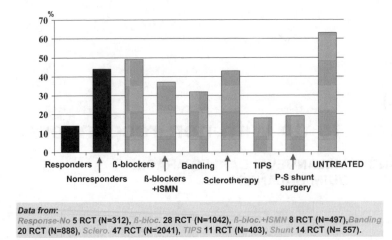

**Figure 1.** Rebleeding rates achieved with different available therapies and those observed in responders and non-responders. The bars represent the pooled means obtained in randomized controlled trials (data from refs 18, 34, 63, 64, 67)

requiring liver transplantation[11]. It should also be emphasized that survival is improved in responders[8,10,11].

## CURRENTLY USED TREATMENTS FOR PORTAL HYPERTENSION. RELATIONSHIP WITH HEMODYNAMIC RESPONSE

Until recently, long-term pharmacologic therapy of portal hypertension was based on the use of non-selective β-blockers which reduce portal pressure by decreasing portal venous inflow[12]. However, the effect of these drugs on portal pressure may be hindered due to an increase in portocollateral and intrahepatic resistance[13]. The association of nitrates may avoid this effect, enhancing the portal hypotensive effect achieved with β-blockers alone[14,15].

At present non-selective β-blockers are the treatment of choice to prevent a first variceal bleeding[16]. β-Blockers alone, or combined with isosorbide mononitrate (ISMN), may be considered as a first-line treatment option to prevent variceal rebleeding[16–18].

### β-Blockers

A major drawback of β-blockers is that 15–20% of patients have contraindications or develop severe side-effects that preclude their use[19]. Another problem is that the risk of bleeding is not abolished, particularly in secondary prophylaxis, a setting in which rebleeding rates of up to 50% are observed with β-blockers[18]. This may be due to the fact that as many as 60–70% of patients are non-responders to this treatment[4,20–23].

It has been shown that rescue therapies do not further decrease portal pressure in responders to β-blockers alone[24,25]; this suggests that no additional treatment is required in responders to β-blockers.

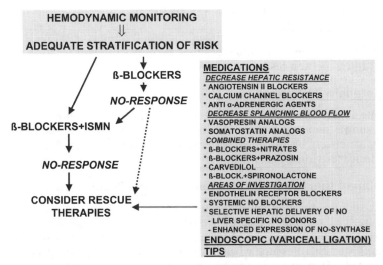

**Figure 2.** Rescue therapies to consider in non-responders. The combination of β-blockers and ISMN should be considered in non-responders to β-blockers alone; however, which treatment may effectively rescue non-responders to this combination should be assessed in randomized controlled trials

## Combination of β-blockers and nitrates

The association of ISMN and β-blockers has yielded a greater reduction in portal pressure than with β-blockers alone[14,15,24], significantly increasing the rate of responders to 40–50% of cases[7,8,14,15,24,25]. Furthermore, this combination does not produce any deleterious effects on renal function or sodium handling[26,27].

For the prevention of variceal rebleeding, combined therapy with β-blockers and ISMN has been compared with β-blockers alone[28,29], with sclerotherapy[7], with variceal ligation[8,30,31], and with shunt surgery[32], showing similar or better efficacy. Based on the results of these trials it has been recommended to use hemodynamic monitoring and to add ISMN in non-responders to β-blockers alone[1]. Such an approach has been supported by the results of a recent study[33]. An alternative strategy consists of using combined therapy with β-blockers and ISMN for the prevention of rebleeding in all patients. This may be supported by the efficacy and safety of such treatment and by the high risk of further hemorrhage in this setting. Hemodynamic monitoring to identify non-responders to this combined therapy will provide prognostic information[10,11]; however, the rescue therapy to be used is at present a matter under investigation (Figure 2)[34].

For the prevention of first bleeding, available evidence does not support the use of β-blockers plus ISMN instead of β-blockers alone[18,19]. This may be because the low residual risk of first hemorrhage achieved with β-blockers makes it difficult to demonstrate any hypothetical improvement[35]. Whether or not the association ISMN may be valuable for the high-risk subset of patients who do not respond to β-blockers alone remains to be clarified.

## PHARMACOLOGIC OPTIONS TO RESCUE NON-RESPONDERS

Several medications used either as single therapy or in combination may be useful to rescue non-responders.

### Angiotensin II blockers

Despite initial expectations from uncontrolled studies[36], subsequent trials have shown that angiotensin II blockade with losartan or irbesartan has negligible effects on portal hypertension, but induces arterial hypotension and decreases glomerular filtration rate[37-39].

### Combined therapy with spironolactone and β-blockers

A low-sodium diet and spironolactone have been shown to reduce portal pressure and variceal pressure in cirrhosis[40,41]. Furthermore, it has been reported that the association of spironolactone and propranolol significantly reduced variceal pressure when propranolol alone had no effect on this parameter[42]. However, this combined treatment does not appear to improve the efficacy of β-blockers in primary prophylaxis[43].

### Carvedilol

Both the acute and chronic administration of carvedilol induced a marked decrease in HVPG. This reduction was greater than that achieved with propranolol, but carvedilol also caused arterial hypotension[44,45]. The long-term administration of carvedilol significantly increased the proportion of hemodynamic responders to 54% of cases[45]; however, chronic treatment with carvedilol, but not with propranolol, was associated with marked arterial hypotension and with a significant increase in plasma volume and body weight[45,46]. Tolerance seems to improve with lower doses (12.5 mg/day instead of 25 mg/day) and a careful titration[46,47].

Whether the portal hypotensive effect of carvedilol will translate into a safe, relevant improvement in clinical practice should be investigated.

### Combined therapy with prazosin and β-blockers

It has been suggested that, in cirrhosis, the synthesis of nitric oxide (NO) by endothelial sinusoidal cells is insufficient to counteract the vasoconstrictor response to α-adrenergic stimuli. This contributes to a further increase in hepatic resistance[48,49], and supports the use of NO donors such as ISMN, and α-adrenergic antagonists such as prazosin.

Prazosin significantly reduces portal hypertension, probably due to a decrease in intraheptic resistance. Nevertheless, it is also associated with side-effects, such as a significant reduction in arterial pressure, activation of endogenous vasoactive systems leading to sodium retention and, in some cases, to the accumulation of ascites[49]. The association of β-blockers and prazosin induces a significantly greater reduction in HVPG than that achieved using combined therapy with β-blockers and ISMN[25]; furthermore, it has been suggested that a careful titration of prazosin dose in patients

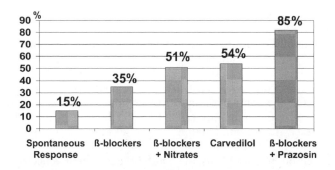

Source: *Spontaneous Response* **2 studies (N=77)**; *β-Blockers* **11 studies (N=378)**; *β-Blockers+ISMN*: **9 studies (N=445)**; *Carvedilol*: **2 studies (N=43)**; *β-Blockers+Prazosin*: **1 study (N=28)**.

**Figure 3.** Rates of hemodynamic response observed with different pharmacological treatments. The bars represent the polled means obtained in randomized controlled trials (data from refs 4, 7, 8, 14, 15, 20–25, 44–47)

already treated with β-blockers may avoid most of the adverse effects of prazosin[25]. However, even in these circumstances such combined therapy induces a greater decrease in arterial pressure than does the combination of β-blockers and ISMN[25]. On the other hand, it should be emphasized that the rate of hemodynamic responders obtained with β-blockers plus prazosin was significantly greater than that achieved with β-blockers plus ISMN, and reached 85% of patients[25]. This constitutes one of the highest proportions of response achieved with medications (Figure 3). Whether this will lead to a greater clinical efficacy should be assessed.

## Other pharmacologic treatments

Several areas of investigation are likely to afford relevant therapeutic advances, such as endothelin receptor blockers and selective hepatic delivery of NO using liver-specific NO donors or enhancing NO-synthase expression[48,50].

## Other aspects of pharmacologic therapy to take into account

Besides a portal hypotensive effect, other aspects of medications may be of additional value, particularly in non-responders.

Meals induce a postprandial splanchnic vasodilation and hyperemia, which in cirrhosis determine a repeated transient increase of portal and collateral blood flow resulting in a transient increase of portal pressure[51,52]. This in turn may lead to a progressive portocollateral dilation, resulting in the development and dilation of varices, and may finally precipitate bleeding and rebleeding[53,54]. Other factors may also induce abrupt increases in portal pressure, such as circadian rhythms, ethanol consumption, exercise, volume restitution or acute changes in intra-abdominal pressure[55,56]. Medications such as somatostatin analogs, ISMN, simvastatin, or even β-blockers, may offer additional beneficial effects by preventing these fluctuations in portal pressure[54,57-59].

Hemodynamic response is usually assessed within 1–3 months from the start of treatment. A recent study has demonstrated that response is usually sustained when it is measured again after a longer follow-up[11]. However, a later gain of response may occur in up to 10% of cases, mainly in abstinent alcoholics. On the contrary, a later loss of initial response may occur in up to 9% of cases, and is mainly related to a reduction in medication dose[11]. This suggests that hemodynamic response may be reassessed in these circumstances.

Some hemodynamic events may not be accurately reflected by HVPG measurements. As an example, in some patients β-blockers cause a more pronounced decrease in gastroesophageal collateral blood flow and variceal pressure than in portal pressure[23]. In keeping with this, it has been suggested that monitoring the variceal pressure response to β-blockers may markedly increase the sensitivity of the prognostic assessment achieved with HVPG monitoring alone[22]. Up to 34% of non-responders, by HVPG measurements, are actually responders according to variceal pressure monitoring[22].

It has also been suggested recently that the HVPG decrease required to define an adequate hemodynamic response may be lower in primary prophylaxis[60]. In this setting the probability of variceal hemorrhage is relatively low with β-blockers, despite the fact that the majority of patients are non-responders.

The above issues are not considered when evaluating hemodynamic response. Their relevance in clinical practice is yet to be established. However, it is clear that hemodynamic monitoring provides valuable prognostic information.

## AN ENDOSCOPIC APPROACH TO RESCUE NON-RESPONDERS

Once esophageal varices are eradicated by endoscopic therapy the mean portal pressure does not change as compared to the baseline value[61,62]. However, in around 30% of patients there is a spontaneous decrease[61,62]. This has been related to the presence of other major collaterals, to abstinence from alcohol and to an improvement in liver function[6,61,62]. A spontaneous hemodynamic response has been observed in up to 16% of patients treated with endoscopic procedures[7,8]. Among patients treated with both sclerotherapy and variceal ligation, spontaneous responders have a significantly lower probability of failure of endoscopic therapy to prevent rebleeding than patients who do not show such a response[7,8]. Furthermore, the association of β-blockers improves the efficacy of sclerotherapy and variceal ligation, possibly as a consequence of an increased rate of hemodynamic responders[63,64]. A spontaneous hemodynamic response may thus account, at least in part, for the efficacy of endoscopic therapy in some patients. Furthermore, it raises caveats regarding the utility of rescue endoscopic therapy for patients who previously have not responded to pharmacological treatment. In a recent study in which treatment was tailored according to hemodynamic response, rebleeding occurred in the majority of non-responders to propranolol and ISMN who were rescued with endoscopic ligation (87%: seven out of eight)[33].

On the other hand, the association of sclerotherapy and β-blockers induces a modest yet significant reduction in the rebleeding risk, with no improvement in survival[63]. This suggests that the local obliterative effect of endoscopic therapy on esophageal varices may enhance the efficacy of the portal hypotensive effect of pharmacologic treatment. Such an additive effect may be particularly apparent in non-responders, given the low residual risk of bleeding in responders. Endoscopic variceal ligation has proven to be superior to sclerotherapy in terms of efficacy and safety[63,64]. However, whether the combination of drug therapy and ligation actually improves the results achieved using medication alone has not been adequately evaluated.

At present it should be emphasized that there is no evidence to support the use of variceal ligation as rescue therapy for non-responders. Whether or not this approach may be valuable should be carefully investigated both for primary and secondary prevention of variceal hemorrhage.

## THE OPTION OF TIPS

Portosystemic shunt procedures are effective in decreasing portal pressure and the risk of variceal hemorrhage, but they also have the disadvantage of enhancing the risk of encephalopathy and worsening liver function[65].

As compared with the combined therapy with propranolol and ISMN, TIPS significantly decreases variceal rebleeding, but increases encephalopathy and has no effect on survival[66]. This combined pharmacologic treatment has also been compared with shunt surgery (and sclerotherapy for Child–Pugh C), showing no significant differences[32].

Non-responders constitute a high-risk group of patients, with a great probability of developing variceal hemorrhage and other complications related to portal hypertension, and with a risk of death above 30% at 2 years of follow-up[8]. TIPS may be effective as a rescue therapy to prevent rebleeding in this high-risk subset of patients[1]; however, this should also be assessed because, despite preventing rebleeding, TIPS may worsen liver function and may not improve survival. This already occurred in trials comparing TIPS and endoscopic therapy for the prevention of variceal rebleeding[67].

## THE ROLE OF LIVER TRANSPLANTATION

At present up to 82% of patients who receive a liver transplantation survive at 2 years of follow-up and 72% at 4 years[68]. These figures are higher than those observed in non-responders to treatment for the prevention of rebleeding (Figure 4), indicating that liver transplantation may perhaps improve outcome in non-responders, and that probably these patients should be listed earlier for transplantation.

## THE ACUTE VARICEAL BLEEDING EPISODE

Several studies have shown that early HVPG measurements during the course of an acute variceal bleeding episode provide useful prognostic infor-

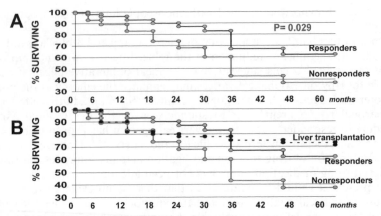

**OLT in cirrhosis:** From European Liver Transplant Registry (*www.eltr.org*).
Updated on October 2003 (N=22907)

**Figure 4.** Probability of survival observed in responders and non-responders, and with liver transplantation. **A**: Probability of survival in responders and non-responders, observed in a large series of patients treated with nadolol and ISMN[11]. **B**: Probability of survival in responders and non-responders, observed in patients treated with nadolol and ISMN[11], and that observed in patients with liver transplantation from 1988 to 2003 (from European Liver Transplant Registry: www.eltr.org)

mation[58,69,70]. In this setting an HVPG above 20 mmHg is associated with a significantly worse outcome[70]. Using this criterion for tailoring therapy, a small study suggested that rescue TIPS significantly improved treatment failure in high-risk patients, as compared with the control group treated with emergency sclerotherapy but not as compared with patients with an HVPG below 20 mmHg[71]. These findings suggest that monitoring portal pressure may improve the management of acute variceal hemorrhage.

## Acknowledgements

We thank the nursing and medical staff of the Gastrointestinal Bleeding Unit and of the Semi-Critics Unit of the Hospital de la Santa Creu i Sant Pau for their cooperation. This study has been supported in part by a grant from the Fundació Investigació Sant Pau and by a grant from the Instituto de Salud Carlos III (CO3/02).

## References

1. Bosch J, Abraldes JG, Groszmann R. Current management of portal hypertension. J Hepatol. 2003;38:S54–68.
2. Garcia-Tsao G. Current management of the complications of cirrhosis and portal hypertension: variceal hemorrhage, ascites, and spontaneous bacterial peritonitis. Gastroenterology. 2001;120:726–48.
3. Groszmann RJ, Bosch J, Grace ND et al. Hemodynamic events in a prospective randomized trial of propranolol versus placebo in the prevention of a first variceal hemorrhage. Gastroenterology. 1990;99:1401–7.

4. Feu F, García-Pagán JC, Bosch J et al. Relation between portal pressure response to pharmacotherapy and risk of recurrent variceal haemorrhage in patients with cirrhosis. Lancet. 1995;346:1056–9.

5. Garcia-Tsao G, Groszmann RJ, Fisher RL, Conn HO, Atterbury CE, Glickman M. Portal pressure, presence of gastroesophageal varices and variceal bleeding. Hepatology. 1985;5:419–24.

6. Vorobioff J, Groszmann RJ, Picabea E et al. Prognostic value of hepatic venous pressure gradient measurements in alcoholic cirrhosis: a 10-year prospective study. Gastroenterology. 1996;111:701–9.

7. Villanueva C, Balanzó J, Novella M et al. Nadolol plus isosorbide mononitrate compared with sclerotherapy for the prevention of variceal rebleeding. N Engl J Med. 1996;334:1624–9.

8. Villanueva C, Miñana J, Ortiz J et al. Endoscopic ligation compared with combined treatment with nadolol plus isosorbide mononitrate to prevent recurrent variceal bleeding. N Engl J Med. 2001;345:647–55.

9. Merkel C, Bolognesi M, Sacerdoti D et al. The hemodynamic response to medical treatment of portal hypertension as a predictor of clinical effectiveness in the primary prophylaxis of variceal bleeding in cirrhosis. Hepatology. 2000;32:930–4.

10. Abraldes JG, Tarantino I, Turnes J, Garcia-Pagan JC, Rodés J, Bosch J. Hemodynamic response to pharmacological treatment of portal hypertension and long-term prognosis of cirrhosis. Hepatology. 2003;37:902–8.

11. Villanueva C, López-Balaguer JM, Aracil C et al. Maintenance of hemodynamic response to treatment for portal hypertension and influence on complications of cirrhosis. J Hepatol. 2004;40:757–65.

12. Boyer TD. Pharmacologic treatment of portal hypertension: past, present and future. Hepatology. 2001;34:834–9.

13. Kroeger RJ, Groszmann RJ. Increased portal venous resistance hinders portal pressure reduction during the administration of beta-adrenergic blocking agnets in a portal hypertensive model. Hepatology. 1985;5:97–101.

14. Garcia-Pagán JC, Feu F, Bosch J, Rodés J. Propranolol compared with propranolol plus isosorbide-5-mononitrate for portal hypertension in cirrhosis. A randomized controlled study. Ann Intern Med. 1991;114:869–73.

15. Merkel C, Sacerdoti D, Bolognesi M et al. Hemodynamic evaluation of the addition of isosorbide-5-mononitrate to nadolol in cirrhotic patients with insufficient response to the b-blocker alone. Hepatology. 1997;26:34–9.

16. De Franchis R. Updating consensus in portal hypertension: report of the Baveno III consensus workshop on definitions, methodology and therapeutic strategies in portal hypertension. J Hepatol. 2000;33:846–52.

17. Groszmann RJ, Garcia-Tsao G. Endoscopic variceal ligation vs. pharmacological therapy for the prevention of recurrent variceal hemorrhage: What makes the difference? Gastroenterology. 2002;123:1388–91.

18. D'Amico G, Pagliaro L, Bosch J. Pharmacological treatment of portal hypertension: an evidence-based approach. Semin Liver Dis. 1999;19:475–505.

19. García-Pagán JC, Villanueva C, Vila MC et al. and Members of the MOVE group. Isosorbide mononitrate in the prevention of first variceal bleed in patients who cannot receive b-blockers. Gastroenterology. 2001;121:908–14.

20. Garcia-Tsao G, Grace ND, Groszmann RJ et al. Short-term effects of propranolol on portal pressure. Hepatology. 1986;6:101–6.

21. Vorobioff J, Picabea E, Villavicencio R et al. Acute and chronic hemodynamic effects of propranolol in unselected cirrhotic patients. Hepatology. 1987;7:648–53.

22. Escorsell A, Bordas JM, Castañeda B et al. Predictive value of variceal pressure response to continued pharmacological therapy in patients with cirrhosis and portal hypertension. Hepatology. 2000;31:1061–7.

23. Feu F, Bordas JM, Luca A et al. Reduction of variceal pressure by propranolol: comparison of the effects on portal pressure and azygos blood flow in patients with cirrhosis. Hepatology. 1993;18:1082–9.

24. García-Pagán JC, Navasa M, Bosch J, Bru C, Pizcueta P, Rodés J. Enhancement of portal pressure reduction by the association of isosorbide-5-mononitrate to propranolol administration in patients with cirrhosis. Hepatology. 1990;11:230–8.

25. Albillos A, García-Pagán JC, Iborra J et al. Propranolol plus prazosin compared with propranolol plus isosorbide-5-mononitrate in the treatment of portal hypertension. Gastroenterology. 1998;115:116–23.
26. Morillas R, Planas R, Cabré E et al. Propranolol plus isosorbide-5-mononitrate for portal hypertension in cirrhosis: long-term hemodynamic and renal effects. Hepatology. 1994;20:1502–8.
27. Merkel C, Gatta A, Donada C et al. Long-term effects of nadolol or nadolol plus isosorbide-5-mononitrate on renal function and ascites formation in patients with cirrhosis. Hepatology. 1995;22:808–13.
28. Gournay J, Masliah C, Martin T, Perrin D, Galmiche JP. Isosorbide mononitrate and propranolol compared with propranolol alone for the prevention of variceal rebleeding. Hepatology. 2000;31:1239–45.
29. Patti R, D'Amico G, Pasta L et al. Isosorbide mononitrate (IMN) with nadolol compared with nadolol alone for the prevention of recurrent bleeding in cirrhosis. A double-blind placebo-controlled randomized trial. J Hepatol. 1999;30:81 (abstract).
30. Patch D, Sabin CA, Goulis J et al. A randomized controlled trial of medical therapy versus endoscopic ligation for the prevention of variceal rebleeding in patients with cirrhosis. Gastroenterology. 2002;123:1013–19.
31. Lo GH, Chen WC, Chen MH et al. Banding ligation versus nadolol and isosorbide mononitrate for the prevention of esophageal variceal bleeding. Gastroenterology. 2002;123:728–34.
32. McCormick PA, Feu F, Sabrin C, Planas R and the Anglo-Spanish variceal rebleeding group. Propranolol and isosorbide mononitrate versus sclerotherapy or shunt surgery for the prevention of variceal rebleeding: a randomized trial. Hepatology. 1994;20:106A (abstract).
33. Bureau C, Péron JM, Alric L et al. "A la carte" treatment of portal hypertension: adapting therapy to hemodynamic response for the prevention of bleeding. Hepatology. 202;36:1361–6.
34. Thalheimer U, Mela M, Patch D, Burroughs AK. Targeting portal pressure measurements: a critical reappraisal. Hepatology. 2004;39:286–90.
35. Burroughs AK, D'Heygere F, McIntyre N. Pitfalls in studies of prophylactic therapy for variceal bleeding in cirrhosis. Hepatology. 1986;6:1407–13.
36. Schneider AW, Kalk JF, Klein CP. Effect of losartan, an angiotensin II receptor antagonist, on portal pressure in cirrhosis. Hepatology. 1999;29:334–9.
37. Schepke M, Werner E, Bieker E et al. Hemodynamic effects of the angiotensin II receptor antagonist irbesartan in patients with cirrhosis and portal hypertension. Gastroenterology. 2001;121:389–95.
38. González-Abraldes J, Albillos A, Bañares R et al. Randomized comparison of long-term losartan versus propranolol in lowering portal pressure in cirrhosis. Gastroenterology. 2001;121:382–8.
39. Debernardi-Venon W, Baronio M, Leone N et al. Effects of irbesartan in reducing portal pressure in cirrhotic patients: comparison with propranolol in a randomised controlled trial. J Hepatol. 2003;38:455–60.
40. Okumura H, Aramaki T, Katsuta Y et al. Reduction in hepatic venous pressure gradient as a consequence of volume contraction due to chronic administration of spironolactone in patients with cirrhosis and no ascites. Am J Gastroenterol. 1991;86:46–52.
41. García-Pagán JC, Salmerón JM, Feu F et al. Effects of low-sodium diet and spironolactone on portal pressure in patients with compensated cirrhosis. Hepatology. 1994;19:1095–9.
42. Nevens F, Lijnen P, VanBilloen H, Fevery J. The effect of long-term treatment with spironolactone on variceal pressure in patients with portal hypertension without ascites. Hepatology. 1996;23:1047–52.
43. Abecasis R, Kravetz D, Fassio E et al. Nadolol plus spironolactone in the prophylaxis of first variceal bleed in nonascitic cirrhotic patients: a preliminary study. Hepatology. 2003;37:359–65.
44. Bañares R, Moitinho E, Piqueras B et al. Carvediol, a new nonselective beta-blocker with intrinsic anti-α-1-adrenergic activity, has greater portal hypotensive effect than propranolol in patients with cirrhosis. Hepatology. 1999;30:79–83.
45. Bañares R, Moitinho E, Matilla A et al. Randomized comparison of long-term carvedilol

and propranolol administration in the treatment of portal hypertension in cirrhosis. Hepatology. 2002;36:1367–73.

46. Stanley A, Therapondos G, Helmy A, Hayes PC. Acute and chronic haemodynamic and renal effects of carvedilol in patients with cirrhosis. J Hepatol. 1999;30:479–84.

47. Tripathi D, Therapondos G, Helmy A, Hayes PC. Haemodynamic effects of acute and chronic administration of long-dose carvedilol, a vasodilating beta-blocker, in patients with cirrhosis and portal hypertension. Aliment Pharmacol Ther. 2002;16:373–80.

48. Wiest R, Gorszmann RJ. The paradox of nitric oxide in cirrhosis and portal hypertension: too much, not enough. Hepatology. 2002;35:478–91.

49. Albillos A, Lledó JL, Rossi I et al. Continuous prazosin administration in cirrhotic patients: effects on portal hemodynamics and on liver and renal function. Gastroenterology. 1995;109:1257–65.

50. Bosch J. Decreasing hepatic vascular tone by liver-specific NO donors: wishful thinking or a promising reality? J Hepatol. 2003;39:1072–5.

51. Lee S, Hadengue A, Moreau R, Sayegh R, Hillon P, Lebrec D. Postprandial hemodynamic responses in patients with cirrhosis. Hepatology. 1988;8:647–51.

52. McCormick PA, Dick R, Graffeo M et al. The effect of non-protein liquid meals on the hepatic venous pressure gradient in patients with cirrhosis. J Hepatol. 1990;11:221–5.

53. Polio J, Groszmann RJ. Hemodynamic factors involved in the development and rupture of esophageal varices: a pathophysiologic approach to treatment. Semin Liver Dis. 1986; 6:318–31.

54. McCormick PA, Jenkins SA, McIntyre N, Burroughs AK. Why portal hypertensive varices bleed and bleed: a hypothesis. Gut. 1995;36:100–3.

55. García-Pagán JC, Santos C, Barberá JA et al. Physical exercise increases portal pressure in patients with cirrhosis and portal hypertension. Gastroenterology. 1996;111:1300–6.

56. Luca A, Cirera I, García-Pagán JC et al. Hemodynamic effects of acute changes in intra-abdominal pressure in patients with cirrhosis. Gastroenterology. 1993;104:222–7.

57. Bellis L, Berzigotti A, Abraldes JG et al. Low doses of isosorbide mononitrate attenuate the postprandial increase in portal pressure in patients with cirrhosis. Hepatology. 2003; 37:378–84.

58. Villanueva C, Ortiz J, Miñana J et al. Somatostatin treatment and risk stratification by continuous portal pressure monitoring during acute variceal bleeding. Gastroenterology. 2001;121:110–17.

59. Zafra C, Abraldes JG, Cortez C et al. Simvastatin ameliorates the increased hepatic vascular tone in patients with cirrhosis. J Hepatol. 2003;38(Suppl. 12):12.

60. Aracil C, López-Balaguer JM, Monfort D et al. Hemodynamic response to beta-blockers and prediction of clinical efficacy in the primary prophylaxis of variceal bleeding in patients with cirrhosis. Hepatology. 2003;38:296A (abstract).

61. Korula J, Ralls P. The effects of chronic endoscopic variceal sclerotherapy on portal pressure in cirrhotics. Gastroenterology. 1991;101:800–5.

62. Lo GH, Liang HL, Lai KH et al. The impact of endoscopic variceal ligation on the pressure of the portal venous system. J Hepatol. 1996;24:74–8.

63. De Franchis R, Primignani M. Endoscopic treatments for portal hypertension. Semin Liver Dis. 1999;19:439–55.

64. Laine L, Cook D. Endoscopic ligation compared with sclerotherapy for treatment of esophageal variceal bleeding. A meta-analysis. Ann Intern Med. 1995;123:280–7.

65. Burroughs AK, Patch D. Transjugular intrahepatic portosystemic shunt. Semin Liver Dis. 1999;19:457–73.

66. Escorsell A, Bañares R, García-Pagán JC et al. TIPS versus drug therapy in preventing variceal rebleeding in advanced cirrhosis: a randomized controlled trial. Hepatology. 2002;35:385–92.

67. Papatheodoridis GV, Goulis J, Leandro G, Patch D, Burroughs AK. Transjugular intrahepatic portosystemic shunt compared with endoscopic treatment for prevention of variceal rebleeding: a meta-analysis. Hepatology. 1999;30:612–22.

68. Adam R, Cailliez V, Majno P et al. Normalised intrinsic mortality risk in liver transplantation: European Liver Transplant Registry Group. Lancet. 2000;356:621–7.

69. Ready JB, Robertson AD, Goff JS, Rector WG. Assessment of the risk of bleeding from esophageal varices by continuous monitoring of portal pressure. Gastroenterology. 1991;100:1403–10.

70. Moitinho E, Escorsell A, Bandi JC et al. Prognostic value of early measurements of portal pressure in acute variceal bleeding. Gastroenterology. 1999;117:626–31.
71. Monescillo A, Martínez-Lagares F, Sierra A et al. Treatment of acute variceal bleeding by the hepatic venous pressure gradient: preliminary results of a randomized trial. Hepatology. 1999;30:220A (abstract).

# 35
# What else we need

JUAN TURNES, JUAN CARLOS GARCÍA-PAGÁN
and JAIME BOSCH

## INTRODUCTION

Available evidence supports the concept that repeat measurements of hepatic venous pressure gradient (HVPG) adequately predict the effectiveness of drug therapy for portal hypertension[1-7]. The HVPG response to continued pharmacologic therapy correlates well with the risk of first variceal bleeding[3,8] or rebleeding[2,4]. Patients who experienced a decrease in HVPG to < 12 mmHg have an extremely low risk of rebleeding ("optimal" hemodynamic response). Even if the final HVPG is not reduced < 12 mmHg, a decrease of over 20% of baseline values is also associated with a marked reduction in the risk of bleeding of about 19.5% vs 45% in non-responders ("good" hemodynamic response) (Table 1). Unfortunately such hemodynamic responses are achieved in only about 30–60% of patients receiving non-selective beta-blockers. Lack of achievement of these targets constitutes the strongest independent predictor of variceal bleeding or rebleeding[2-4,10]. Therefore, ideally, the treatment of portal hypertension should be guided by measuring the individual portal pressure response to therapy. This allows us to predict whether the treatment is likely to offer optimal or adequate protection from the risk of bleeding on follow-up[10,11].

However, measurements of HVPG, although safe and relatively simple, are invasive and require specific training[5]. This makes it unlikely that repeat measurements of HVPG could be used routinely out of the context of clinical research. So it would be extremely useful to have a valid non-invasive surrogate that can be used to monitor drug therapy. Unfortunately, such a "splanchnic sphygmomanometer" is not yet available. However, it is useful to keep in mind the ideal requirements for such a method (Figure 1).

## NON-INVASIVE TECHNIQUES (WHAT WE NEED)

Because of the above-mentioned limitations for generalized use of HVPG monitoring, there has been much interest in developing potential non-invasive methods to monitor the hemodynamic response.

**Table 1.** Risk of variceal bleeding depending on the HVPG response to continued pharmacologic therapy (adapted from ref. 9)

| Reference | Non-responders reduction in HVPG <20% or to >12 mmHg; bleeders/total (%) | All responders (reduction in HVPG >20% or <12 mmHg); bleeders/total (%) | "Optimal response" (final HVPG <12 mmHg); bleeders/total (%) | "Good response" (reduction in HVPG >20% but not <12 mmHg); bleeders/total (%) |
|---|---|---|---|---|
| Feu et al.[2] | 23/44 (52%) | 2/25 (8%) | 0/8 (0%) | 2/17 (11.7%) |
| Villanueva et al.[47] | 8/18 (44%) | 1/13 (7.7%) | 0/9 (0%) | 1/4 (25%) |
| McCormick et al.[65] | 4/16 (25%) | 12/28 (43%) | 7/23 (30%) | 5/5 (100%) |
| Merkel et al.[3] | 7/19 (36.8%) | 2/30 (6.7%) | 0/12 (0%) | 2/18 (11.1%) |
| Escorsell et al.[25] | 13/28 (46.4%) | 1/19 (5%) | 0/9 (0%) | 1/10 (10%) |
| Villanueva et al.[48] | 16/24 (66.6%) | 4/25 (16%) | 0/7 (0%) | 4/18 (22.2%) |
| Bureau et al.[10] | 9/14 (64%) | 2/20 (10%) | 0/8 (0%) | 2/12 (16.6%) |
| Abraldes et al.[4] | 20/45 (44.4%) | 6/28 (21.4%) | 1/11 (9%) | 5/17 (29.4%) |
| Turnes et al.[8] | 14/46 (30%) | 2/25 (8%) | 1/8 (12.5%) | 1/17 (6%) |
| All | 114/254 (45%) | 32/213 (15%) | 9/95 (9.5%) | 23/118 (19.5%) |

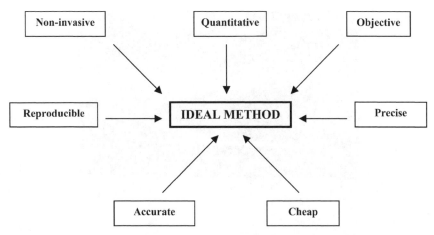

**Figure 1.** Characteristics of the ideal method to monitor the effects of drug therapy for portal hypertension

## Variceal pressure measurements

Besides HVPG (the gold standard) the method in which there is more experience is the measurement of variceal pressure at endoscopy. Variceal pressure is a direct determinant of the tension in the wall of the varix, which has been identified as the key factor in determining variceal rupture[12]. Previous studies have shown that variceal pressure can be accurately measured at endoscopy by puncturing the varices or by means of pressure gauges or low-resistance balloons[13-17]. The endoscopic pressure gauge (Varipress) is the method used most commonly in prospective studies, since variceal puncture can be justified only while performing endoscopic injection sclerotherapy. The Varipress consists of a pressure-sensitive capsule, attached to the tip of an endoscope that permits measurement of variceal pressure merely by placing it over a varix. The capsule has a small chamber covered by a thin latex membrane, which is continuously perfused with a constant flow of nitrogen by means of a non-compliant perfusion system (Figure 2). It is assumed that when the gauge is applied to the varix, the pressure needed to perfuse the gauge, measured on-line by a quartz pressure transducer, equals the pressure inside the varix[13,14,18,19].

Variceal pressure correlates significantly with portal pressure[14]. Despite this correlation, variceal pressure is significantly lower than portal pressure, probably because a significant resistance along the collaterals feeding the varices causes a pressure drop from the portal vein to the varix[18]. Variceal pressure is of clinical interest because patients who have bled from varices have significantly greater variceal pressure than those who have not (but who are matched for a similar portal pressure); this finding suggests an independent prognostic value of variceal pressure[18,20,21]. In addition, variceal pressure is usually greater in patients with large varices than in those with small varices, who are known to have a lower risk of bleeding[14,20,22].

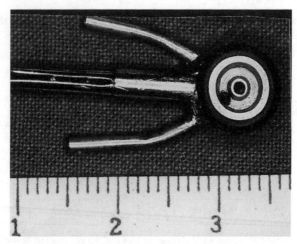

**Figure 2.** The small pressure-sensitive capsule is attached to the tip of the endoscope, allowing measurement of the variceal pressure merely by placing it over a varix

Several clinical studies have demonstrated that variceal pressure measurements using the Varipress have strong prognostic value with regard to the evolution of an acute variceal bleeding episode[23], the development of the first variceal hemorrhage[24], and on the risk of variceal rebleeding in patients receiving pharmacologic therapy[25]. Variceal pressure measurement adequately reflects the effects of pharmacologic treatment[21,25,26]. A reduction of variceal pressure after pharmacologic therapy of at least 20% from baseline has been shown to be associated with a low actuarial probability of variceal bleeding on follow-up (7% at 3 years vs 46% in those not showing this reduction)[25]. Moreover, the results of this study showed that the prognostic value of the variceal pressure response was as powerful as that of the HVPG response. The two methods identified different populations of patients with a favorable outcome, therefore they should be considered complementary rather than mutually exclusive[25].

Unfortunately, measurements of variceal pressure are difficult and prone to artifacts due to esophageal peristalsis. The technique is not feasible in every patient; about 25% of patients initially scheduled to have variceal pressure measurements must be excluded because of technical difficulties, especially patients with small varices[25]. Additionally, endoscopic measurements are not exactly non-invasive, though certainly less so than HVPG measurements. Finally, the variability of the measurement and the training required for correct measurements by far exceed those of HVPG. Because of these limitations it is highly unlikely that it might be used in routine clinical practice.

## Doppler ultrasonography

Doppler ultrasonography has been widely explored to evaluate changes in portal blood flow, blood flow velocity, superior mesenteric artery blood flow

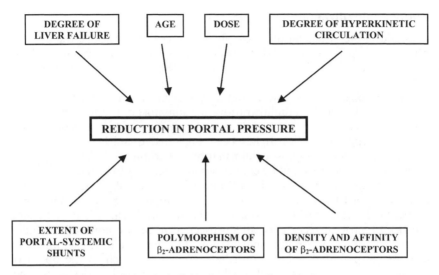

**Figure 1.** Factors modulating the individual response to beta-blockers

velocity and pulsatility index after pharmacologic therapy with beta-blockers. Although it is totally non-invasive and reasonably cheap, unfortunately it is not accurate enough to be used as a surrogate measurement of changes in portal/variceal pressure[27,28]. Critical issues such as angle of insonation, assumptions in the calculation of "mean" blood flow velocity, and "optimal" sampling point introduce variations due to observer and to equipment. Ultrasonography is subject to excessively high interobserver variability in addition to observer dependency, which hampers accurate measurements[29,30]. Moreover, the method estimates blood flow velocity. Blood flow is calculated from the product of blood flow velocity and cross-sectional area of the portal vein, which is estimated from the measurement of portal vein diameter (which adds an extra 10% error), which adds uncertainty to the calculations. On the other hand, even if Doppler ultrasonography could be improved so as to allow observer-independent accurate measurements of changes in blood flow, its applicability would be limited to assessing the effects of agents that decrease portal pressure by reducing splanchnic blood flow (vasopressin, beta-blockers, etc.). Even in this situation changes in blood flow do not translate into equal changes in portal pressure, due to the fact that a concomitant increase in portal–collateral resistance hinders the fall in portal pressure caused by vasoconstrictors[31]. Moreover, the effects of vasodilators (alone or in combination with beta-blockers) on portal pressure cannot be detected by measuring parameters related only to portal or mesenteric artery blood flows[32].

On the other hand, the portal pressure response (or lack of response) to beta-blockers is a multifactorial phenomenon, which makes it unlikely that a single test could predict it, besides the measurement of HVPG (Figure 3).

## Endoscopic ultrasonography (EUS)

This allows the visualization of esophageal and gastric varices, the perieso-phageal and perigastric collateral veins, the portal venous system, and the azygos vein. In addition, recent data suggest that endoscopic ultrasonogra-phy may be used for minimally invasive estimations of azygos blood flow[33]. Furthermore, EUS was able to detect transient changes in azygos blood flow after the acute administration of somatostatin and octreotide[33], although it is unlikely that such measurements could give reproducible results in separate studies. It has been suggested that EUS does not add further important prognostic information regarding the risk of variceal bleeding over that provided by conventional endoscopy (which also identifies red color signs in the variceal wall) and ultrasonography[34]. Currently, the clinical use of EUS is restricted to two main applications: the diagnosis of gastric fundal varices when endoscopy offers doubtful results[35], and assessing the risk of variceal recurrence after varices have been eradicated by endo-scopic sclerotherapy or banding ligation. Further studies are required to explore the potential unique contributions of EUS, such as the objective measurement of variceal wall thickness diameter and variceal volume, parameters which are direct determinants of variceal wall tension and that therefore have a good potential to correlate with the risk of bleeding.

## Other non-invasive techniques

Other non-invasive imaging techniques such as computed tomographic scan and magnetic resonance imaging (MRI) may allow visualization of the portal venous system and observer-independent measurements of portal and collateral (azygos) blood flow. Promising results have been obtained measur-ing portal and azygos blood flow using phase-contrast MR angiography[36,37] and recently with dynamic contrast material-enhanced MRI[38]. These are preferable to Doppler ultrasound since they are quantitative and observer-independent. Despite these promising results, its potential to assess the effects of drug treatment for portal hypertension has not been adequately evaluated. As with Doppler ultrasound, it should be kept in mind that changes in blood flow do not reflect the hemodynamic changes at the varices caused by vasodilators, and because of this limitation might not be adequate to assess the effect of drugs different from beta-blockers.

## Systemic hemodynamic parameters

Although routinely used in the clinical setting, easily accessible systemic hemodynamic parameters such as heart rate reduction or changes in arterial pressure do not predict the hemodynamic effect of propranolol on portal hypertension[1,39-41]. The common practice of titrating beta-blocker therapy against heart rate merely shows the degree of $\beta_1$-adrenergic blockade, which does not correlate with the fall in portal pressure. It has been suggested that patients should receive the maximal tolerated dose of beta-blockers indepen-dently of the percentage fall in heart rate in order to increase the rate of hemodynamic response[1,4].

Other methods have been used to assess both $\beta_1$ and $\beta_2$-adrenergic blockade in a non-invasive manner. Propranolol reduces arterial blood flow to the extremities by a mechanism involving a reduction in the cardiac output due to $\beta_1$-adrenoceptor blockade and a constriction of the peripheral arteries by blockade of the $\beta_2$-adrenoceptors. Initial studies evaluated the use of dual-beam Doppler, a technique that allows measurements of total blood flow independent of the angle of isonation and not requiring measurement of the cross-sectional area of the vessel. Such measurements of femoral blood flow after acute propranolol administration identified 94% of the patients with a poor HVPG response to propranolol, but had low power to detect those with a good response (57% positive predictive value)[42]. Similar results were found when the effect of beta-blockers was assessed from changes in forearm blood flow, measured by strain-gauge plethysmography[43].

## Others

It has been suggested that the lack of response to beta-blockers could be related to a down-regulation of $\beta$-adrenoceptors[44]. This finding has attracted interest, since it provided the rationale for trying to predict the portal pressure response to propranolol with a blood test. However, a subsequent study clearly showed that non-response to propranolol cannot be explained on the basis of a decreased density or affinity of $\beta_2$-adrenoceptors or to circulating levels of cathecholamines[45].

It is likely that other factors, such as $\beta_2$-adrenoceptor polymorphisms[46], may be involved in the unpredictable response to beta-blockers, but this has not been explored so far.

## IMPROVING HEMODYNAMIC RESPONSE WITH BETTER DRUGS (WHAT WE HOPE)

Another approach to this problem is the use of better drugs, that could achieve a "clinically effective" reduction of portal pressure (below 12 mmHg or of more than 20% of baseline values) in a vast majority of patients, so there is no need to measure the individual portal pressure response.

Overall, non-selective beta-blockers achieve a modest reduction in HVPG in cirrhotic patients with esophageal varices[1,47]. However, their effects are heterogeneous, and the prevalence of responders varies in different series in a range of 30–60%[2,3,8,25,48,49]. Generally, well-compensated patients (without ascites, jaundice or previous bleeding episodes) more frequently exhibit a good response than do those with more advanced cirrhosis.

Several drugs or drug combinations have been shown to allow greater falls in portal pressure than propranolol or nadolol alone (Table 2). The combination of beta-blockers plus isosorbide-5-mononitrate (*ISMN*) has been shown to cause a greater reduction in HVPG than either drug alone, specially in propranolol non-responders[47,50] (Table 2).

*Vasodilators* (ISMN[51,52], clonidine[53], prazosin[54,55], losartan[56], irbesartan[57–59] and molsidomine[60–62]) have been explored as single agents but abandoned either because they are ineffective or because of systemic hypotension and worsening of sodium retention.

355

**Table 2.** Drugs and drug combinations tested showing the mean decrease on HVPG and proportion of responders

| Drugs and references | Mean reduction on HVPG (%) | Responders (%)* |
|---|---|---|
| Propranolol[1,2,8,39] | 10–13.4% | 33–36% |
| ISMN[50] | 7.5% | Not available |
| Propranolol[46]/nadolol[47,48] + ISMN | 19%–21.4% | 42–51% |
| Prazosin[54] | 19.5% | Not available |
| Propranolol + prazosin[62] | 24.2% | 82% |
| Carvedilol[63] | 19% | 58% |
| Clonidine[52] | 15.4% | Not available |
| Losartan[55] | 2% | Not available |

*Defined as HVPG reduction over 20% from baseline or to less than 12 mmHg.

The association of propranolol plus the $\alpha_1$-adrenergic antagonist *prazosin*, was significantly more effective in reducing HVPG than the association of propranolol plus isosorbide-5-mononitrate[63] (Table 2). However, this combination caused a greater decrease in arterial pressure and was less well tolerated than propranolol plus ISMN.

*Carvedilol* is a non-selective beta-blocker with intrinsic anti $\alpha_1$-adrenergic activity. Recent randomized studies have demonstrated that carvedilol causes a significantly greater mean reduction in HVPG than propranolol (Table 2). Moreover, the proportion of patients achieving target reductions in HVPG (a decrease of $\geq 20\%$ from baseline values or to $\leq 12$ mmHg) was significantly higher with carvedilol than with propranolol (58% vs 23%)[64]. On the contrary, carvedilol was associated with a significant decrease in mean arterial pressure and with an increase in plasma volume, suggesting that it may increase the need for diuretics and that it should be used with care in patients with ascites.

Whether the greater hemodynamic effects achieved with some of these combinations translate into better clinical results should be verified by randomized controlled studies.

## ACUTE RESPONSE TO PROPRANOLOL

Another way of minimizing the requirements for repeat measurements of HVPG is by determining the acute effect of therapy on HVPG. Several investigations have shown an acceptable correspondence between the acute and chronic effects of propranolol on HVPG[1,41,65]. The correlation between the acute response to an oral dose of 40–80 mg of propranolol and the response to continued drug therapy was 74%[1].

Interestingly, a recent study that evaluated the acute HVPG response 20 min after an intravenous propranolol administration (of 0.15 mg/kg) disclosed that the acute response correlated with the incidence of bleeding during follow-up[65]. If these results are confirmed it could be of clinical relevance, since it would be possible to obtain prognostic information on the bleeding-risk reduction afforded by therapy in a single hepatic vein catheterization study.

## SUMMARY

All available evidence supports the concept that repeat measurements of HVPG adequately predict the effectiveness of drug therapy for portal hypertension. Therefore, ideally, the treatment of portal hypertension should be guided by measuring the individual portal pressure response to therapy. However, to achieve this, the ideal method should be totally non-invasive (or minimally invasive), quantitative, precise, accurate and objective.

Besides HVPG (the gold standard) the method in which there is more experience is the measurement of variceal pressure at endoscopy. This has been shown to give prognostic information and to adequately reflect the effects of pharmacologic treatment. However, measurements of variceal pressure are difficult, prone to artifacts due to esophageal peristalsis and cannot be considered as totally non-invasive.

Doppler ultrasonography has been widely evaluated, but unfortunately it is not accurate enough to be used as a surrogate measurement of portal/variceal pressure. Other non-invasive imaging techniques (CT, MRI) may allow visualization of the portal venous system and observer-independent measurements of portal and collateral (azygos) blood flow, but their potential to assess the effects of drug treatment for portal hypertension has not been adequately evaluated.

Changes in arterial blood pressure, heart rate, cardiac output, femoral blood flow, plasma catecholamines or lymphocyte $\beta_2$-adrenoceptors do not correlate with the portal pressure response to beta-blockers.

Another approach to this problem is the use of better drugs, that could achieve a "clinically effective" reduction of portal pressure (below 12 mmHg or of more than 20% of baseline values) in a vast majority of patients, so there is no need to measure the individual portal pressure response. Several drugs or drug combinations have been shown to allow greater falls in portal pressure than propranolol or nadolol.

Another way of minimizing the requirements for repeat measurements of HVPG is by determining the acute effect of therapy on HVPG. Several investigations have shown an acceptable correspondence between the acute and chronic effects of propranolol on HVPG. More importantly, the acute HVPG response 20 min after intravenous propranolol administration has recently been shown to correlate with clinical efficacy on follow-up.

### Acknowledgements

Dr J.T. is the recipient of a grant from the Ministerio de Sanidad y Consumo (CM0300123). The work was supported in part by grants from the Instituto de Salud Carlos III (CO3/02 and PI 020739).

### References

1. Groszmann RJ, Bosch J, Grace ND et al. Hemodynamic events in a prospective randomized trial of propranolol versus placebo in the prevention of a first variceal hemorrhage [See comments]. Gastroenterology. 1990;99:1401–7.
2. Feu F, Garcia-Pagan JC, Bosch J et al. Relation between portal pressure response to pharmacotherapy and risk of recurrent variceal haemorrhage in patients with cirrhosis. Lancet. 1995;346:1056–9.

3. Merkel C, Bolognesi M, Sacerdoti D et al. The hemodynamic response to medical treatment of portal hypertension as a predictor of clinical effectiveness in the primary prophylaxis of variceal bleeding in cirrhosis. Hepatology. 2000;32:930–4.

4. Abraldes JG, Tarantino I, Turnes J et al. Hemodynamic response to pharmacological treatment of portal hypertension and long-term prognosis of cirrhosis. Hepatology. 2003;37: 902–8.

5. Groszmann RJ, Wongcharatrawee S. The hepatic venous pressure gradient: anything worth doing should be done right. Hepatology. 2004;39:280–2.

6. Boyer TD. Changing clinical practice with measurements of portal pressure. Hepatology. 2004;39:283–5.

7. Thalheimer U, Mela M, Patch D, Burroughs AK. Targeting portal pressure measurements: a critical reappraisal. Hepatology. 2004;39:286–90.

8. Turnes J, García-Pagán JC, Abraldes JG et al. Pharmacological reduction of portal pressure and long term risk of first variceal bleeding in patients with cirrhosis. Hepatology. 2003;38: 62A.

9. García-Pagán JC, Bosch J. Monitoring hepatic venous pressure gradient during pharmacological therapy. Hepatology. 2004 (In press).

10. Bureau C, Peron JM, Alric L et al. "A la carte" treatment of portal hypertension: adapting medical therapy to hemodynamic response for the prevention of bleeding. Hepatology. 2002;36:1361–6.

11. Bosch J, Garcia-Pagan JC. Prevention of variceal rebleeding. Lancet. 2003;361:952–4.

12. Polio J, Groszmann RJ. Hemodynamic factors involved in the development and rupture of esophageal varices: a pathophysiologic approach to treatment. Semin Liver Dis. 1986;6:318–31.

13. Mosimann R. Nonaggressive assessment of portal hypertension using endoscopic measurement of variceal pressure. Preliminary report. Am J Surg. 1982;143:212–14.

14. Bosch J, Bordas JM, Rigau J et al. Noninvasive measurement of the pressure of esophageal varices using an endoscopic gauge: comparison with measurements by variceal puncture in patients undergoing endoscopic sclerotherapy. Hepatology. 1986;6:667–72.

15. Polio J, Hanson J, Sikuler E et al. Critical evaluation of a pressure-sensitive capsule for measurement of esophageal varix pressure. Studies *in vitro* and in canine mesenteric vessels. Gastroenterology. 1987;92:1109–15.

16. Polio J, Leonard R, Groszmann RJ, Vogel G. An improved pressure-sensitive capsule for endoscopic measurement of esophageal variceal pressure. Dig Dis Sci. 1988;33:737–40.

17. Gertsch P, Fischer G, Kleber G, Wheatley AM, Geigenberger G, Sauerbruch T. Manometry of esophageal varices: comparison of an endoscopic balloon technique with needle puncture. Gastroenterology. 1993;105:1159–66.

18. Rigau J, Bosch J, Bordas JM et al. Endoscopic measurement of variceal pressure in cirrhosis: correlation with portal pressure and variceal hemorrhage. Gastroenterology. 1989;96: 873–80.

19. Escorsell A, Bordas JM, Feu F et al. Endoscopic assessment of variceal volume and wall tension in cirrhotic patients: effects of pharmacological therapy. Gastroenterology. 1997;113:1640–6.

20. Nevens F, Sprengers D, Feu F, Bosch J, Fevery J. Measurement of variceal pressure with an endoscopic pressure sensitive gauge: validation and effect of propranolol therapy in chronic conditions. J Hepatol. 1996;24:66–73.

21. Feu F, Bordas JM, Luca A et al. Reduction of variceal pressure by propranolol: comparison of the effects on portal pressure and azygos blood flow in patients with cirrhosis. Hepatology. 1993;18:1082–9.

22. Ueno K, Hashizume M, Ohta M, Tomikawa M, Kitano S, Sugimachi K. Noninvasive variceal pressure measurement may be useful for predicting effects of sclerotherapy for esophageal varices. Dig Dis Sci. 1996;41:191–6.

23. Ruiz del Arbol L, Martin de Argila C, Vázquez M et al. Endoscopic measurement of variceal pressure during hemorrhage from esophageal varices. Hepatology. 1992;16:147.

24. Nevens F, Bustami R, Scheys I, Lesaffre E, Fevery J. Variceal pressure is a factor predicting the risk of a first variceal bleeding: a prospective cohort study in cirrhotic patients. Hepatology. 1998;27:15–19.

25. Escorsell A, Bordas JM, Castaneda B et al. Predictive value of the variceal pressure response to continued pharmacological therapy in patients with cirrhosis and portal hypertension. Hepatology. 2000;31:1061–7.

26. Bosch J, Bordas JM, Mastai R et al. Effects of vasopressin on the intravariceal pressure in patients with cirrhosis: comparison with the effects on portal pressure. Hepatology. 1988;8:861–5.
27. Iwao T, Oho K, Sakai T et al. Noninvasive hemodynamic measurements of superior mesenteric artery in the prediction of portal pressure response to propranolol. J Hepatol. 1998;28:847–55.
28. Merkel C, Sacerdoti D, Bolognesi M, Bombonato G, Gatta A. Doppler sonography and hepatic vein catheterization in portal hypertension: assessment of agreement in evaluating severity and response to treatment. J Hepatol. 1998;28:622–30.
29. Sabba C, Weltin GG, Cicchetti DV et al. Observer variability in echo-Doppler measurements of portal flow in cirrhotic patients and normal volunteers. Gastroenterology. 1990;98:1603–11.
30. Sacerdoti D, Gaiani S, Buonamico P et al. Interobserver and interequipment variability of hepatic, splenic, and renal arterial Doppler resistance indices in normal subjects and patients with cirrhosis. J Hepatol. 1997;27:986–92.
31. Kroeger RJ, Groszmann RJ. Increased portal venous resistance hinders portal pressure reduction during the administration of beta-adrenergic blocking agents in a portal hypertensive model. Hepatology. 1985;5:97–101.
32. Merkel C, Sacerdoti D, Bolognesi M et al. Hemodynamic evaluation of the addition of isosorbide-5-mononitrate to nadolol in cirrhotic patients with insufficient response to the beta-blocker alone. Hepatology. 1997;26:34–9.
33. Nishida H, Giostra E, Spahr L, Mentha G, Mitamura K, Hadengue A. Validation of color Doppler EUS for azygos blood flow measurement in patients with cirrhosis: application to the acute hemodynamic effects of somatostatin, octreotide, or placebo. Gastrointest Endosc. 2001;54:24–30.
34. de Franchis R. Updating consensus in portal hypertension: report of the Baveno III Consensus Workshop on definitions, methodology and therapeutic strategies in portal hypertension. J Hepatol. 2000;33:846–52.
35. Caletti GC, Brocchi E, Ferrari A, Fiorino S, Barbara L. Value of endoscopic ultrasonography in the management of portal hypertension. Endoscopy. 1992;24(Suppl. 1):342–6.
36. Debatin J, Zahner B, Meyenberger C et al. Azygos blood flow: phase contrast quantitation in volunteers and patients with portal hypertension pre- and postintrahepatic shunt placement. Hepatology. 1996;24:1109–15.
37. Wu MT, Pan HB, Chen C et al. Azygos blood flow in cirrhosis: measurement with MR imaging and correlation with variceal hemorrhage. Radiology. 1996;198:457–62.
38. Annet L, Materne R, Danse E, Jamart J, Horsmans Y, Van Beers BE. Hepatic flow parameters measured with MR imaging and Doppler US: correlations with degree of cirrhosis and portal hypertension. Radiology. 2003;229:409–14.
39. Bosch J, Mastai R, Kravetz D et al. Effects of propranolol on azygos venous blood flow and hepatic and systemic hemodynamics in cirrhosis. Hepatology. 1984;4:1200–5.
40. Garcia-Tsao G, Grace ND, Groszmann RJ et al. Short-term effects of propranolol on portal venous pressure. Hepatology. 1986;6:101–6.
41. Vorobioff J, Picabea E, Villavicencio R et al. Acute and chronic hemodynamic effects of propranolol in unselected cirrhotic patients. Hepatology. 1987;7:648–53.
42. Luca A, Garcia-Pagan JC, Feu F et al. Noninvasive measurement of femoral blood flow and portal pressure response to propranolol in patients with cirrhosis. Hepatology. 1995;21:83–8.
43. Albillos A, Perez-Paramo M, Cacho G et al. Accuracy of portal and forearm blood flow measurements in the assessment of the portal pressure response to propranolol. J Hepatol. 1997;27:496–504.
44. Gerbes AL, Remien J, Jungst D, Sauerbruch T, Paumgartner G. Evidence for down-regulation of beta-2-adrenoceptors in cirrhotic patients with severe ascites. Lancet. 1986;1:1409–11.
45. Garcia-Pagan JC, Navasa M, Rivera F, Bosch J, Rodes J. Lymphocyte beta 2-adrenoceptors and plasma catecholamines in patients with cirrhosis. Gastroenterology. 1992;102:2015–23.
46. Dishy V, Sofowora GG, Xie HG et al. The effect of common polymorphisms of the beta2-adrenergic receptor on agonist-mediated vascular desensitization. N Engl J Med. 2001;345:1030–5.
47. Garcia-Pagan JC, Feu F, Bosch J, Rodes J. Propranolol compared with propranolol plus isosorbide-5-mononitrate for portal hypertension in cirrhosis. A randomized controlled study. Ann Intern Med. 1991;114:869–73.

48. Villanueva C, Balanzo J, Novella MT et al. Nadolol plus isosorbide mononitrate compared with sclerotherapy for the prevention of variceal rebleeding. N Engl J Med. 1996;334:1624–9.
49. Villanueva C, Minana J, Ortiz J et al. Endoscopic ligation compared with combined treatment with nadolol and isosorbide mononitrate to prevent recurrent variceal bleeding. N Engl J Med. 2001;345:647–55.
50. Garcia-Pagan JC, Navasa M, Bosch J, Bru C, Pizcueta P, Rodes J. Enhancement of portal pressure reduction by the association of isosorbide-5-mononitrate to propranolol administration in patients with cirrhosis. Hepatology. 1990;11:230–8.
51. Garcia-Pagan JC, Feu F, Navasa M et al. Long-term haemodynamic effects of isosorbide 5-mononitrate in patients with cirrhosis and portal hypertension. J Hepatol. 1990;11:189–95.
52. Hayes PC, Westaby D, Williams R. Effect and mechanism of action of isosorbide-5-mononitrate. Gut. 1988;29:752–5.
53. Albillos A, Banares R, Barrios C et al. Oral administration of clonidine in patients with alcoholic cirrhosis. Hemodynamic and liver function effects. Gastroenterology. 1992; 102:248–54.
54. Albillos A, Lledo JL, Banares R et al. Hemodynamic effects of α-adrenergic blockade with prazosin in cirrhotic patients with portal hypertension. Hepatology. 1994;20:611–17.
55. Albillos A, Lledo JL, Rossi I et al. Continuous prazosin administration in cirrhotic patients: effects on portal hemodynamics and on liver and renal function. Gastroenterology. 1995;109:1257–65.
56. Gonzalez-Abraldes J, Albillos A, Banares R et al. Randomized comparison of long-term losartan versus propranolol in lowering portal pressure in cirrhosis. Gastroenterology. 2001;121:382–8.
57. Schepke M, Werner E, Biecker E et al. Hemodynamic effects of the angiotensin II receptor antagonist irbesartan in patients with cirrhosis and portal hypertension. Gastroenterology. 2001;121:389–95.
58. Debernardi-Venon W, Barletti C, Alessandria C et al. Efficacy of irbesartan, a receptor selective antagonist of angiotensin II, in reducing portal hypertension. Dig Dis Sci. 2002;47:401–4.
59. Debernardi-Venon W, Baronio M, Leone N et al. Effects of long-term Irbesartan in reducing portal pressure in cirrhotic patients: comparison with propranolol in a randomised controlled study. J Hepatol. 2003;38:455–60.
60. Vinel JP, Monnin JL, Combis JM, Cales P, Desmorat H, Pascal JP. Hemodynamic evaluation of molsidomine: a vasodilator with antianginal properties in patients with alcoholic cirrhosis. Hepatology. 1990;11:239–42.
61. Ruiz dA, Garcia-Pagan JC, Feu F, Pizcueta MP, Bosch J, Rodes J. Effects of molsidomine, a long acting venous dilator, on portal hypertension. A hemodynamic study in patients with cirrhosis. J Hepatol. 1991;13:179–86.
62. Garcia-Pagan JC, Escorsell A, Feu F et al. Propranolol plus molsidomine vs propranolol alone in the treatment of portal hypertension in patients with cirrhosis. J Hepatol. 1996;24:430–5.
63. Albillos A, Garcia-Pagan JC, Iborra J et al. Propranolol plus prazosin compared with propranolol plus isosorbide-5-mononitrate in the treatment of portal hypertension. Gastroenterology. 1998;115:116–23.
64. Banares R, Moitinho E, Matilla A et al. Randomized comparison of long-term carvedilol and propranolol administration in the treatment of portal hypertension in cirrhosis. Hepatology. 2002;36:1367–73.
65. Aracil C, López-Balaguer J, Monfort D et al. Hemodynamic response to beta-blockers and prediction of clinical efficacy in the primary prophylaxis of variceal bleeding in patients with cirrhosis. Hepatology. 2003;38:296A.

# Index